# THE HANDY DIABETES ANSWER BOOK

# About the Authors

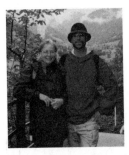

Patricia Barnes-Svarney is a nonfiction science and science-fiction writer. Over the past few decades, she has written or coauthored more than thirty-five books, including *When the Earth Moves: Rogue Earthquakes, Tremors, and Aftershocks* and the award-winning *The New York Public Library Science Desk Reference*, and she has written hundreds of magazine articles on science and sundry other subjects.

Thomas E. Svarney is a scientist and naturalist. His books, with Patricia Barnes-Svarney, include Visible Ink Press' *The Handy Geology Answer Book*, *The Handy Ocean Answer Book*, *The Handy Math Answer Book*, and *The Handy Nutrition Answer Book*, along with several revisions, such as second editions of *The Handy Biology Answer Book*, *The Handy Dinosaur Answer Book* and *The Handy Anatomy Answer Book*. In addition, they have written several other books, including *Skies of Fury: Weather Weirdness around the World* and *The Oryx Guide to Natural History*. You can read more about their writing at www.pattybarnes.net.

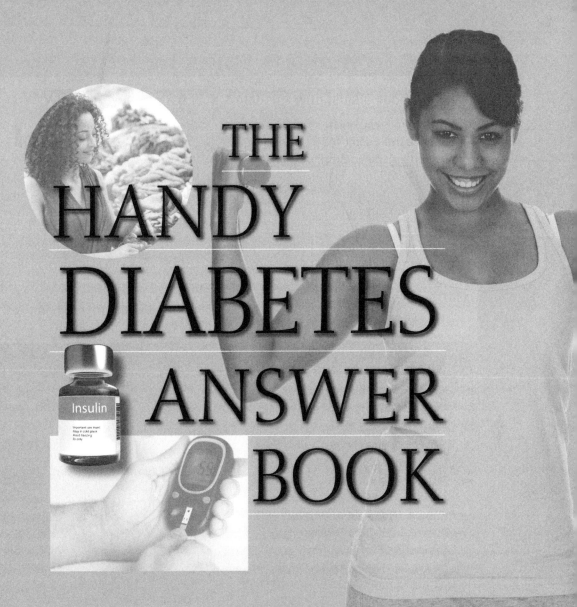

# THE
# HANDY
# DIABETES
# ANSWER
# BOOK

**Patricia Barnes-Svarney and Thomas E. Svarney**

VISIBLE
INK
PRESS

Detroit

# ALSO FROM VISIBLE INK PRESS

*The Handy Math Answer Book,*
  2nd edition
by Patricia Barnes-Svarney and
  Thomas E. Svarney
ISBN: 978-1-57859-373-6

*The Handy Military History Answer*
  *Book*
by Samuel Willard Crompton
ISBN: 978-1-57859-509-9

*The Handy Mythology Answer Book*
by David A. Leeming, Ph.D.
ISBN: 978-1-57859-475-7

*The Handy New York City Answer*
  *Book*
by Chris Barsanti
ISBN: 978-1-57859-586-0

*The Handy Nutrition Answer Book*
by Patricia Barnes-Svarney and
  Thomas E. Svarney
ISBN: 978-1-57859-484-9

*The Handy Ocean Answer Book*
by Patricia Barnes-Svarney and
  Thomas E. Svarney
ISBN: 978-1-57859-063-6

*The Handy Personal Finance Answer*
  *Book*
by Paul A. Tucci
ISBN: 978-1-57859-322-4

*The Handy Philosophy Answer Book*
by Naomi Zack, Ph.D.
ISBN: 978-1-57859-226-5

*The Handy Physics Answer Book,*
  2nd edition
by Paul W. Zitzewitz, Ph.D.
ISBN: 978-1-57859-305-7

*The Handy Politics Answer Book*
by Gina Misiroglu
ISBN: 978-1-57859-139-8

*The Handy Presidents Answer Book,*
  2nd edition
by David L. Hudson
ISB N: 978-1-57859-317-0

*The Handy Psychology Answer Book,*
  2nd edition
by Lisa J. Cohen, Ph.D.
ISBN: 978-1-57859-508-2

*The Handy Religion Answer Book,*
  2nd edition
by John Renard, Ph.D.
ISBN: 978-1-57859-379-8

*The Handy Science Answer Book,*
  4th edition
by The Carnegie Library of Pittsburgh
ISBN: 978-1-57859-321-7

*The Handy State-by-State Answer*
  *Book: Faces, Places, and Famous*
  *Dates for All Fifty States*
by Samuel Willard Crompton
ISBN: 978-1-57859-565-5

*The Handy Supreme Court Answer*
  *Book*
by David L Hudson, Jr.
ISBN: 978-1-57859-196-1

*The Handy Technology Answer Book*
by Naomi E. Balaban and James Bobick
ISBN: 978-1-57859-563-1

*The Handy Weather Answer Book,*
  2nd edition
by Kevin S. Hile
ISBN: 978-1-57859-221-0

PLEASE VISIT THE "HANDY ANSWERS" SERIES
WEBSITE AT WWW.HANDYANSWERS.COM.

# THE HANDY DIABETES ANSWER BOOK

Visible Ink Press®
43311 Joy Rd., #414
Canton, MI 48187–2075

Visible Ink Press is a registered trademark of Visible Ink Press LLC.

Most Visible Ink Press books are available at special quantity discounts when purchased in bulk by corporations, organizations, or groups. Customized printings, special imprints, messages, and excerpts can be produced to meet your needs. For more information, contact Special Markets Director, Visible Ink Press, www.visibleink.com, or 734–667–3211.

Managing Editor: Kevin S. Hile
Art Director: Mary Claire Krzewinski
Typesetting: Marco Divita
Proofreaders: Brian Buchanan and Shoshana Hurwitz
Indexer: Larry Baker
Cover images: Shutterstock.

ISBN: 978-1-57859-597-6

**Library of Congress Cataloging–in–Publication Data**

Names: Barnes–Svarney, Patricia L., author. | Svarney, Thomas E., author.
Title: The handy diabetes answer book / by Patricia Barnes-Svarney and Thomas E. Svarney.
Description: Canton, MI : Visible Ink Press, [2018] | Series: Handy answers series | Includes indexes.
Identifiers: LCCN 2017015273| ISBN 9781578595976 (pbk. : alk. paper) | ISBN 9781578596638 (epub) | ISBN 9781578596621 (pdf)
Subjects:  LCSH: Diabetes–Miscellanea.
Classification: LCC RC660 .B287 2018 | DDC 616.4/62–dc23
LC record available at https://lccn.loc.gov/2017015273

Printed in the United States of America.

10 9 8 7 6 5 4 3 2 1

# Table of Contents

## INTRODUCTION TO DIABETES ... 1

## WHO GETS DIABETES? ... 23

## TYPE 1 DIABETES ... 45

## PREDIABETES AND TYPE 2 DIABETES ... 59

## OTHER TYPES OF DIABETES ... 73

## DIABETES AND BODY CONNECTIONS ... 89

# Photo Sources

# Disclaimer

Information in this book is not meant as a replacement for the medical treatment of diabetes or other aliments, nor is it intended to substitute for the advice of your physician. It is meant for educational and information purposes only. If you have any questions about diabetes or any other medical problem, please seek help from a health care professional.

(*Note*: Because some people are sensitive to the term "diabetic," the word will be used sparingly in this text. The preferred phrase is "people with diabetes" (and we will refrain from using the annoying acronym "PWDs" or "People with Diabetes"). Also note, type 1 and type 2 diabetes are written as such throughout this text, although they are often written in the media as "Type 1," "Type I," or "T1D," and "Type 2," "Type II," or "T2D," respectively. Also, some health care professionals prefer to call diabetes a "syndrome," not a "disease." Because most references refer to diabetes as a "disease," this text will also use that term.)

# Acknowledgments

We, the authors, would like to thank everyone who "wages the war on diabetes"—from the doctors, nurses, and dieticians who help people cope with diabetes to the researchers and scientists who are constantly trying to mitigate the many forms of this disease.

Thanks to Roger Jänecke, our publisher, who asked us to write this book and let us take it in a more scientific direction. Thanks to Kevin Hile, our fabulous editor, for all his help and suggestions, not to mention realizing that Patricia writes best with plenty of chocolate. We'd also like to thank typesetter Marco Divita, page and cover designer Mary Claire Krzewinski, indexer Larry Baker, and proofreaders Shoshana Hurwitz and Brian Buchanan. And, as always, thanks to Agnes Birnbaum, our good friend and agent who puts up with our many questions—and always has the answers. You're the best, and always will be, Agnes.

A special (and huge) thanks goes to Gail Bykonich (who has had type 1 diabetes since she was ten) for all her help with this book. She is also one of the bravest people we've ever known, along with being a good friend. And, of course, thanks to brother James Barnes, sister Karen Barnes, and aunt and uncle Janet and John Barnes.

Finally, thanks to all the wonderful people who told us their (good and bad) experiences with diabetes. You all give people who cope with diabetes something special: hope.

# Introduction

Both of us have known many people—friends, family, and acquaintances—who have had (or currently have) some form of diabetes. Patricia's paternal grandmother died after 72 hours with uremia-acidosis (kidney problems exacerbated by her type 2 diabetes) and other complications of the disease at the tender age of 66. Her mother was diagnosed with type 2 diabetes at 68, and three years later she experienced her first heart attack. Her mother's attending physician nodded and stated, "Diabetes and heart problems. No surprise there."

And after writing this book, and knowing people who have the disease, we can both say, "No surprise there."

There are other stories. One night in June, there was the gentleman who rammed his truck into the front of a nearby house, the vehicle's nose landing right in the front part of the kitchen. He had no idea what was going on, including that he had also rammed a car down the street on his way up the hill, causing the car to flip over into a ditch (with no injuries). The EMTs were finally able to take his blood glucose (sugar) levels. The meter revealed a reading of 29 (normal hovers around 100), which is a dangerously low blood sugar level.

Amazingly, no one was hurt and there was only house and car damage. The sheriff told us the gentleman in the truck was lucky. He also mentioned how hard it was for a policeman or emergency personnel to determine if a person was drunk or had low blood sugar, a condition called hypoglycemia. Apparently and tragically, he also mentioned that this happens quite frequently.

One of the reasons for so many such stories is that diabetes (especially type 2) has almost become an epidemic. It is extremely pervasive not only in the United States but in other countries around the world. In 2016, it was no surprise when the World Health Organization announced that 422 million adults had diabetes, with 3.7 million deaths per year due to diabetes and its complications.

And there are reasons. First and foremost, medical research has greatly advanced in the past fifty years, and more is known about the causes and effects of the disease. Thus, it is studied and mentioned more in the medical literature and media. Second, more people are going to their doctors for checkups—and being tested for diabetes—than five decades ago. When Patricia's grandmother was diagnosed, there were no diabetic centers to go to for information, no Internet to check for information from the National Institutes of Health, the American Diabetes Association, and other diabetes interest groups. And above all, there was no "fit the treatment to the individual" attitude that is prevalent in many health care facilities today. There are more devices and medications than ever before to help those with type 1 and 2 diabetes, and even more treatments for the lesser-known forms of the disease.

And of course, another reason for the seeming epidemic of diabetes is that many more people are truly developing the disease.

Presented in this book is the latest about diabetes—from what causes the disease and why people develop it to how to best cope with diabetes at this time (we have no doubt treatment of diabetes will continue to metamorphose and improve). We present much of the science behind the disease, along with the details of how diabetes affects the various systems of the human body. We offer the history of diabetes research, who gets diabetes (including some animal research), and statistics surrounding diabetes. We even mention some celebrities who have diabetes—people who have bravely stepped forward (some after many years of hiding the disease) to help and educate others about how to cope and understand it.

There are suggestions for readers as to why exercise, along with better, healthier eating habits, can actually help people with the disease. And for those with prediabetes, we offer ways to help possibly stave off, or at least slow down, the disease. There are also book, Internet, and app resources to assist the reader (and, hopefully, to help them seek out more information), as well as a glossary of terms.

We also mention the promise of help in the future. For example, there is the current testing of an artificial pancreas for people with type 1 diabetes, along with monitors that don't require stabbing a person's finger over and over to test blood glucose levels. For people with type 2 diabetes, there are many studies that propose various ways to reverse the disease, along with possible ways never to contract type 2 diabetes (much if it in obesity research). And, of course, along with all the changes, research, and inventions, there are plenty of discussions (many of them heated) of the best ways to treat the disease.

This book is especially for those who have just learned they have diabetes. It is also for those who have a family member or friend with the disease. We discovered it is truly important for those who live, work, or play with a person with diabetes to know not only the signs of a diabetic emergency, but also when to contact emergency medical help. It can often save a family member or good friend. We know because we've been there many times.

One of the most difficult parts of having diabetes is coping. It's not easy when a person gets their first diagnosis of having diabetes. It's not easy for a person with diabetes to constantly be aware of their blood glucose (sugar) levels. It's not easy trying to watch what they consume—while others consume "forbidden" foods around them—and to understand how foods and beverages affect the person with diabetes. And it's especially difficult to watch a young child—or anyone, especially those close to us—cope with the disease.

We hope this book helps you to understand diabetes and lets you know how much of an effort is now placed in finding ways to help those with the disease, or at least ways to slow down the progression of diabetes. (We hesitate to say "cure," as not everyone can be helped with newer treatments, although one day, there may be a "cure" to mitigate the disease for many in the future.) We also hope you walk away knowing there are people who care, who can help you, and who are truly trying to understand this disease.

We found that many times it's not easy for a person to admit to others they have diabetes. But having diabetes is nothing to be "ashamed" of or to fear. Maybe this book will help a person with diabetes explain to others what it's like to cope with diabetes—to get over the fear of being (what some of our friends with diabetes say) "different." And we hope this book answers many of your questions about diabetes and helps you find the assistance you need.

To the brave people who have to deal with diabetes every day, we salute you.

# INTRODUCTION TO DIABETES

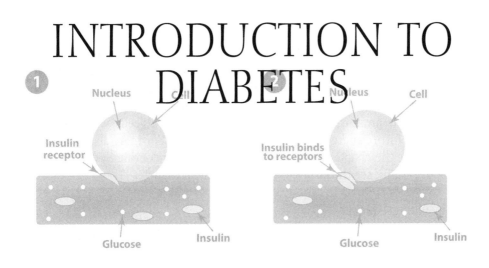

## What is a general definition of diabetes?

Diabetes is considered a complex group of diseases with a variety of causes. It is also often called a syndrome, or a combination of associated conditions. In most cases, people with diabetes have a high amount of glucose (a sugar) in their blood, also referred to as high blood glucose (or sugar) levels or, in the case of extremely high glucose levels, hyperglycemia. It is a disease that occurs when for various reasons the body's cells are unable to absorb excess glucose from the blood, which causes an overabundance of the sugar in the body. This is a very basic definition, as there are several types of diabetes, including type 1, type 2, and gestational diabetes.

For simplicity, and because most media mentions that diabetes is a disease (after all, it does include a collection of diseases with various causes), the remainder of this text will mention diabetes as a "disease" not a "syndrome."

## What is the medical term for the condition caused by the body's inability to produce or use insulin?

*Diabetes mellitus* is the medical term for the disease associated with the body's inability to naturally produce or use insulin. There are two major types—one is considered an autoimmune disease (type 1), and the other is a disorder of the body's metabolism, or the way the body processes food for energy (type 2). In general, diabetes occurs when the pancreas either produces little or no insulin, or when the cells do not respond appropriately to the insulin that is produced. Because of either of these conditions, glucose (sugar) builds up in the bloodstream (causing high blood glucose levels) and overflows into the urine. This excess amount of glucose is why a health care professional will tell patients newly diagnosed with diabetes that they have "high blood glucose levels."

## What is insulin?

Insulin is a hormone produced by the beta cells in the pancreas, an approximately six-inch-long organ found behind the stomach and below the liver. After a meal is eaten, insulin is released from the pancreas in response to rising blood glucose levels (most foods cause a person's blood glucose level to rise). The insulin then helps the passage of the glucose, along with amino acids and fatty acids, into the body's cells, which helps facilitate storage for future energy needs and cellular growth. (For more about insulin and the pancreas, see the chapter "How Diabetes Affects the Endocrine System"; for more details about insulin, see the chapter "Taking Charge of Diabetes.")

## What is insulin resistance?

Insulin resistance is a condition most associated with type 2 diabetes. It occurs when the body's natural hormone insulin is less effective in reducing a person's blood glucose

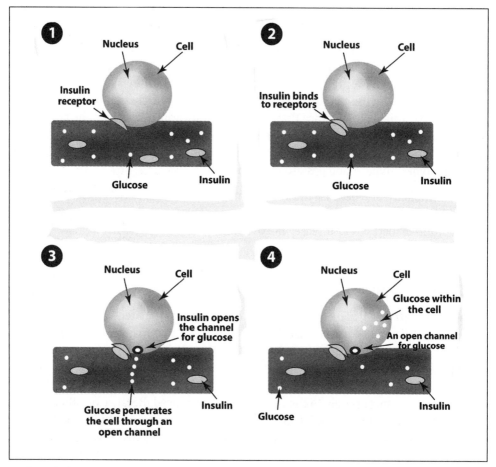

Insulin is the hormone that allows cells in our bodies to absorb sugar.

levels. This is caused by the body's cells being resistant to insulin's action, and/or not enough insulin is made in the pancreas. Either situation makes the glucose levels rise and, if severe enough, can lead to type 2 diabetes and other health problems. (For more about insulin resistance, see the chapter "Prediabetes and Type 2 Diabetes.")

## What is glucose?

During digestion, the fats, carbohydrates, and proteins consumed are eventually broken down into smaller components that can be used by the body's cells. One of the components is glucose, a six-carbon sugar that is a fuel providing energy the body's cells need. It is the imbalance of this glucose in the body—mainly too much glucose—that can lead to diabetes. (For more about glucose and the digestive tract, see the chapter "How Diabetes Affects the Digestive System.")

## What is the difference between "sugar" and "glucose" in discussing diabetes?

The terms "sugar" and "glucose" are often used interchangeably in relation to diabetes. Both terms are actually correct, as glucose is a form of sugar. But the term "sugar" is more commonly used by the public, which is why many people will say they "have sugar" when they are diagnosed with any type of diabetes.

## What is glucagon?

Glucagon is a hormone produced by the pancreas's alpha cells. This hormone is responsible for increasing the concentration of glucose in the blood. It is secreted from the pancreas when the blood glucose levels fall below normal. Glucagon actually stimulates the liver to convert glycogen to glucose, which causes the person's blood glucose level to rise. It does this by stimulating the production of glucose from amino acids and lactic acid in the liver and stimulates the release of fatty acids from fat (also called adipose) tissues. And when blood glucose levels sufficiently rise in the blood, the secretion of glucagon decreases as part of what is called a negative feedback system. (For more about glucagon and the pancreas, see the chapter "How Diabetes Affects the Endocrine System.") Glucagon can also be made synthetically and often comes in what is called a "glucagon kit," which is often used when a person with diabetes experiences a severe hypoglycemic episode, which is when blood sugar gets too low. (For more about glucagon kits, see the chapter "Taking Charge of Diabetes.")

## What does "plasma-glucose level" mean?

Plasma-glucose level is what is referred to by most people—and throughout this book—as blood glucose level. The term plasma refers to the liquid part of the blood that remains after the blood cells have been removed. This is the part of the blood, too, that is analyzed when a person has his or her blood glucose levels checked in a laboratory or doctor's office. All blood glucose meters are calibrated to measure the plasma-glucose level within a blood sample, although most people still say "blood glucose level."

### Is blood the only part of the body that contains glucose?

No, there are many "liquids" associated with the human body that contain glucose, not just the blood. For example, saliva, sweat, and tears contain glucose, as was known as far back as the 1930s. And of course, all the body's cells contain glucose because they need that component for energy.

### What are the most common types of diabetes?

Diabetes is commonly divided into several categories, depending on the severity, initial occurrence of the disease, and the cause of the diabetes. The most common types are prediabetes, type 1 and type 2, and gestational diabetes. (For more details about prediabetes, types 1 and 2 diabetes, gestational, and the many other forms of diabetes, see their respective chapters.) The following lists the general conditions for these forms of diabetes:

- *Prediabetes (also called impaired glucose tolerance [IGT] or impaired fasting glucose [IFG], depending on the test used)*: When a person has blood glucose (sugar) levels above the normal range but not high enough to be diagnosable as diabetes, he or she is considered prediabetic.
- *Type 1 (also seen as type I, type 1, or T1D)*: Also referred to as immune-mediated diabetes mellitus—formerly called insulin-dependent diabetes mellitus or juvenile diabetes. People with type 1 diabetes do not make enough insulin, the protein hormone made by the pancreas that helps the body use (and store) glucose from food.

---

### Does eating sugar cause type 1 or type 2 diabetes?

No, eating sugar does not cause type 1 or type 2 diabetes. Neither does eating fruit or vegetables that contain various types of sugars. In fact, if a person has a healthy pancreas, eating a modest amount of sugar in its various forms can help that organ produce more insulin for the body to use.

That being said, it is thought that there are several reasons that a person develops type 2 diabetes, and many are connected to sugar. Indirectly, the disease can often be "helped along" by the ingestion of the various types of sugar. For example, if the person's pancreas is diseased or does not function well, it can cause the body to process sugars incorrectly, which can lead to diabetes. If a person eats too many sweets, the pancreas can eventually have a difficult time handling the excess sugar, and a person can develop type 2 diabetes. If a person has a genetic predisposition to type 2 diabetes and/or overeats (often by eating too many sweets), becoming obese, this can lead to diabetes. Thus, sugar has been known to affect a person and can help lead to diabetes, but it is not the cause of the disease. (For more about sugar and diabetes, see the chapter "Diabetes and Eating.")

---

- *Type 2 (also seen as type II, type 2, or T2D)*: Also called insulin-resistant diabetes mellitus or adult-onset diabetes by some (although many do not use these terms anymore), type 2 diabetes usually occurs for two reasons. A person can develop type 2 diabetes when the body becomes less responsive to insulin, also known as insulin resistance. Or it can occur when the pancreas supplies too little insulin to keep up with the increased demand when a person has insulin resistance.

- *Gestational diabetes*: Also called gestational diabetes mellitus, it occurs during some pregnancies, but not all. It is a form of diabetes that affects between 5 and 9 percent of pregnant women (depending on the study) in the United States. There are usually no symptoms or the symptoms are mild, and it is usually found during a fasting blood glucose test.

## Why are there so many misconceptions when it comes to understanding diabetes?

One of the main reasons for misconceptions concerning diabetes is that it comes in several different but related forms. Someone who has type 1 diabetes develops the disease differently from a person with type 2 diabetes. But because many of the symptoms of the disease are similar and often overlap, many people confuse the true causes behind the two types.

Many other misconceptions about diabetes originated from how the disease was treated over the past century. For example, even the common phrase "I have sugar"—usually meant to indicate that a person has diabetes—is why most people think eating too much sugar will cause the disease, but this is definitely a myth (see sidebar).

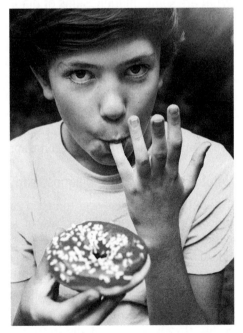

## If a person is overweight or obese, will he or she always develop type 2 diabetes?

No, not everyone who is overweight or obese will develop type 2 diabetes. In fact, some people who are normal weight or even moderately overweight can develop the disease. But having such extra weight often means the person has a higher risk for the disease. There also are other factors, such as family history (genetics), age (older people are more at risk to develop the disease), and ethnicity, that can also mean a higher risk of developing type 2 diabetes. (For more about diabetes and obesity, see the chapter "Diabetes and Obesity.")

Eating sugar doesn't cause diabetes, but there are indirect links between sugar and the disease, such as how it affects the health of the pancreas.

### In general, what is the difference between the causes of type 1 (or type I) and type 2 (or type II) diabetes?

Type 1, once (and still often) called insulin-dependent diabetes mellitus (IDDM), and type 2, once (and still often) called non-insulin-dependent diabetes mellitus (NIDDM), are the two most well-known types of diabetes. In general, insulin is deficient in a person with type 1 diabetes. With type 2 diabetes, a person's insulin secretion may be normal, but the target cells for insulin are less responsive than normal, or the insulin secretion may become abnormal. (For more details about type 1, see the chapter "Type 1 Diabetes," and for type 2 diabetes, see the chapter "Prediabetes and Type 2 Diabetes.")

### Are there divisions within divisions of type 1 and type 2 diabetes?

Yes, research has shown that both type 1 and type 2 diabetes—especially in the past decade—are truly not specific diseases but syndromes (although most health care professionals, researchers, and media still refer to diabetes as a disease). This means that within type 1 and type 2 diabetes profiles there are many subtypes and subdivisions. In fact, it is hoped that in the near future, health care professionals will be offering their patients with diabetes a wider range of therapy plans to treat—and in some cases, possibly mitigate—the effects of this syndrome. It may also mean that everyone who has diabetes will have a more personalized treatment to help cope with their specific type of diabetes.

### What are some "hidden" signs of diabetes?

Not all signs of the major types of diabetes are evident. They also may mimic other health problems and are often misinterpreted. Some of the more "hidden" signs of type 1 diabetes—and to a lesser extent type 2 diabetes—include red, tender, or swollen gums and tooth decay; high blood pressure; digestive problems; excessive thirst; mental confusion and fatigue; wounds that heal slowly; and numbness, burning pain, or tingling in the hands and feet. Because some of these symptoms are also signs of other major diseases, it is important to see a health care professional to test for diabetes or other health problems if these symptoms become apparent.

### What are some ways to diagnose early signs of diabetes?

Two of the best-known ways to detect early signs of any type of diabetes is to check for glucose in the urine (an "older" way of detecting glucose) and/or test for high blood glucose levels (a "newer" way of detecting glucose). Normally, the hormone insulin is produced by the pancreas, allowing the body to remove glucose from the blood and use it as fuel for cells. If a person has diabetes, the blood glucose in the body rises to unhealthy levels because the glucose is not removed at all or is not removed quickly enough.

When there is too much glucose—or when it reaches a certain level in a person's body—the glucose essentially spills over into the urine. Although not used as much, and usually only if a test for blood glucose is not available, a special test strip exposed to a person's urine can detect if blood sugar is high (but it cannot measure if the level is too low). The second, more reliable way (and one used by most health care professionals today) is to measure a person's blood sugar with a blood glucose test, such as the fasting blood glucose test. (For more about blood glucose tests, see the chapter "Taking Charge of Diabetes.")

## What is the effect of diabetes on the kidneys?

There is often a connection between diabetes and kidneys for a person with diabetes. Called diabetic kidney disease, or diabetic nephropathy, it is the most common kidney disease caused by diabetes. Even when it is controlled, diabetes can lead to chronic kidney disease (CKD) and eventual kidney failure. In fact, it is estimated that more than 40 percent of people who have diabetes can expect to develop CKD. Because of this statistic, in the United States it is often said that diabetes is the most common cause of kidney failure. (For more about kidneys and diabetes, see the chapter "How Diabetes Affects the Urinary System.")

## What is the major effect of diabetes on the heart?

Diabetes and heart problems are often said to go hand in hand. After all, according to Harvard Medical School, once a person has diabetes the risk for heart disease is four to five times greater. Furthermore, it is estimated that about 65 percent of people with diabetes will die from heart disease or stroke. (For more about the heart and diabetes, see the chapter "How Diabetes Affects the Circulatory System.")

## Does diabetes run in families?

Although most people believe diabetes runs in families, whether it does or not actually depends on the type of diabetes. In general, about 80 to 90 percent of people with type

---

### Can aspirin affect a person with diabetes?

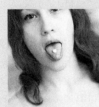

Yes, an aspirin can affect a person with diabetes—especially by lowering their blood glucose levels below a healthy range, but only with prolonged use and if taken in large amounts (eight or more 325-milligram [mg] tablets per day). Therefore, most doctors believe the occasional aspirin is generally safe for most people with diabetes. (But, as always, patients should check with their doctor to determine whether there is any problem with taking an aspirin and for the correct dosage of aspirin for their condition.) Most doctors usually suggest that people with diabetes check their blood glucose levels while taking the drug. Doctors should also inform patients if they need to be monitored while taking aspirin for any extended period.

> ## Can the weather affect a person with diabetes more than a person without diabetes?
>
> Yes, weather can affect a person with diabetes more than a person without diabetes. For example, in extreme humidity, there is always a risk of heat exhaustion. If a person with diabetes has poor glucose management—which can affect that person's ability to sweat in the first place—he or she may have more of a tendency to overheat. And because higher blood glucose levels make people urinate more, they can also become dehydrated faster in hot, humid weather. (For more about diabetes and extreme temperatures, see the chapter "Coping with Diabetes.")

1 diabetes have no family history of the disease, while the majority of people with type 2 diabetes do have a family history of the disease.

# EARLY STUDIES OF DIABETES

### How long has diabetes been known as a disease?

Symptoms of diabetes (though it was not called diabetes) were known around 3,500 years ago and were first recorded by the Egyptians. By the mid-seventh century, the Chinese physician Chen Ch'üan (c. 640 C.E.) also noted the symptoms of diabetes, including excessive thirst and sweet urine. In the first century, the celebrated Greek physician Aretaeus of Cappadocia (81–138 C.E.) called it *diabainein,* from the Greek *dia* ("to pass through") and *bainein* ("to go"), referring to the excessive urination associated with the disease. He further noted the horrible way in which the patients with the disease met their demise, writing that, as far as he could tell, it was the "melting down of the flesh and limbs into urine." And around the early eleventh century, the Persian physician Avicenna (980–1037) supposedly described the disease and its many consequences.

### Where does the term "diabetes" come from?

The term as "diabetes" was first mentioned in 1425 (as *diabete*), from the Latin. This, in turn, comes from the ancient Greek words *dia* meaning "to pass through" and *betes* meaning a "water tube," thus the loose translation that is often seen as "water siphon." The word *mellitus* was added probably around 1670 (see below), from the Latin for "like honey" or "sweetened with honey" to reflect the sweet smell (and taste) of the patient's urine.

### Who was Thomas Willis?

Thomas Willis (1621–1675) was an English physician who is most remembered for his rationalist approach to the human brain and nervous system. Although many historians consider his contributions to diabetes minor (others centuries before had noted the symptoms; see above), he did rediscover that urine from people with diabetes tasted sweet and is credited with referring to the condition as *diabetes mellitus,* or "honey diabetes," around 1670. (There is some disagreement as to this date, with some references suggesting that the scientific term *diabetes mellitus* was first used in 1860.) He is often called the "first modern Western physician" to rediscover the sweet urine–diabetes connection. But instead of sugar, he attributed the sweetness of urine to salts and acids. He also thought this disease was a rare condition before his time and believed diabetes in *his* time was from excessive living. He also associated the disease with depression, stating that "diabetes is caused by melancholy."

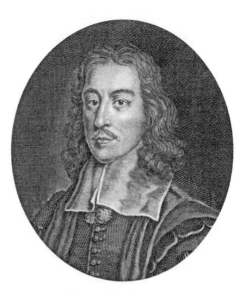

English physician Thomas Willis was the first Western doctor to figure out the connection between diabetes and sugar in the urine.

## How did early doctors "test" for diabetes in patients?

Around 1670, Thomas Willis announced the rediscovery of the connection between diabetes and the sweetness of the patient's urine, although the symptoms of the disease had already been noted earlier by the Egyptians, Chinese, Greeks, and Indians. Doctors who knew about the disease—it had yet to be understood—would then diagnose the disease by tasting a patient's urine. This is because when the blood glucose levels in a person rise, the body takes out water from the cells' tissues and eliminates the sugar through the urine. As time went on, not all doctors used the modern tests, often discovering the disease in a patient through tasting the urine. It was even, as some reports mentioned, noticed by observation. For example, one report stated that in the 1800s, an incontinent person with diabetes and on his or her deathbed would often attract black ants.

## Who was Matthew Dobson?

English physician and experimental physiologist Matthew Dobson (1732–1784) was the first to discover, in 1775, that sugar was the sweet substance in the patients with diabetes (caused by hyperglycemia). His work, *Experiments and Observations on the Urine in Diabetics* (1776), did not have a great impact on the medical community. He also noted that diabetes was not associated with the kidneys, as many physicians believed at that time.

## What is polyuria?

Polyuria is when a patient urinates excessively, usually producing dilute urine. This excessive urination is often one of the first symptoms of uncontrolled diabetes, especially of type 1 and type 2 diabetes, in both children and adults. This symptom was known by many early physicians before the main reasons for diabetes were understood.

## Who was Michel Chevreul?

In 1815, Michel Eugène Chevreul (1786–1889), a French chemist, showed that the sugar or sweetness in the urine of a person with diabetes came from what he termed "grape sugar." It is what is now known as glucose. In Chevreul's time, the finding was an important step toward understanding diabetes.

## What did early doctors think caused diabetes?

Diabetes was not well understood until the early 1900s. Before then, there were many suggestions as to the cause. For example, many doctors believed the disease was just an imbalance in the body. They believed the reason for a patient's experiencing excessive urination, profuse sweating, and often vomiting was that the body was trying to get back into balance again.

## What were some early common treatments for patients with diabetes?

Because diabetes was so misunderstood, there were many treatments that seem bizarre and even dangerous by today's standards. One of the most popular treatments was commonly used for almost all diseases in the 1800s—the practice of bleeding the patient. Others included having the person fast (many times to near starvation), having him or her eat excessive amounts of sugar, giving the person only the meat and fat of animals to eat, or feeding him or her specific herbs that were thought to cleanse the body of diabetes.

## Who were Jean De Meyer and Edward Sharpey-Schäfer?

English physiologist Edward Albert Sharpey-Schäfer (1850–1935) was the first scientist to suggest that the pancreas was connected to blood sugar levels in the body. He was also the first person to discover adrenaline and inferred the existence of "insuline," the term he used for what is now called insulin. Several years before, Belgian clinician and physiologist Jean-Egide-Camille-Philippe-Hubert De Meyer (1878–1934) worked on pancreatic secretions and also suggested the name "insuline"—the original French—13 years before the hormone was isolated. Sharpey-Schäfer was apparently unaware of De Meyer's work.

As early as 1895, Sharpey-Schäfer theorized that glucose came from the pancreas and originated in the islets of Langerhans. He also suggested several ideas about the nature of insuline, including that it may be an enzyme that the body uses to metabolize glucose. The theory he preferred was that insuline may inhibit the breakdown of glycogen, and if the liver did not have this "inhibitor," it would no longer store glucose, causing it to spill into the body's circulation.

## Who discovered the connection between the islets of Langerhans and diabetes?

American physician and pathologist Eugene Lindsay Opie (1873–1971) was the first to discover the relationship between the islets of Langerhans (found in the pancreas) and diabetes. After examining postmortem patients who had developed diabetes, he correctly assumed that degenerative changes in the tissues of the pancreas (or islets of Langerhans) caused the diabetes. Along with his diabetes-and-pancreas discoveries, Opie was also known for his research on the causes, transmission, and diagnosis of tuberculosis (TB) and worked on immunization against the disease. He was also the first to suggest that an obstruction at the junction of the bile and pancreatic ducts was responsible for acute pancreatitis.

## Which researchers are credited with discovering insulin?

The credit for the discovery of insulin most often goes to Canadian physician Frederick Grant Banting (1891–1941), Scottish biochemist and physiologist John James R. Macleod (1876–1935), and Canadian medical scientist Charles Best (1899–1978). Although earlier researchers had suggested that the pancreas secreted a substance that controlled the metabolism of the body's blood sugar, it was not proven until 1922, when Banting, Macleod, and Best announced their discovery. In 1921, they had begun experimenting on dogs, removing the animals' pancreases, essentially making the dogs diabetic. They would then grind down the animals' organs and extract a solution they called isletin. Injecting the solution into other animals resulted in a drop in blood sugar levels. By January 1922, they formulated an extract—this time from cattle pancreases—to try on humans with type 1 diabetes (see Leonard Thompson, below). When Thompson had an allergic reaction, Canadian biochemist James Bertram Collip (1892–1965) worked for about 11 straight days, making the injection more "pure" for humans. The new solution worked, and after several more patients were treated successfully, insulin eventually became one of the best treatments for people with diabetes.

## Did any other researchers come close to discovering insulin?

Yes, several other researchers came close to discovering, extracting, and developing insulin. The list is long and often confusing. Some people claim that certain researchers came close but did not understand what they were witnessing. Other historians believe certain researchers should have been given more credit for their discoveries. And there is also a political, social, and infighting aspect of science in the early days before, during, and even after the first insulin trials. The following lists some of the more well-known cases in the history of insulin (and some of these events are often highly debated by historians):

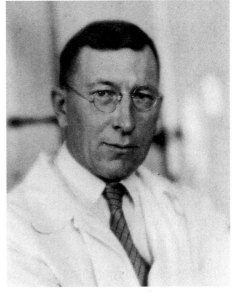

Canadian physician and Nobel laureate Frederick Banting was co-discoverer of insulin.

- In 1889, two European researchers, German physiologist and pathologist Oskar Minkowski (1858–1931) and German physician Joseph Freiherr von Mering (1849–1908), working at an institute in Strasbourg headed by an authority on diabetes, German pathologist Bernhard Naunyn (1839–1925), discovered that when the pancreas was removed from dogs, the animals would develop symptoms of diabetes. The researchers suggested that the pancreas was crucial to the body's sugar regulation and metabolism.
- American physiologist Ernest Lyman Scott (1877–1966) conducted blood-sugar experiments on dogs. If a dog's pancreas was removed, he noticed the animal's blood sugar would rise. He then isolated secretions from the pancreas (what is now known as insulin) and injected the dog, causing its blood sugar level to lower. Thus, he is often credited as the first person actually to extract insulin (in 1911; insulin for medical use was introduced in 1923). In addition, he is most well known for developing the standard blood test for diabetes in 1914.
- Romanian physiologist and professor of medicine Nicolas Constantin Paulescu (also seen as Paulesco; 1869–1931) worked to identify the active pancreatic substance that Minkowski and von Mering suggested could be used to treat diabetes. In 1916, he isolated the substance and called it "pancrein," or what is now called insulin. Thus, Paulescu is often suggested as the discoverer of insulin (and why some researchers believe Paulesco and Scott should have been credited with discovering insulin).
- But in the end, the Nobel Prize in Physiology or Medicine in 1923 was awarded to Banting and Macleod, as they were the first known actually to develop insulin for human use. (Banting shared his half of the prize with Best, while Macleod shared his half of the prize with Collip.)

## Who was Elizabeth Evans Hughes?

Elizabeth Evans Hughes (later Gossett; 1907–1981) developed type 1 diabetes at age 11. She was the daughter of Charles Evans Hughes (1862–1948), a former governor of New York, an associate justice of the Supreme Court of the United States, and a presidential candidate (he was defeated by Woodrow Wilson), among other political accomplishments. At the time Elizabeth was diagnosed, most people who had untreated type 1 diabetes only lived about a year after diagnosis. In addition, most treatments included a starvation diet. Elizabeth was put on such a diet, going from around 75 pounds (34 kilograms) to 45 (20.4 kilograms) in three years. Eventually, Frederick Banting agreed to take Elizabeth on as a private patient. Determined to get well even though the disease was destroying her health, she became one of the first patients treated with the "new" medication for diabetes—insulin. She recovered quickly and was eating a normal diet within two weeks. (For more about Banting and insulin, see above.)

## Who was Leonard Thompson?

In January 1921, Leonard Thompson (1908–1935) was the first person with type 1 diabetes to receive an injection of insulin. He was 14 years old at the time and weighed a mere 65 pounds (27 kilograms). The insulin was created by Macleod, Banting, and Best (see above) and was reported to be "a murky, light brown liquid containing much sediment," a far cry from what insulin is like today. Thompson had an allergic reaction to the first shot. But after James Collip (1892–1965) removed many of the contaminants, the cattle-extracted solution was successful, resulting in Thompson's sugar levels returning to "normal." Thompson would continue taking insulin for the rest of his life. He died at age 27 of pneumonia, thought to be a complication from his diabetes.

## Why was it so difficult to make insulin long ago?

Overall, insulin was difficult to manufacture in large quantities, and there was also a problem with contamination of the insulin. In addition, at that time, there were about one million Americans with type 1 diabetes. Not only was there a low quantity and quality of insulin, there were also problems matching a correct dosage to a person.

## Which company made the first commercial insulin?

The company responsible for making the first commercial insulin was Eli Lilly. In 1922, in collaboration with MacLeod, Banting, Best, and Collip (who realized they could not commercially produce their insulin in large quantities), the company put the new drug through more than 100,000 tests. By April 1923, the company was producing more than 180,000 units of insulin per week, although the overall preparations were difficult (they used cattle and porcine pancreas glands).

## Who was the first person to crystallize (purify) insulin?

Because the first human insulin preparations were so impure, there was a need to isolate a pure form of the hormone. The first person to develop such a pure insulin—also called crystallized insulin—was American biochemist John Jacob Abel (1857–1938) in 1926. Abel was also the first person to purify adrenaline (originally discovered by Edward Sharpey-Schäfer; see above), a substance he called epinephrine, and first to invent a primitive artificial kidney.

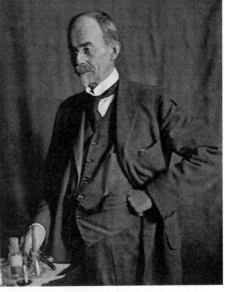

## Who was Sir Harold Himsworth?

Sir Harold Percival Himsworth (1905–1993) is thought by many historians to be the first to describe diabetes as a syndrome. Other earlier physicians had men-

American pharmacologist John Jacob Abel was the first scientist to purify insulin.

tioned the possible connection between late-onset diabetes and obesity, hypertension, and arterial diseases. But Himsworth was the first to mention the syndrome in his 1949 *Lancet* paper "The syndrome of diabetes mellitus and its causes."

## Who was Elliot Joslin?

Elliot Joslin (1869–1962) is credited as one of the first diabetes researchers to uncover the association between obesity and diabetes and one of the first physicians to specialize in diabetes. In addition, in the 1930s, he was the first to note the association between diabetes, hypertension, and arterial disease. He was the founder of the Joslin Institute, a premier research institute specializing in diabetes. (For more about the Joslin Institute, see the chapter "Resources, Websites, and Apps.")

## When was the true structure of insulin determined?

The full structure of insulin, called a peptide hormone, was discovered in 1955 by British biochemist Frederick Sanger (1918–2013). It was the first protein to be fully sequenced (or determining DNA bases in a genome; for more about genomes and DNA, see the chapter "Other Types of Diabetes"). Sanger won the Nobel Prize in Chemistry in 1958 for his research on insulin (he also won a Nobel Prize in Chemistry in 1980, one of only two people ever to have done so in the same category).

## What were the steps to developing synthetic insulin?

Research shows that once a protein's sequence is known, it is possible (in theory) to make the same thing synthetically. Thus, in 1963, insulin was the first protein to be chemically synthesized in the laboratory. But it was still difficult to produce enough of the insulin for the million or more people with diabetes. By 1978, insulin became the first human protein to be manufactured through biotechnology. It was first synthesized by American geneticist Arthur Riggs (1939–) and Japanese molecular biologist and chemist Keiichi

### Why did so many people hide their diabetes diagnosis long ago?

It is hard to say why so many people once hid their diagnosis of diabetes. In fact, it was often called an "invisible" disease because most people showed no symptoms, and many chose to hide their condition. Some of the reason was no doubt cultural (often called the "stiff upper lip" syndrome), and many people with the disease did not want others to know they were not healthy. Before the availability of insulin, having the disease often meant a quick death. Other times, because the disease was not well understood, many people did not know whether the disease would spread. All this, and no doubt more, led people to hide their diagnosis of diabetes. Through research and education in the last half century, the disease—although still not fully understood—does not have the same stigma as in earlier times.

Itakura (1942–) using *E. coli* bacteria with recombinant DNA technology. The City of Hope National Medical Center (to date, Keiichi Itakura still works at the center), along with the biotechnology company Genentech, synthesized the first human insulin in a process that could produce insulin in large amounts. In order to do this, the researchers inserted a gene for human insulin into bacterial DNA and used the bacteria as minifactories to make the A and B chains of the protein separately. Then a chemical process combined them. This procedure created a more "human-user-friendly" type of insulin, which was much more stable than animal insulin. Most insulin-dependent people with diabetes now use recombinant human insulin instead of animal insulin.

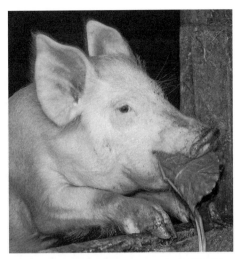

Before synthetic insulin was invented, pigs like this one had been used to produce insulin for humans with diabetes, since their insulin is quite similar to a person's.

## Which animals were used for insulin in the past?

Long before synthetic insulin was available, insulin for human use was usually derived from animals, especially pigs and cattle. For example, the amino-acid sequence of pig and human insulin are almost identical, but not exact: pigs' insulin differs from humans' by one amino acid, and cattle (bovine) insulin differs by three amino acids. But in the 1920s, no one knew the details of genetic sequencing. Thus, the researchers were fortunate that the various animal species' insulin used were almost the same as in humans (although sometimes there were adverse reactions to the animal-extracted insulin, such as skin rashes).

## What is Humalog®?

Humalog® is a commercially available—by prescription—modified human insulin. It was approved by the Food and Drug Administration in 1996 and was specifically developed to be active quickly after injection by quickly lowering levels of blood glucose (thus it is called a rapid-acting insulin). It is mostly used to treat type 1 diabetes in adults and usually given with long-acting insulin. Humalog® (also referred to as "insulin lispro injection") is manufactured much like Humulin®, as it is produced by recombinant DNA technology (using a strain of *E. coli* or *Escherichia coli*).

## When was the first synthesized human insulin available?

The first human insulin to be synthesized was called Humulin®, manufactured by a technique known as recombinant DNA (or the inserting of human genetic instructions into a bacterium that then produces the drug). It was approved by the Food and Drug Administration in 1982 but was not marketed—and thus was not widely available—until 1983. It is almost, but not exactly, identical to the insulin produced by the human pancreas, and for the most part, it acts in the same way as the body's own natural insulin. Humulin® is also considered a rapid-acting insulin (it takes a relatively short time to become active in a person's bloodstream after taking it, compared to some other types of insulin; for more about the various types of insulin, see the chapter "Taking Charge of Diabetes").

# STATISTICS AND DIABETES

## What are the ten leading causes of death in the United States?

According to the U.S. Centers for Disease Control and Prevention (CDC), the top leading causes of death in the United States were as follows as of 2014 (listed in a report in 2015)—and included diabetes:

1. Heart disease (also called ischemic heart disease)
2. Cancer (malignant neoplasms)
3. Chronic lower respiratory disease
4. Accidents (unintentional injuries)
5. Stroke (cerebrovascular diseases)
6. Alzheimer's disease
7. Diabetes (diabetes mellitus)
8. Influenza and pneumonia

9. Kidney disease (nephritis, nephritic syndrome, and nephrosis)

10. Suicide (intentional self-harm)

Annually, and on average, these ten causes account for nearly 75 percent of all deaths in the United States. In fact, this list has not changed much in several years.

## Is diabetes truly the seventh leading cause of death in the United States?

Yes, it is, but in some ways, it should be considered the third leading cause of death. The numbers—seventh or third—are true, but they are dependent on whether people who die from related cardiovascular disease are included. In other words, just diabetes alone accounts for the listing as seventh, whereas diabetes and the often-resulting cardiovascular disease (heart problems in particular) would make diabetes third on the list.

## What percentage of people have prediabetes in the United States?

According to the Centers for Disease Control and Prevention (CDC), in 2014, almost 80 million Americans were thought to have prediabetes (also written as pre-diabetes). By 2016, it was estimated that the number had grown to 86 million, but only about 11 percent of pre-diabetic people realize they have prediabetes. The CDC also suggests that 70 percent of those who have prediabetes (and know it) will go on to develop type 2 diabetes if they do not take care of themselves. In other words, many Americans are ignoring the signs and symptoms of prediabetes and will eventually develop type 2 diabetes. This outcome will, in turn, put a major strain on public health and the health care system—not to mention inflict a possible emotional and most likely economic toll on people and their families.

## How many people have diabetes in the United States?

According to Harvard Medical School, to date, there are nearly 26 million Americans with diabetes (mainly type 1 and type 2)—a number that has almost doubled in just over a decade. It is estimated that another 86 million adults have elevated blood sugar levels and are at a higher-than-normal risk for developing diabetes (prediabetes). Thus, overall, it is estimated that one in three Americans has diabetes or has a high risk for developing it.

## What percentage of the United States population has type 1 diabetes?

According to the International Diabetes Federation, to date, around 5 percent of the people in the United States with diabetes have type 1 diabetes. Because it is estimated that there are around 26 million Americans with diabetes, "5 percent" means that over 1 million people have type 1 diabetes in the United States (another estimate is that 1.25 million Americans have type 1 diabetes).

According to several statistics from various diabetes organizations, more than 40,000 cases of type 1 diabetes are reported per year in the United States, and that number continues to grow. It is also estimated that by the year 2050, there will be 5 million people in the United States with type 1 diabetes, with nearly 600,000 of them less than 20 years of age.

### How many American children and adults are thought to have type 1 diabetes?

Although type 1 diabetes is most often associated with children, it also can affect adults (for more about adult type 1 diabetes, see the chapter "Type 1 Diabetes"). According to the JDRF (formerly the Juvenile Diabetes Research Foundation), of the 1.25 million Americans who have type 1 diabetes, 200,000 are young (under 20 years old) and over a million are adults (20 and older).

### How fast has the number of diabetics in the United States increased over the past 25 years?

According to Harvard Medical School, statistics have shown that the number of Americans with diabetes (all types) has grown sharply—some estimates say doubled in number in just over a decade. It is also estimated that more than 90 percent of the people who have diabetes have type 2 diabetes.

### Which one of the largest U.S. cities has the highest diabetes rate?

According to a study conducted at Drexel University in 2014, Philadelphia has the highest diabetes rate among the nation's largest cities. In addition, the county where Philadelphia is located is considered to have one of the worst health conditions of any county in the state. A study from the journal *Advances in Preventive Medicine* found in surveying more than 17,000 participants in the Philadelphia area that living in a disadvantaged neighborhood seemed to play a major role in a person's risk of developing diabetes. Researchers said focusing on the individual to curtail the number of people with the disease in this region would not be as effective as concentrating on the education— and thus the health—of the overall community.

### How much is spent on diabetes care each year in the United States?

According to the most recent data (2012), it is thought that spending on diabetes and its care costs more than $245 billion per year in the United States alone—a record high (and it is no doubt even higher as of this writing). Of that, $176 billion went for such diabetes-

---

### What are the four leading causes of death worldwide?

According to the World Health Organization, in 2012 (the most recent data was updated in 2014), ischemic heart disease, stroke, lower respiratory infections, and chronic obstructive lung disease were the top major killers worldwide. In fact, this four-causes list has remained the same for the past decade. (The lung-related ailments were listed at around 3.1 million deaths per year.) Even though this short list does not include diabetes, heart disease is often found in connection with diabetes. (Diabetes was listed as the eighth leading cause at 1.5 million deaths per year.)

associated items as medications and emergency care. In fact, in 2010, almost 10 percent of all emergency-room visits in the United States were by people with diabetes-related conditions, such as nerve damage, eye trouble, and kidney and circulatory problems.

## How many people around the world are thought to have prediabetes?

According to the International Diabetes Federation, in 2013 (the latest data from IDF), around 316 million people have what is called impaired glucose intolerance (or impaired fasting glucose), or prediabetes. This number has grown significantly in the past decade.

## Has the number of deaths from diabetes increased worldwide?

Yes, according to data from the World Health Organization (WHO), diabetes caused around one million deaths in the year 2000. In 2012 (updated in 2014), the number increased, with diabetes causing around 1.5 million deaths. (Note: These numbers do not distinguish between people with type 1 or type 2 diabetes.)

## How many people die of diabetes-related complications around the world each year?

The statistics concerning how many people die of diabetes-related complications around the world each year would fill many pages of this book. Such information can be found on several diabetes-education websites, such as the International Diabetes Federation (www.idf.org). For example, in 2013, the IDF estimated that 5.1 million people died of diabetes-related complications worldwide.

## Why is it difficult to estimate the number of people with diabetes around the world or for specific countries?

Probably the main problem when estimating how many people have diabetes is that there is no national registry or database for the disease in most countries or even an international database (unlike for some infectious diseases or even for such conditions as Lyme disease). In addition, many reports of deaths from diabetes are actually couched in terms of secondary diseases, such as heart or kidney failure (which can be from diabetes but are listed only as heart or kidney failure). Thus, many organizations that present statistics on how many people have diabetes may be underestimating the disease.

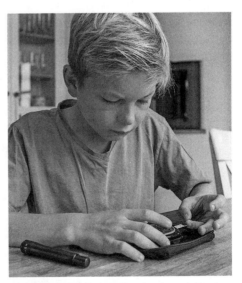

Over half a million children worldwide have type 1 diabetes.

19

### How many children around the world have type 1 diabetes?

It is estimated that 542,000 children worldwide have type 1 diabetes. Of this number, about 200,000 live in the United States, according to the JDRF (formerly called the Juvenile Diabetes Research Foundation). And it is thought that the numbers will keep rising around the world. For example, according to the International Diabetes Federation, more than 79,000 children developed type 1 diabetes in 2013. This number was up from 77,800 in 2011.

### Which continent has the highest number of children with type 1 diabetes?

According to the International Diabetes Federation, the European continent has the highest number of children with type 1 diabetes. It is not known why this is so, but some researchers suggest that it may be due to one or more environmental, genetic, or dietary factors.

### How many people have diabetes in the United Kingdom?

As of this writing, it is estimated that 3.2 million people in the United Kingdom have diabetes. It is estimated that the number will reach 5 million people by the year 2025.

---

## Why do some researchers believe sugar may have a direct link to diabetes in other countries?

In a study conducted in 2013, researchers suggested that the amount of sugar sold in a country may have a close link to diabetes. In particular, the study examined data of global sugar availability and diabetes rates from 175 different countries over the past ten years. They found that as the sugar in certain countries' food supplies increased (and therefore, consumption increased), there were higher type 2 diabetes rates. In addition, they found that the longer a population was exposed to excess sugar, the higher the diabetes rate. The study's statistical methods controlled for factors such as obesity rates, calories available per day, percentage of the population age 65 or older (as age is associated with increased diabetes risk), and so on. Thus, because of this study, some researchers suggest that sugar may affect the liver and pancreas in ways that other types of foods or obesity do not.

Of course, not all researchers agree. Many believe that obesity has a direct and major effect on a person's predisposition toward type 2 diabetes, along with total calorie intake. This study, too, does not prove that sugar causes diabetes—either type 1 or 2. But it does add more data to the quandary faced by many researchers who are trying to understand why there has been such an increase in the number of people worldwide who have diabetes. (For more about sugar in the diet and diabetes, see the chapter "Diabetes and Eating.")

## What is the estimate as to how many people with diabetes die of heart disease or stroke?

According to the American Diabetes Association, it is estimated that more than 65 percent of people with diabetes die of heart disease or stroke. But the association also notes that if people with diabetes manage their blood pressure and cholesterol—along with their blood glucose levels—they can greatly reduce their risk of both heart disease and stroke.

## How many people are afflicted by diabetes around the world—and will be affected in the future?

In 2015, the International Diabetes Federation estimated that there were 415 million adults with diabetes around the world, or one person in 11 has the disease. This is merely an estimate, as it is thought that one in two adults (or around 46.5 percent) with diabetes is undiagnosed. The organization also estimates that by the year 2040, around 642 million people—or about one person in ten—will have the disease.

Of course, like many statistics, numbers reported depend on the organization. For example, in 2016 the UN World Health Organization released its figures: 422 million adults around the world—or one in 11 people or 8.5 percent of the population—have diabetes. WHO also reported that in 2012, 1.5 million deaths were caused by diabetes, with higher-than-optimal blood glucose levels causing an additional 2.2 million deaths that year, mainly by the increased risk of cardiovascular and other diseases.

## What are some of the reasons for the higher levels of type 2 diabetes around the world?

There is probably no one reason for the high levels of type 2 diabetes around the world, and many researchers mention several factors. For example, type 2 diabetes seems to be associated with higher levels of urbanization; an aging population; more sedentary lifestyles; and unhealthful diets (which often include a high sugar intake). In addition, according to the International Diabetes Federation, around 75 percent of people with diabetes live in low- and middle-income countries (but IDF does not list type 1 and type 2 diabetes separately).

## Are treatments for diabetes available around the world?

Although most wealthy countries have a good supply of insulin available for people with diabetes, several do not. For example, according to the World Health Organization, essential diabetes medicines and technologies, including insulin, that are needed for treatments are mainly available in only one in three of the world's poorest countries.

## On average, how much is spent on diabetes around the world?

According to the International Diabetes Federation, in 2015, 12 percent of global health expenditures were spent on diabetes. By the year 2040, with the increase in the number of people with diabetes, it is estimated that the amount of global health expenditures for the disease will be around $802 billion (U.S.) per year.

# WHO GETS DIABETES?

## Do type 1 and type 2 diabetes run in families?

According to the American Diabetes Association and research on genetics, type 1 diabetes does seem to have a genetic component. In other words, a person's particular genetic makeup means that he or she is more likely to develop type 1 diabetes, especially under certain conditions. Research also indicates that many people with type 2 diabetes have a genetic predisposition to the disease—more so than a person with type 1 diabetes. The risk of developing diabetes is also based on such factors as aging; whether the person has an inactive lifestyle; and/or if he/she becomes overweight or obese. (For more about genetics and diabetes, see the chapter "Other Types of Diabetes.")

## What are some statistical chances of getting diabetes within families?

Like most data in science, the statistics about a person's chance of developing type 1 or type 2 diabetes is often dependent on the research study. For example, one organization states that if a brother, sister, son, or daughter has diabetes, the chance of an immediate relation contracting type 1 diabetes is 10 percent; if the mother has type 1, the chance is 2 percent, and if the father does, 6 percent. For type 2, if a brother or sister has type 2, the chances of a relation's having type 2 diabetes is 25 percent; a mother or father having it gives a chance of 12 percent; both the mother and father, the chance is 50 percent; and if an identical twin has type 2 diabetes, the chance is 90 percent.

But not everyone agrees. Still another group, the Harvard School of Public Health, states that if a parent, sister, son, or daughter has type 1 diabetes, the risk of an immediate relation developing type 1 diabetes is 10 to 20 times that of the general population, with the risk going from one in 100 to one in ten depending on which family member has diabetes and when he or she developed it. In addition, their studies indicate that if a mother has diabetes, the risk of a child developing type 1 diabetes is lower than if the father has the disease (around 10 percent chance of getting type 1 diabetes if the father has it). But if the mother has type 1 diabetes and is age 25 or younger when the child is born, the risk is reduced by 4 percent; if the mother is over age 25, the risk drops to one in 100, or around the same as the average American. Thus, statistics and chances of developing type 1 and type 2 are extremely dependent on the conditions surrounding the person who develops the disease—and especially the scientific group or study!

## Which ethnic, racial, or cultural groups are more prone to type 1 and type 2 diabetes in the United States?

There is a difference among groups who seem to be more prone to type 1 and type 2 diabetes. In particular, it is thought that white people of northern European heritage are more prone to type 1 diabetes than members of other ethnic and racial groups. Other groups also have their share of diabetes diagnoses. According to the American Diabetes Association, the following ethnic, racial, or cultural groups in the United States have various percentages of diagnosed diabetes:

- Ethnic or racial backgrounds: 7.6% of non-Hispanic whites; 9.0% of Asian Americans; 12.8% of Hispanics; 13.2% of non-Hispanic blacks; 15.9% of American Indians or Alaskan Natives.
- Asian Americans: 4.4% of Chinese; 11.3% of Filipinos; 13% of Asian Indians; 8.8% of other Asian Americans.
- Hispanic background (adults): 8.5% of Central and South Americans; 9.3% of Cubans; 13.9% of Mexican Americans; 14.8% of Puerto Ricans.

## Which countries have the most cases of diabetes, and which have the highest rates as a percentage of the countries' overall population?

Many organizations present various numbers and results concerning diabetes around the world. And no matter which organizations find what results, the underlying message is clear: Diabetes is very prevalent all over the world. For example, according to the International Diabetes Federation, China, India, and the United States have the most cases of diabetes. Several islands in the Pacific Ocean have the most rates of prevalence, or in other words, the highest rates of diabetes cases as a percentage of the country's overall population. For instance, around 37.5 percent of the population of Tokelau (northeast of Fiji) has diabetes; Saudi Arabia, Qatar, Kuwait, and Micronesia all have higher-than-average rates of diabetes cases. In addition, Southeast Asia has nearly one-fifth (20 percent) of the global diabetes cases (and it is estimated that almost 50 percent of the population has not been formally diagnosed). Many of these countries are growing, and the availability and consumption of foods has changed (including more imported foods being eaten). As a result, many researchers believe diabetes is prevalent in these countries because of a growing obesity problem.

Of course, as with all statistics, other organizations find different results in their studies. For example, the World Health Organization notes that in 2014, half of adults

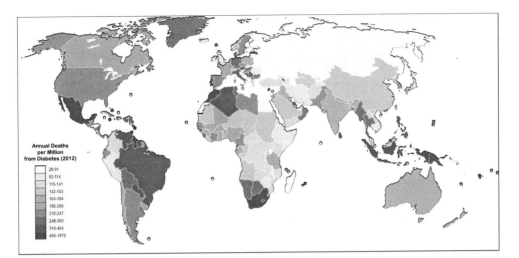

A map of the world showing the prevalence of diabetes by country, according to a World Health Organization 2012 study.

around the world with diabetes lived in five countries: China, India, the United States, Brazil, and Indonesia, and noted that the rates doubled for men in India and China between the years 1980 to 2014. They also found that northwestern Europe has the lowest rates of diabetes among both women and men, with age-adjusted prevalence lower than 4 percent for women and around 5 to 6 percent for men in Switzerland, Austria, Denmark, Belgium, and the Netherlands.

### Why is it sometimes difficult for health care professionals to treat a person who has diabetes?

For health care professionals (and even friends and family who try to help a person with the disease), it is often difficult to help a person with diabetes. The difficulty is not because of the disease itself, but because so many people are in denial and unwilling to accept that they have diabetes. Often, it is because there can be few symptoms, so the person does not believe the risks from diabetes actually exist. Other times, they don't have (or don't know how to find) the support they need to cope with the disease, both physically and emotionally. And still others are not willing to—or cannot without help—make lifestyle changes to manage their diabetes. (For suggestions on coping and getting help for diabetes, see the chapter "Coping with Diabetes," and for those with and without access to the Internet and apps, see the chapter "Resources, Websites, and Apps.")

### Who should be tested for diabetes?

Everyone should be tested for diabetes, especially if there are any symptoms of the disease or if someone in the family has diabetes—no matter what age. Overall, the American Diabetes Association recommends that all adults be tested beginning at age 45.

# DIABETES IN INFANTS AND CHILDREN

## Can a baby have type 1 diabetes?

According to the most recent data, children under the age of three can have type 1 diabetes. Although no one agrees on the actual numbers, some research suggests that less than 1 percent of all children less than a year old develop type 1 diabetes; another statistic states that less than 2 percent of children under three years develop type 1 diabetes. The most recent data also suggests that there is a significant upward trend of type 1 diabetes at such young ages for some unknown reason. There may be several reasons, including and especially that there is a better understanding of the disease in infants (and therefore more diagnoses).

## Why is it often a challenge to diagnose and treat an infant who may have type 1 diabetes?

There are several reasons that it is difficult to diagnose and treat a young infant who has diabetes. Initially, babies do not often have the "classic diabetic" early symptoms and signs of the disease. If they are diagnosed with type 1 diabetes, it is often a challenge to set up a therapeutic treatment for the infant (especially in terms of insulin dosage as the child grows), including if the mother is breastfeeding. Managing the child's diabetes is also difficult because the child is growing and developing and is not able to take care of

---

### What is the youngest child known to develop type 2 diabetes?

As of this writing, and according to a study presented at the 2015 meeting of the European Association for the Study of Diabetes, the youngest child to develop type 2 diabetes was a three-and-a-half-year-old Hispanic female from Texas. Her initial symptoms were excessive urination and thirst, but her other medical history showed virtually nothing. In addition, although both parents were reported to be obese, there was no history of diabetes. But the child was in the top 5 percent of children her age in weight and height, putting her in the body mass index (BMI) obesity range (for more about BMI, see the chapter "Diabetes and Obesity"). Her blood tests also showed a high HbA1c level (also seen as A1C or A1c) but negative for antibodies that would mean she would have had type 1 diabetes. After treatment for six months with metformin (a common type 2 diabetes drug) at various levels and a change in diet and lifestyle, the girl had normal blood glucose levels and a "normal" HbA1c level. She stopped taking metformin. According to most researchers, this was a good sign. It may mean that type 2 diabetes is reversible in many young children—as long as they are diagnosed early and with certain modifications in eating, exercise, and lifestyle.

his or her needs. Thus, the parents, and often other members of the family, must be involved in the baby's treatment. And finally, there is the psychological impact of how diabetes affects not only the child but also the child's family, as the daily work of managing the disease is often difficult.

## What is hyperinsulinism (hyperinsulinemia) in a newborn baby?

Hyperinsulinism (hyperinsulinemia) is just as the term implies—an excessive amount of insulin in the bloodstream. There are various types of hyperinsulinism, including congenital hyperinsulinism, a rare condition in which there is severe, persistent hypoglycemia in a newborn baby. In the United States, it is estimated that one in 50,000 newborns is affected by hyperinsulinemia, with symptoms ranging from sweating and lethargic behavior to irritability, jitteriness, and respiratory distress, all of which can mimic other conditions, which is why it is often difficult to diagnose.

## Why is diabetes thought to be one of the most common chronic illnesses of young people?

According to several organizations that specialize in diabetes, diabetes is one of the most common chronic illnesses of young people. This is because it is estimated that 5 percent of all new diabetes cases are type 1, and most of those affected are children and adolescents. It is also estimated that more than 18,000 people under age 20 are diagnosed with type 1 diabetes each year. The numbers are also high in terms of type 2 diabetes—with estimates of more than 5,000 new cases of type 2 diabetes in young people each year. At this writing, these figures are often translated as meaning that one of every 350 children has diabetes, although some recent studies show this trend may be slowing.

## What are the challenges of treating a toddler (one to three years old) who has type 1 diabetes?

The challenges associated with treating a toddler ages one to three who has type 1 diabetes is similar to that of an infant less than a year old. In addition, as children get older, they tend to refuse to eat certain foods, meaning there is a chance of hypoglycemia. Discipline and temper tantrums are also known to be issues at the toddler stage, possibly making it difficult for the parent to measure the child's blood glucose levels. The best way to overcome such challenges is for the parent or guardian to better understand the disease

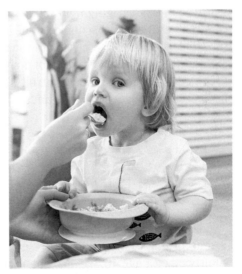

One challenge of having a toddler with diabetes is getting them to eat foods low in sugars.

27

(through education) and to get the overall support of a diabetes team and the child's health care professional.

### What are some challenges of preschool and early school-aged children (three to seven years old) to school-aged children (eight to 12 years old) who have type 1 diabetes?

A child (ages three to seven) with type 1 diabetes still needs help managing injections and blood glucose readings. But in many cases, children in this age group are ready to participate in certain activities that will help them manage their diabetes. In particular, many parents ask their child to participate in the testing and keeping records of the child's glucose measurements, along with helping to make meals for the child. These responsibilities often make a child gain confidence in helping to manage diabetes.

For school-aged children (ages eight to twelve) with type 1 diabetes, the challenges are somewhat different, especially if they have been diagnosed with the disease at a later age. If the child has had diabetes for a while, the tasks include continuing to manage blood glucose levels with injections and maintaining nutritional balance. For those who are diagnosed at an older age, the challenge becomes learning to cope with not only a different way of eating but also taking medication each day. There is also the psychological challenge of managing the disease every day, dealing with their peers' understanding (and misunderstanding) of diabetes, and realizing the disease will not go away.

### Why is it often difficult for children (ages six to twelve) with type 1 diabetes while at school?

One of the most difficult challenges for children ages six to twelve with diabetes—type 1 or type 2—is managing their blood glucose levels while they attend school. Younger children's challenges at school include assistance in administering insulin (including if the child uses an insulin pump) and supervision in managing glucose levels. For older children, school becomes more of a challenge as they increase their activities while keeping their glucose under control. In addition, there are often problems stemming from peers, many who may not understand diabetes and what challenges it entails.

# DIABETES AND TEENS
# THROUGH YOUNG ADULTS

### Has type 2 diabetes increased in teens and young adults?

Yes, according to most diabetes research, type 2 diabetes, which usually develops in adulthood past age 40, has become increasingly common in children and teenagers. Some studies also indicate that along with this rise in type 2 diabetes cases is an increased number of teenagers and young adults who are also obese. Although one study indicated that a rise in obesity was slowing down, there are still enough teens and young adults who are at risk to become obese and develop type 2 diabetes to prompt concern.

## What are some challenges faced by parents or guardians of adolescents and young adults with diabetes?

The parents or guardians of adolescents and young adults with diabetes can face several challenges. One of the biggest challenges is in helping a young person gain the independence and confidence he or she will need in the future—without too much parental involvement that may alienate the young person. Parents must also realize that the young person (especially an adolescent) will need help now and then with the management and decision making of diabetes (for example, with insulin adjustments and eating habits).

Psychologically, peer pressure may be hard on a young person with diabetes. In such cases, parents need to be understanding, give guidance, and even obtain counseling if necessary to help the young person. Plus, it is good to know that parents and the young person are not alone. There are others who can help a young person with diabetes, including teachers, health care professionals, dietitians, and diabetes educators.

## Why is a Diabetes Medical Management Plan (DMMP) important to a student with diabetes?

A Diabetes Medical Management Plan (DMMP) consists of the medical orders or diabetes care plan developed by the student's personal diabetes health care team. The main reason for having such a plan is that every student who has diabetes needs different methods of treatment. Because of this, a student's doctor orders for school care need to be specifically designed for that student. According to the American Diabetes Association, along with the National Diabetes Education Program (under the National Institutes of Health), there is now a DMMP that can be customized for every student who has diabetes, whether it be type 1 or type 2. (To obtain this template, visit the American Diabetes Association website at http://www.diabetes.org/living-with-diabetes/parents-and-kids/diabetes-care-at-school/written-care-plans/diabetes-medical-management.html.)

## What are some ways to help adolescents and young adults with diabetes eat right—especially at school?

There are several ways to help adolescents and young adults with diabetes cope with eating right, especially while they're at school. According to the National Institute of Diabetes and Digestive and Kidney Diseases (under the National Institutes of Health), several approaches will help a student plan meals and take care of his or her blood glucose levels during school. The following lists some of those ways (for more about diet and diabetes, see the chapter "Diabetes and Eating"):

*Carbohydrate (carb) counting*—This is a popular meal-planning approach for children and adolescents with diabetes. It involves calculating the number of grams of carbohydrates (also called carbs), or choices of carbohydrate, eaten at meals or snacks.

29

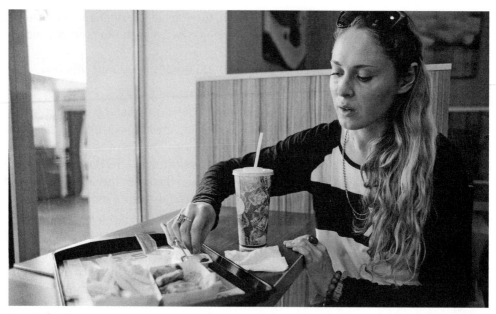

It can be hard to keep an active teen away from high-carb foods like French fries and sodas. They also need to know about other sources of carbs that seem unlikely, including sandwich wraps, raisins, smoothies, bagels, and bananas.

*Changing-carb-intake meal plan*—This is a method of meal planning used by students who take multiple daily insulin injections or have an insulin pump. Students who use this method do not have to eat the same amount of carbs at every meal or snack, but they must adjust their insulin doses (with either rapid- or short-acting insulin) to cover the amount of carbs they consume (they often use this method in conjunction with a basal/bolus insulin plan; for more about basal and bolus insulin treatments, see the chapter "Taking Charge of Diabetes").

*Consistent-carb-intake meal plan*—This is a meal plan in which students aim for a set amount of carbohydrates at each meal and snack but do not adjust their mealtime insulin for the amount of carbohydrate intake. These students follow a traditional or fixed insulin-dose plan.

Overall, these methods can be used in conjunction with the student's Diabetes Medical Management Plan (DMMP; see above) developed by the student's personal diabetes health care team.

# DIABETES AND MIDDLE–AGED ADULTS

### What is the average life expectancy of a person with type 1 diabetes?

According to a study conducted in 2012, men with type 1 diabetes had an average life expectancy of about 66 years versus 77 years among men without it. Women with type

## What study connected type 2 diabetes with female puberty?

In research conducted in 2013, scientists studied more than 15,000 middle-aged women from eight countries in Europe, asking when the women started their periods. On the basis of their statistics, they determined that women who began menstruating between the ages of 8 and 11 years had a 70 percent greater chance of developing type 2 diabetes in adulthood than those who started their periods at the average age of 13. When the women's BMI (body mass index; for more about BMI, see the chapter "Diabetes and Obesity") was taken out of the equation, only about 42 percent had a greater risk of developing type 2 diabetes if they began menstruating at an early age. Although the researchers believe that early puberty in women somehow affects the women's diabetes risk (no matter what the weight), it seems this study also does not factor in lifestyles or medical histories—thus the results are highly debated.

1 diabetes had an average life expectancy of about 68 years compared with around 81 years for those without type 1 diabetes. Of course, these are merely statistics, as many men and women with type 1 diabetes live well into their eighties, nineties, and even past the century mark.

## What percentage of adults develop type 1 diabetes?

Although type 1 diabetes is commonly diagnosed in childhood, around 25 percent of people with type 1 diabetes are diagnosed as adults, some even into their nineties. If an adult develops type 1 diabetes, the symptoms usually occur suddenly and are similar to those symptoms in children who develop the disease. These include weight loss, nausea, constant thirst, and urination. (For more about type 1 diabetes in adults, see the chapter "Type 1 Diabetes.")

## Does type 2 diabetes occur suddenly in middle-aged adults?

No, a person develops type 2 diabetes gradually over a number of years—at middle age or any age. Internally, it usually begins when muscle and other cells in the body stop responding to insulin. The reason it seems to occur more often in middle-aged adults is that it develops gradually and because more middle-aged people develop problems with weight gain, blood pressure, and other conditions that can lead to type 2 diabetes.

## What is the average age a person is diagnosed with type 2 diabetes?

According to the Centers for Disease Control and Prevention (CDC), there were a total of 1.7 million new total diabetes cases in 2012 (the latest data available). In addition, adults (both male and female) ages 45 to 64 were the most-diagnosed age group for type 2 diabetes.

31

### How does type 2 diabetes affect the life expectancy of a person with the disease?

According to several studies, type 2 diabetes cuts about eight and a half to ten years off the life of the average 50-year-old person (male and female) compared with a 50-year-old without the disease. (These numbers often differ for type 2 diabetes because of gender, how healthy the person is before the diagnosis, and lifestyle differences, such as smoking, blood pressure, etc.) Of course, these are merely statistics, as many men and women with type 2 diabetes live well into their eighties, nineties, and beyond.

### Is there a connection between diabetes and the metabolic syndrome?

Many health care professionals believe there is a definite connection between diabetes (especially type 2) and what is called the metabolic syndrome. This condition is found mostly in adults, usually beginning at middle age. The syndrome includes several symptoms, including large waist measurement, abnormal blood fats, elevated blood pressure, and glucose intolerance—all of which usually start to appear in middle age. (For more about the metabolic syndrome, see the chapter "Prediabetes and Type 2 Diabetes.")

## DIABETES AND SENIORS

### How does a person's response to diabetes change as he or she ages?

As people with diabetes age, their bodies change along with their response to diabetes. For example, sometimes the method of monitoring blood glucose levels or administering insulin must change as a person gets older, especially if he or she is having difficulty with cognitive function. For some older people, aging with diabetes may mean a new routine, such as changing from using a syringe for insulin injections to an insulin pen. Or it can mean a major lifestyle change, such as engaging in more physical activity to keep blood glucose levels under control.

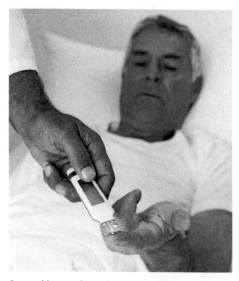

Some older people might require additional assistance with monitoring their glucose levels or taking their medications.

### Why is it often difficult to determine how aging affects a person with diabetes?

There is one major reason why researchers and health care professionals find it difficult to determine how aging affects a person with diabetes: We don't have enough data (such as a good cross-section of older people who have had the disease for very long) to understand what happens. It is true that insulin has been available for less than a century. But, as of this writing, few elderly people have been on insulin long enough for scientists to collect long-term data of how older people live with diabetes. There is a positive aspect even though there is less data about aging and diabetes. Managing diabetes has changed since the mid-twentieth century, with more technology and medications to treat diabetes no matter at what stage of life—and there is also a better understanding of the disease.

## Do menopausal women have more type 1 or type 2 diabetes?

In general, most statistics show that most menopausal women who develop diabetes have type 2. This is because many menopausal women tend to gain weight after their childbearing years. The more a woman weighs, the more risk for developing type 2 diabetes, especially if it runs in her family.

## How is menopause connected to diabetes in women?

If a woman is menopausal, she faces challenges even if she does not have diabetes, and if she does, bodily changes complicate the illness, especially its management. Bodily changes occur because two major hormones—estrogen and progesterone—are not stable. (In fact, a higher level of estrogen usually improves insulin sensitivity, while higher levels of progesterone cause resistance.) According to the Mayo Clinic, the following lists several possible effects on a woman's body that can increase the risk of diabetes (for those who do not have the disease or are prediabetic) or exacerbate the problems associated with a menopausal woman who has diabetes:

*Gaining weight*—If a menopausal woman gains weight during the transition and after menopause, she may also cause an increase in blood glucose levels. This could increase the need for insulin or oral diabetes medications.

*Blood glucose level changes*—The two major female hormones, estrogen and progesterone, both affect how a woman's cells respond to the natural insulin in her body. After menopause, the levels of these hormones change and thus can cause fluctuations in the woman's blood glucose levels. This may also cause changes in how her

### What is menopause in women?

In women, menopause is the cessation of ovulation and menstrual periods; after the period has stopped completely, the woman is considered to be post-menopausal. The supply of follicles in the ovaries is depleted, increasing the amount of follicle-stimulating hormone (FSH), while decreasing the amount of estrogen and progesterone. The process may take one to two years and usually occurs between the ages of 45 and 55, with the average age in the United States being 51 to 52. The few years preceding the final menstrual period are known as perimenopause.

body responds to glucose and insulin, which in turn can lead to a higher risk of diabetes and its complications.

*Infections of the urinary and reproductive tracts*—Because of the fluctuations in blood glucose levels after menopause—especially the high glucose levels—a woman can more easily develop urinary and vaginal infections. In fact, the drop in estrogen levels in a menopausal woman allows bacteria and yeast to thrive in the urinary tract and vagina, increasing the risk of infections.

*Sleep problems*—Many women experience trouble sleeping after menopause, most often because of hot flashes and night sweats. Because of the lack of sleep, along with the stresses associated with having hot flashes and night sweats, many women with diabetes find it more difficult to manage their blood glucose levels. Even women who do not have diabetes can be affected by lack of sleep, as the stress causes blood glucose levels to rise.

### Is there an osteoporosis–menopause connection in women?

Yes, there is often thought to be a connection between osteoporosis (see sidebar) and menopause in women. In particular, after a woman reaches menopause, and if she has a more sedentary lifestyle, she is at increased risk for osteoporosis. There is also an increased risk of the disease if the woman is thin or has a small frame, if she has a family history of the disease, or if she takes certain medications or has certain illnesses that leach or stop the absorption of calcium in the body. In women after menopause, osteoporosis is called primary type 1 or post-menopausal osteoporosis; after age 75, it is often called primary type 2 or senile osteoporosis.

### Can type 1 and/or type 2 diabetes affect a menopausal woman's bone density?

Yes, there seems to be a connection between menopause in a woman with type 1 diabetes and lower bone density, but no one is sure why. Some researchers believe that it may be because insulin, which is deficient in women with type 1 diabetes, may help promote bone growth and strength. Others believe cytokines (substances produced in many cells

---

### What is osteoporosis?

Osteoporosis (from the Greek, meaning "porous bones") is a disease in which a person's bone-mineral density decreases because of the lack of certain elements in the body, including calcium and vitamin D. This causes the bone to break down and increases the risk of fractures and breaks, usually in older adults (female and male) and especially in post-menopausal women. (For more on osteoporosis and diabetes, see the chapter "How Diabetes Affects Bones, Joints, Muscles, Teeth, and Skin," and for more about vitamins and minerals, see the chapter "Diabetes and Nutrition.")

of the body's immune system that have an effect on other cells) may play a role not only in the development of type 1 diabetes but also in osteoporosis.

There is one additional statistic that researchers are examining: Although women with type 1 diabetes are at a higher risk overall for osteoporosis, the risk seems to be even more pronounced for overweight women with type 2 diabetes. It is thought that increased body weight can reduce the risk of osteoporosis, but it also increases the risk of type 2 diabetes. But studies have shown that although bone density increased in women with type 2 diabetes, fractures also increased.

Some suggest that people with type 1 diabetes also experience more fractures—and that these may be due to an increased number of falls because of poor vision and nerve damage caused by the disease. Others suggest that diabetes may damage bone structure and quality, causing a decrease in bone density.

## How many Americans over age 60 are thought to have insulin resistance?

It is estimated that 40 percent of Americans over age 60 have some insulin resistance. This means that the cells in the body become less sensitive to the hormone and need larger amounts of insulin to metabolize certain compounds in the body, such as proteins, fats, and carbohydrates. And it is not only people with diabetes who are affected by insulin resistance. It also can affect those who suffer from obesity and hypertension and those with impaired glucose tolerance. (For more about insulin resistance, see the chapters "Introduction to Diabetes" and "Prediabetes and Type 2 Diabetes.")

## Can older people's sense of taste and smell affect their eating habits—and their diabetes?

Yes, older people (with or without diabetes) do not have as keen a sense of smell or taste as when they were young—and these factors may affect their eating habits. In general,

it is thought that a person's sense of smell peaks between ages 30 and 60. After 60, a person's ability to smell and taste declines. With further aging, especially over age 80, people lose even more of their sense of smell and their ability to discriminate between smells (medically called olfactory impairment). Research has shown that more than 75 percent of people over 80 have some decline in smell.

Overall, the reason for a decline usually has to do with the normal aging process, drug use (possibly including some medications associated with diabetes), infections (especially upper respi-

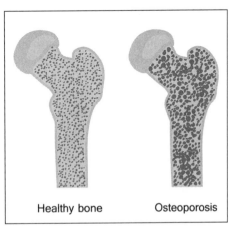

Healthy bone          Osteoporosis

Osteoporosis is a disease in which bone density decreases, making fractures and breaks more likely.

ratory), changes in the mouth (such as dentures or tooth loss), and even the reduction of saliva. Thus, because smell and taste are so intertwined with a person's perception of foods and eating habits, a large proportion of elderly people who lose their smell don't eat well and become nutrient deficient, and for older people with diabetes, this can be a problem, as it may cause them to eat poorly, which can affect their ability to control blood glucose levels. (For more about diabetes, smell, and taste, see the chapter "Diabetes and Inside the Human Body.")

### What are some other eating challenges that can affect an older person with diabetes?

Seniors with diabetes face many challenges, especially taking in enough nutrients to stay healthy. This can be for a multitude of reasons, including a loss of appetite (from medications or illness), problems with chewing and swallowing (difficulty with dentures or lack of teeth), and a need to reduce the intake of fats and sugars that are associated with certain chronic conditions (sugars and fats provide energy but also add weight that can lead to other diseases). All these conditions can (and often do) create problems with an older person's blood glucose levels.

### Is there a connection between complications from diabetes and dementia?

Although more studies need to be conducted, according to research published in 2015 in the Endocrine Society's *Journal of Clinical Endocrinology & Metabolism,* people who have diabetes and experience high rates of complications are more likely to develop dementia as they age than people who have fewer diabetic complications. In particular, the researchers noted that when blood glucose levels remain high because of uncontrolled diabetes, complications such as blindness, kidney failure, and decreased blood flow in the extremities can occur. These complications, in turn, seem to be connected with the development of dementia as the person ages. (For more about dementia—including Alzheimer's disease—see the chapter "How Diabetes Affects the Nervous System.")

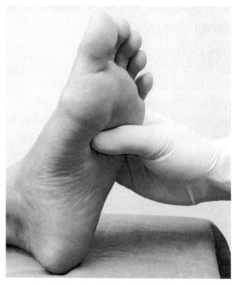

### What are peripheral neuropathy and orthostatic hypertension, often complications of diabetes and aging?

Peripheral neuropathy is nerve damage affecting the long nerves that run from the

One possible complication of diabetes is peripheral neuropathy, which affects the nerves leading to extremities such as the feet, but it can also affect hands, arms, legs, facial muscles, and internal organs.

spine to the arms, legs, and hands. Orthostatic hypertension is a form of autonomic (occurs unconsciously) neuropathy that affects a person's balance. Both are often complications of type 1 and type 2 diabetes and the aging process. (For more about peripheral and autonomic neuropathies, see the chapter "How Diabetes Affects the Nervous System.")

## Who are some famous historical figures who have had diabetes?

Many historical figures have had diabetes—some with complications that greatly affected their lives and even their decisions over time. The following are only a few examples:

- American Thomas Edison (1847–1931), inventor and businessman, managed to produce a prolific amount of patents while suffering from diabetes (this was before insulin was introduced)—including the phonograph, motion-picture camera, and the long-lasting, practical lightbulb.

- George R. Minot (1885–1950) received the Nobel Prize (with two others) for studies in anemia. He was also diagnosed with diabetes in 1921 and was one of the first patients to be treated with the "new drug" insulin by Banning and Best (see above for more information). He had developed complications from diabetes by 1940, had a serious stroke in 1947, and died in 1950.

## Who are some famous authors who have had or have diabetes?

The list of famous people who have had diabetes is long—and authors are among them. They include some of the following famous writers:

- American writer Ernest Hemingway (1899–1961) had diabetes, but some researchers suggest that Hemingway may have had hemochromatosis (also called "bronze diabetes"). This disease—also known as iron overload—along with other health problems such as depression, diabetes, and alcoholism, probably contributed to his suicide in 1961. (For more about bronze diabetes, see the chapter "Other Types of Diabetes.")

- English writer H.G. Wells (1866–1946), often called the "father of science fiction," was diagnosed with "mild diabetes" in his early 60s. He was instrumental in helping fund a diabetes center, and because of public response, Wells further involved himself in diabetes education by advocating an association specifically for diabetes charity (for research and awareness of the disease) in 1934. The result was the Diabetic Association, which developed into the British Diabetic Association in 1954 and was renamed Diabetes UK in 2000.

- Novelist Anne Rice (1941–), most famous for her vampire novels, was diagnosed with type 1 diabetes in 1998. At the time of diagnosis, her blood sugar was around 800, and her health was fragile. If her husband had not called 911, the diabetic coma she was experiencing might have been fatal. After losing and then gaining more weight, Rice underwent gastric bypass surgery, losing 100 pounds (45.3 kilograms) and is in better control of her diabetes.

## Who are some famous contemporary people who have made special contributions to their field of interest— and who have diabetes?

Many famous people in various fields of interest have had or have diabetes. The following are only a few examples:

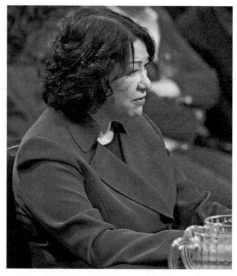

U.S. Supreme Court Justice Sonia Sotomayor is one of many luminaries in America who struggle with diabetes but manage to lead productive lives anyway.

- U.S. Supreme Court Justice Sonia Sotomayor (1954–) is the first person with type 1 diabetes ever to serve on the high court. Sotomayor was diagnosed with type 1 at age seven after fainting in church and always being extremely thirsty and urinating a great deal. She still takes insulin and is an advocate of diabetes education.

- Nicole Johnson Baker (1974–), a former Miss America (1999) and Miss Virginia (1998), became the first Miss America with diabetes (type 1) and the first contestant to publicize an insulin pump. She is also an advocate of diabetes awareness and education and helps others understand how to cope with the disease.

- Cynthia Ice (1959–2008) was an accessibility expert at IBM, specializing in Lotus Notes. She was diagnosed with type 1 diabetes at age seven and lost her eyesight to diabetic retinopathy in her twenties. Even though she lost her eyesight, she was instrumental in making certain programs accessible to the blind and disabled (among other computer-oriented contributions) in order to help them find employment and connect with the world.

## Who are some famous musicians who have had or have diabetes?

Many musicians have had or have diabetes. The following lists only a few of them:

- Blues singer and bass player B. B. King (1925–2015) was called "The King of Blues." He was diagnosed with type 2 diabetes 20 years before his death and became an advocate of diabetes education, as he had watched both of his parents suffer from complications of the disease when he was a child. He died at age 89 from complications of diabetes.

- American guitarist, singer, and songwriter Jerry Garcia (1942–1995) was a rock musician with the Grateful Dead. Later in life, Garcia was sometimes ill because of type 2 diabetes and in 1986 went into a diabetic coma that nearly cost him his life. Although his overall health improved somewhat after that, he still struggled with drug addictions. In 1995 he died of a heart attack while staying at a California drug-rehabilitation facility.

- American singing great Ella Fitzgerald (1917–1996), known as the "First Lady of Song," was one of many people's favorite singers, and she pushed herself to exhaustion in her performing years. By the 1980s, Fitzgerald was having serious health problems. She had heart surgery in 1986 and was diagnosed with diabetes. Eventually, the diabetes left her blind, and she had to have both legs amputated in 1994. Never fully recovering from her surgery, she died in 1996.

- American jazz musician Dizzy Gillespie (1917–1993) pioneered the 1940s movement that changed the shape of traditional jazz into bebop. Gillespie was hospitalized in 1992 with uncontrolled diabetes and an intestinal blockage, which required surgery. He died in 1993 of pancreatic cancer.

- Country singer Johnny Cash (1932–2003), called the "Man in Black," was considered one of the most influential musicians of the twentieth century. Cash was diagnosed with type 2 diabetes in his fifties and eventually died of complications from diabetes.

- Pop singer and actress Patti LaBelle (1944–). Patti LaBelle is her stage name; she was born Patricia Louise Holt-Edwards. She has type 2 diabetes, but it was not until she passed out onstage during a concert that she finally took charge of her health. (She was diagnosed in 1995.) The disease is also in her family, as her mother died of type 2 diabetic complications at age 58.

- American rock-'n'-roll singer Bret Michaels (1963–), known for his work as lead singer for the band Poison, was diagnosed with type 1 diabetes when he was six years old. After an onstage collapse because of a low blood glucose level and rumors about drug use, he finally went public about his disease. Since then, he has become more active in diabetes education.

## Who are some famous politicians who have had or have diabetes?

Many well-known politicians have had or have diabetes. The following lists only a few of those people:

- American politician Fiorello LaGuardia (1882–1947), the former (and 99th) New York City mayor and namesake of LaGuardia Airport in New York, was a diabetic.

- Mikhail Gorbachev (1931–) was the general secretary of the Soviet Union from 1985–1991 and a Nobel Peace Prize winner (1990). He was also instrumental, along with U.S. President Ronald Reagan in ending the Cold War between the United States and the Soviet Union. In 2014 he was diagnosed with "an acute form" of diabetes.

- Yuri Andropov (1914–1984) was the general secretary of the Communist Party of the Soviet Union from November 1982 until his death 15 months later. Toward the end of his life, he had several health problems, including hypertension and diabetes, which were connected to chronic kidney deficiency. He eventually died from toxicity in his blood (mainly due to renal failure he had experienced the year before).

39

## Who is Theresa May?

In 2016, after the United Kingdom voted to leave the European Union and Prime Minister David Cameron resigned, Theresa May, 59 at that time, became Britain's 76th prime minister. She is also thought to be one of the first major world leaders with type 1 diabetes. May was diagnosed with diabetes later in life, seeking medical attention in 2012 for sudden weight loss, fatigue, and thirst. At first, she was misdiagnosed with type 2 diabetes, but then she was surprised to learn she had actually developed type 1. (Like many people, she assumed that at her age, she would not get the disease, but it can develop at any age; for more about adults and type 1 diabetes, see the chapter "Type 1 Diabetes.") Since that time, she has been open about her diabetes, indicating that she has been able to effectively manage her condition and her responsibilities as prime minister. According to several reports, she does admit that she has to be a little more careful about what she eats and has to take injections, but that situation, she has said, is something that millions of people have. In fact, many people who have type 1 (and type 2) diabetes look to May as an example of what can be accomplished as long as they manage their diabetes sensibly.

## Who are some famous sports personalities who have had or have diabetes?

Many famous sports personalities have had or have diabetes, including the following:

- Tennis legend Billie Jean King (1943–), a six-time Wimbledon champion and four-time U.S. Open champion, was diagnosed with type 2 diabetes in 2007. She has attributed her developing the disease to a fluctuating weight and sometimes unhealthful eating habits while on the tennis circuit.

- American professional baseball player Jack Roosevelt "Jackie" Robinson (1919–1972) was the first African American to play Major League Baseball in the modern era. After his retirement in 1957, Robinson was diagnosed with diabetes (after complaining of numerous ailments). Although he took insulin, the medication did not stop Robinson's physical deterioration from the disease. Complications from heart disease and diabetes weakened Robinson and made him almost blind by middle age. He died of a heart attack in 1972.

- Ty Cobb (1886–1961), the baseball legend, considered one of the best baseball players of all time, had type 1 diabetes while he played for the Detroit Tigers and the Philadelphia Athletics. After he retired, he became overweight and along with diabetes had high blood pressure, both contributing to heart and kidney damage. He died in 1961 from cancer, complications of diabetes, and heart disease.

- English rugby player Chris Pennell (1987–) was diagnosed with type 1 diabetes when he was 19 years old. He has become an advocate for diabetes education, especially for young people who may develop the disease.

• American race-car driver Charles Newton "Charlie" Kimball (1985–) was the first licensed driver with diabetes in the history of IndyCar racing (he competes in the IndyCar Series).

## How does Ryan Reed cope with racing and his diabetes?

In 2011, Ryan Reed (1993–), a stock-car racing driver who competes on NASCAR's Xfinity Series circuit, was diagnosed with type 1 diabetes at age 17. Told he would be unable to race again, Reed found a way of treating his diabetes and racing. To do this, he installed a drink system in his race car, along with a blood glucose monitor. The monitor communicates with a wireless device attached to Reed's stomach (for more about monitors, see the chapter "Taking Charge of Diabetes"), with the readout on the car's dashboard, allowing him to keep track of his blood glucose levels. If he needs adjustment, Reed receives the necessary insulin (or whatever he needs) during his pit stops. He is one of two professional race-car drivers who have diabetes and has become a diabetes advocate, starting his own nonprofit foundation called Ryan's Mission.

## Who are some movie and television personalities with diabetes?

Many movie and television personalities—from about 1900 to the present—have or have had diabetes. Some of the more famous actors and actresses include the following:

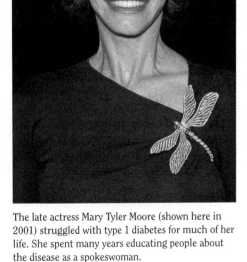

• Mary Jane "Mae" West (1893–1980), nicknamed "Diamond Lil," was a popular actress, singer, and comedian in the 1940s and 1950s. She suffered from diabetes (type unknown) for 15 years before her death at age 87 (she had had a stroke that was thought to be a complication of her diabetes).

• Talk-show host Larry King (1933–) had a major heart attack in 1987, after which he gave up smoking and changed his lifestyle. But even with the changes—and probably owing to a family history of the disease—he was diagnosed with type 2 diabetes in 1998.

• Actress Mary Tyler Moore (1936–2017) was diagnosed with type 1 diabetes after being hospitalized with a miscarriage—when a blood test re-

The late actress Mary Tyler Moore (shown here in 2001) struggled with type 1 diabetes for much of her life. She spent many years educating people about the disease as a spokeswoman.

41

vealed a blood glucose level of 750. She was put on insulin therapy in her early thirties (while she was in the early years of *The Mary Tyler Moore Show*). After that, she became a major spokesperson for the disease, serving as the international chairman of the JDRF (formerly Juvenile Diabetes Research Foundation) for several years.

• Actor Tom Hanks (1956–) reported once that he had elevated blood glucose levels for years before he was definitely diagnosed with diabetes. He may have developed the disease because of yo-yo dieting to fill certain roles in his movies (for example, he gained 30 pounds (13.6 kilograms) and lost 50 pounds (22.7 kilograms) for *A League of Their Own* and *Cast Away,* respectively, among other roles that required weight changes). He made his diagnosis public in 2013 and has since spoken candidly about his disease in several interviews.

# DIABETES' EFFECTS ON ANIMALS

### Do all animals experience diabetes?

No, not all animals get diabetes. Those that do include pigs, apes, sheep, cats, dogs, and horses. In particular, all mammals produce insulin and will develop what humans often refer to as diabetes (high blood glucose levels) if the beta cells in their pancreases are removed. But in the case of animals that can develop diabetes-type problems, there are various classifications, usually depending on the species. For example, veterinarians divide dog (canine) diabetes into insulin-deficiency diabetes and insulin-resistance diabetes, which are somewhat similar to human type 1 and type 2 diabetes, respectively. In addition, female dogs can develop a canine form of gestational diabetes; other dogs can develop a form of autoimmune diabetes that is similar to a human's latent autoimmune diabetes in adults (LADA). Even cats are not immune, often developing feline diabetes that is similar to a human's type 2 diabetes.

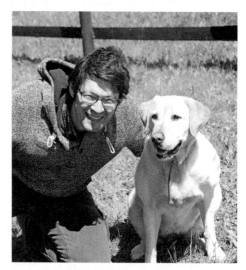

### How do some dogs—and cats—help humans who have diabetes?

One of the more amazing talents of some animals—especially dogs and some cats— is knowing when their owner is experiencing a diabetic event. These "therapy dogs" (and some cats) often alert a person with diabetes that he or she will soon experience a diabetic episode. The reason for the ability is thought to be a dog's powerful

Dogs can be trained to recognize when their owners are having a diabetic event; they can then alert others to the emergency.

ability to smell: Many people with diabetes have a certain smell when blood glucose levels are too high.

## Can cats develop diabetes?

Yes, cats can develop diabetes. As with humans, diabetes is a common disease in cats, in which the cat's body does not produce or does not use insulin properly (similar to human type 2 diabetes). The insulin in cats is also produced in the pancreas and, as with humans, is responsible for regulating the flow of glucose from the bloodstream and to various cells in the body. Also similar to humans, the classic signs of diabetes in cats are increased (and often ravenous) appetite, weight loss, increased thirst, and increased urination. And as of this writing, there are treatments but no cure for feline diabetes.

Feline diabetes is generally divided into two types: insulin-dependent diabetes mellitus (IDDM) and non-insulin-dependent (NIDDM) diabetes mellitus. Statistically, half to three-quarters of diabetic cats have IDDM, which requires injections of insulin as soon as the disease is diagnosed. The rest have NIDDM and can be treated with oral medications and diet, and some cats (especially if the diabetes is a result of being obese) may not need insulin months or years after the diagnoses once the obesity is controlled. But if obesity or some other connected disorder is not a factor, the diabetes will probably not go away, and such cats will often eventually require insulin injections to control the disease. Without treatment, a cat with diabetes will have a shorter lifespan. In addition, other related disorders will cause the cat to become progressively weaker, including from diabetic neuropathy; several fatal conditions may develop, including ketoacidosis.

## What are some risk factors associated with diabetes in cats?

The risk factors for diabetes in cats are very similar to human diabetes risk factors. According to the Cornell University Feline Health Center, risk factors for cats include obesity (the biggest risk and most often in older cats), age, gender (male cats are more commonly afflicted than females), chronic pancreatitis, medications (such as corticosteroids), and concurrent disease or infections.

## Can dogs develop diabetes?

Yes, as with most animals that develop the disease, diabetes in a dog is a disorder of carbohydrate, protein, and fat metabolism (how the body digests and uses food, mainly for energy) caused by an absolute or relative insulin deficiency. The process of metabolism is largely dependent on a sufficient amount of insulin in the body—and if a dog is deficient, it may develop diabetes. There are several symptoms of the disease, including weight loss, increase in urination, a change in appetite (eating more or eating less), drinking more water, fruity-smelling breath, dehydration, lethargy, and often urinary tract infections.

## How do smaller and larger animals differ when it comes to diabetes?

Besides cats and dogs, many other small animals—mammals, mostly—can develop their own forms of diabetes. But there are differences. For example, ferrets develop insuli-

## Why are dolphins of interest to diabetes researchers?

Researchers are interested in the bottlenose dolphin as that animal can have what could be called type 2 diabetes but with a big difference. Bottlenose dolphins can turn their type of diabetes "on and off" in a process that helps them keep enough glucose in their bodies even though they eat sugar-sparse diets (mostly high-protein fish and little sugar). The researchers believe this on-and-off process may have to do with the animals' brains. Humans have relatively large brains as compared with their size, and dolphins are second only to humans in the ratio of brain to body size. In humans, it takes a great deal of sugar (glucose) to keep the brain functioning. Thus, researchers believe dolphins may have evolved their on-and-off diabetic-like states as an adaptation to maintain glucose for their bigger brains. This is only a theory, so more studies are needed.

noma, or the opposite of what is common in humans with diabetes (lack of insulin). Afflicted ferrets have too much insulin because their beta cells are out of control, causing blood glucose levels to drop too low (hypoglycemia), which often causes nodules to form on the pancreas. Symptoms can often be inactivity (most healthy ferrets are active unless they are asleep), vomiting, drooling, and loss of appetite and weight. Larger animals, on the other hand, are less apt to develop diabetes than smaller animals, but diabetes has been reported in cattle, pigs, sheep, horses, and bison.

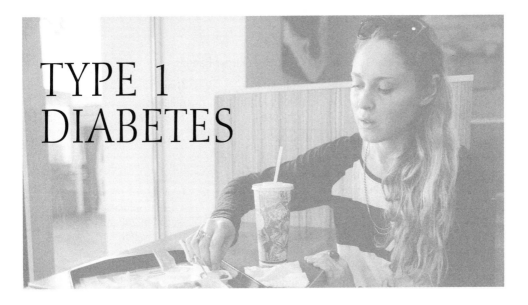

# TYPE 1 DIABETES

## BLOOD GLUCOSE LEVELS

### How is a person's blood glucose level measured?

Blood glucose levels are measured with four major tests, including the fasting plasma blood glucose, random plasma blood glucose, oral glucose tolerance, and glycated hemoglobin (HbA1c) tests. The first three tests measure a person's blood glucose in terms of milligrams per deciliter (seen as mg/dl or mg/dL), whereas the HbA1c (or A1c) test is measured in percentages.

### What are considered to be "normal" blood glucose levels?

Although everyone's blood glucose levels change during the day, when a person's blood glucose levels are measured, there are some standards advocated by health care professionals. The following chart shows the target ranges most health care professionals use to make a diagnosis of diabetes or no diabetes—based on four types of tests (for more details about these tests, see the chapter "Taking Charge of Diabetes").

### What are considered general blood glucose level targets for a person with diabetes?

Although there are exceptions to every rule, the following lists the general blood glucose level targets for a person who has diabetes (note: these numbers may not apply to all people with diabetes):

- Fasting or before-meal glucose level—90 to 130 mg/dl
- After-meal glucose (or two hours after the start of the meal) level—greater than (>) 180 mg/dl
- Bedtime glucose—100 to 140 mg/dl

## Diabetes Diagnosis Target Ranges

| Test Result Is | Fasting blood glucose | Random blood glucose | Oral glucose tolerance | HbA1c |
|---|---|---|---|---|
| Normal | ≤ 100 mg/dl | | ≤ 140 mg/dl | < 6.0% |
| Impaired fasting glucose | ≥ 100 mg/dl and ≤ 126 mg/dl | | | |
| Impaired glucose tolerance | | | a 2-hour glucose level is ≥ 140 mg/dl and ≤ 200 mg/dl | |
| Diabetes | ≥ 125 mg/dl on two consecutive blood tests | ≥ 200 mg/dl and have diabetes symptoms | A 2-hour glucose level is ≥ 200 mg/dl | > 6.5% |

*These test-result numbers sometimes change because of new discoveries in the study of diabetes, and some do not apply to all people with diabetes.

## Have standard levels for blood glucose levels changed over the years?

A main goal for a person with or without diabetes is to maintain certain blood glucose levels that sustain his or her health. And over the past two decades, the numbers that indicate "normal," "prediabetes," and "diabetes" have changed, mainly because of advancements in medical research and technology.

# TYPE 1 (OR TYPE ONE OR TYPE I) DIABETES

## What are the early warning signs of type 1 diabetes?

There are several warning signs of type 1 diabetes. It is thought to be caused by the immune system attacking and destroying the body's own pancreatic cells (those that produce the necessary insulin for the body). The following lists some of the traditional type 1 diabetes warning signs:

- The onset is apparently sudden, although for many people (especially children) it may seem to occur slowly as some of the symptoms mimic other conditions.
- The person urinates frequently, as the body tries to rid itself of the excessive amounts of blood glucose.
- The person has excessive thirst, as the person urinates more frequently.
- As the disease develops, the person may become progressively hungry, as the body burns its own fat for energy.

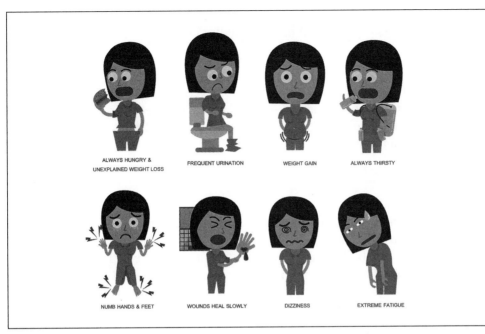

Some common symptoms of diabetes to watch for.

- Even though the person may be hungry and eat more, there may also be sudden weight loss, as the body continues to burn its own fat.
- Although they are not as much of a sign as the others mentioned above, nausea and vomiting can accompany the disease in some people.

## Is type 1 diabetes more harmful to women than to men?

According to a recent study in *The Lancet Diabetes & Endocrinology,* it appears that type 1 diabetes is truly more harmful to women than to men. The researchers looked at 26 studies that included more than 200,000 participants and found that women with type 1 diabetes had more than twice the risk of men of dying from heart disease, a 37 percent higher risk of dying from stroke, and a 44 percent greater risk of dying from kidney disease. Some scientists believe that the fluctuating hormone levels in women may affect their sensitivity to insulin. Furthermore, women's blood vessels may experience more damage than men's vessels when blood glucose levels are higher. Overall, the researchers recommend close monitoring of blood glucose levels in women with type 1 diabetes—and paying more attention to the risk factors (such as high blood pressure) that can raise women's chances of cardiovascular events.

## What is LADA?

LADA is a form of type 1 diabetes mellitus. It is referred to by many names, including latent autoimmune diabetes in adults (LADA), late-onset autoimmune diabetes of adult-

## What is polydipsia?

**P**olydipsia is the medical term for abnormal thirst. It is also considered an early symptom of diabetes, especially type 1. This thirst occurs because the body, as it suffers from elevated blood glucose (sugar) levels, responds by eliminating the excess glucose through urination. And as the person urinates more, the body demands more water, which is why a person with diabetes often experiences excessive, abnormal thirst.

hood or aging, slow-onset type 1 diabetes, or type 1.5 diabetes. In this disease, the type 1 diabetes diagnosis is made when the person is an adult. It comes on more slowly in adults, with the person not usually being overweight (as in type 2 diabetes) and having low or no insulin resistance. Overall, for a person who develops type 1.5 diabetes, insulin may not be needed for months or, in some cases, years (one report stated that insulin is, on the average, required five to ten years after diagnosis). No one knows how many adults truly have LADA because many health care professionals use the term LADA only for super-slow-to-develop cases, not all type 1 adult cases.

### Why do some adults develop LADA?

As in young children who develop type 1 diabetes, LADA diabetes apparently occurs in adults because of autoantibodies, or the antibodies that attack the insulin-producing cells in the pancreas. LADA can also form because of a person's genetics or if someone in the person's family (most likely a parent and/or sibling) has diabetes. (For more information about autoantibodies, see this chapter.)

# POSSIBLE REASONS FOR TYPE 1 DIABETES

### What causes most cases of type 1 diabetes?

It is thought that there are several reasons for the development of type 1 diabetes, but most of them are debated or still need to be studied. The most commonly mentioned one involves the body's own immune system attacking beta cells in the pancreas, causing the organ to stop producing insulin. The development of the disease is thought to be part genetic, but scientists (to date) agree that no one characteristic seems to bring about type 1 diabetes.

### How long does it take for type 1 diabetes to develop?

There is no real set "schedule" for a person to eventually develop type 1 diabetes. According to research and statistics, the body's autoimmune system can attack a person's beta cells over months or even years, eventually resulting in type 1 diabetes.

## What are some of the definitions of "type 1.5 diabetes"?

The term "type 1.5 diabetes" has been used to describe several different types of conditions. In some research, it is also called LADA, or latent autoimmune diabetes in adults. Type 1.5 diabetes has also been used to describe the condition of a person who has both type 1 and 2 diabetic features. In particular, the body not only fails to make its own insulin but also resists injected insulin (it has also been called "double diabetes").

## Do only young children develop type 1 diabetes?

No, it is a misconception that only children develop type 1 diabetes. Although the majority of type 1 diabetics are children—which is why so many people erroneously believe any adult-onset diabetes must be type 2—an adult can develop a slow-onset form of type 1 diabetes called latent autoimmune diabetes in adults (or LADA; for more about LADA, see above).

## Can exposure to chemicals or drugs cause type 1 diabetes?

A few studies suggest that there may be a connection between type 1 diabetes and exposure to chemicals or drugs. But it is unlikely that such an environmental factor (such as exposure to a chemical or drug) alone can cause diabetes. It may be that if a person with a genetic susceptibility (inheriting a particular set of genes) is exposed to a certain chemical or environmental "triggering" factor, he or she may develop type 1 diabetes. But overall, this concept is highly debated.

## What are the chances of developing type 1 diabetes because someone in the person's family has the disease?

According to several studies, including one from the Joslin Diabetes Center, if a father has type 1 diabetes, the child has a 7 percent chance of developing the disease; if the mother has type 1 diabetes, the child has a 2 percent chance of developing type 1 diabetes. Other research suggests that the risk for developing type 1 diabetes is between 1 and 10 percent for people with a parent or sibling with the disease. Overall, the average chance of a child's developing type 1 diabetes is 0.3 to 0.4 percent.

## Why does heredity play a part in type 1 diabetes?

Although the genetic component of type 1 diabetes is not as strong as for type 2 diabetes, there is a reason for the higher risk of the disease being passed from generation to generation. Research has shown that DNA, or deoxyribonucleic acid—the set of instructions that tells the cells in the body how to grow, live, and function—mutates, increasing the risk for the disease.

49

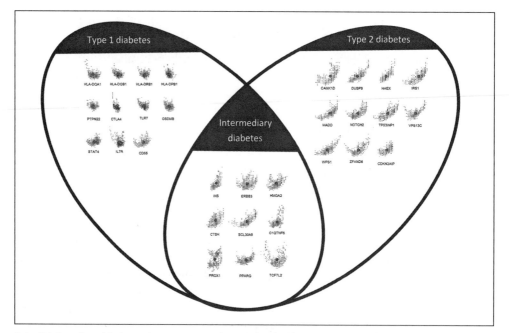

Scientists have found that certain genes seem to be associated with type 1, type 2, and intermediary diabetes.

## What are antibodies and autoantibodies?

Certain white blood cells of a person's immune system are mainly responsible for protecting the body from germs and foreign invaders, including T cells (they attack foreign cells directly) and B cells (they produce antibodies, or special proteins that can recognize the surface shapes of molecules that attack the body).

Autoantibodies—usually found in people with autoimmune disorders—are B cells that sometimes make their own antibodies and recognize a person's own cells. In the case of type 1 diabetes, it is thought that the autoantibodies identify the insulin-producing cells of the pancreas (beta cells) as cells to be attacked, and from there, the T cells destroy the beta cells.

## What autoantibodies are common in people with type 1 diabetes?

There appear to be three autoantibodies that are common in people with type 1 diabetes. In the pancreas, these autoantibodies recognize and attack the islet cells (of which beta cells are one type), insulin, and glutamic acid decarboxylase (a protein made by the beta cells in the pancreas, also called GAD or the 64 K protein). The autoantibodies seem to be markers in the body and contribute to the destruction of the pancreas' beta cells by identifying which cells should be attacked by the immune system. Ultimately, this causes the immune system's T cells to destroy the insulin-producing cells of the pancreas.

Overall, of the people who are newly diagnosed with type 1 diabetes, 70 to 80 percent have autoantibodies to islet cells, 30 to 50 percent have autoantibodies to insulin, and 80 to 95 percent have autoantibodies to GAD. These autoantibodies often appear before the symptoms of type 1 diabetes show up. Thus, some researchers suggest that people who are at higher risk of developing type 1 diabetes be screened for these autoantibodies.

## Can a virus cause type 1 diabetes?

Through the many years of research on type 1 diabetes, several reports have suggested that the disease may be caused by a virus. To date, no such virus—or even indirect evidence of such a virus—exists. Here are several of the viral-diabetes connection suggestions:

- One suggestion is that people who develop type 1 diabetes, according to some reports, often have had a recent viral infection before they are diagnosed. It has also been reported that many diagnoses of type 1 diabetes occur after a major viral outbreak.

- Another suggestion comes from research suggesting that viruses that cause mumps and German measles, along with the Coxsackie family of viruses (related to the virus that causes polio), may play a role in the development of type 1 diabetes. The researchers note that a certain autoantibody (see above) is almost identical to a region of a protein found in the virus Coxsackie B4. And because both are similar, the immune system's T cells may not be able to tell the difference, thus destroying the "invading" cell, but in reality destroying the body's own beta cells.

- Still another virus suggestion is that type 1 diabetes is a relatively new disease caused by a slow-acting virus, causing the immune system to attack proteins in the pancreas. To date, no such virus has been found.

# INSULIN AND TYPE 1 DIABETES

## Why does a person with type 1 diabetes need to take insulin?

A person with type 1 diabetes will need to take insulin for the rest of his or her life. In this case, the person's immune system mistakenly has attacked and destroyed the pancreas' beta cells that are responsible for producing insulin. Without insulin to aid blood glucose to be used by the body's cells, the person's blood glucose levels rise. There must be some type of replacement—thus, a person with type 1 diabetes must take insulin (usually by injection) every day.

## What is insulin shock?

Insulin shock occurs if a person's blood glucose levels are extremely low, causing him or her to lose consciousness. Such a severe low blood glucose level is considered a medical emergency.

## Do people with type 2 diabetes ever have to take insulin injections?

Yes, some people with type 2 diabetes may eventually have to take injections of insulin to stabilize their blood glucose levels, especially if they take oral medications (like met-

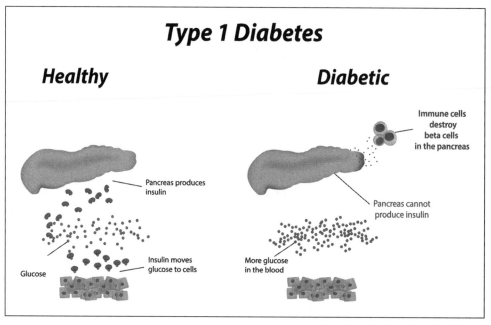

## Type 1 Diabetes

**Healthy**

**Diabetic**

Immune cells destroy beta cells in the pancreas

Pancreas produces insulin

Pancreas cannot produce insulin

Insulin moves glucose to cells

More glucose in the blood

Glucose

In type 1 diabetes the pancreas doesn't produce insulin, and therefore, glucose builds up in the body.

formin) for a long time. (For more about type 2 diabetes and insulin, see the chapter "Prediabetes and Type 2 Diabetes.")

### What are the various types of insulin a person with type 1 diabetes (and sometimes eventually a person with type 2 diabetes) takes?

There are several types of insulin you can take, each serving a different purpose for a person with type 1 diabetes (and sometimes eventually a person with type 2 diabetes). Some are used one at a time, while others can be taken in combination. They include rapid-acting, regular or short-acting, intermediate-acting, long-acting, or pre-mixed. (For more about the various types of insulin, see the chapter "Taking Charge of Diabetes.")

## RISKS AND COMPLICATIONS FOR PEOPLE WITH TYPE 1 DIABETES

### What are ketones?

Ketones are naturally occurring fatty acids produced in the body. There are three ketone bodies, known as acetone, aceo-acetone, and beta-hydroxybutyrate (important to diabetes; see below), which are produced from fat and certain amino acids. An excessive amount of ketones is also often produced by the body during an uncontrolled diabetic event (see DKA, below).

## Why does the body need ketones?

The body cannot store glucose for more than 24 hours, which is why it is important to maintain glucose levels for energy. And of course, this is also why humans must consume various foods to maintain the levels. In particular, the human brain (and other cells in the body) functions with the help of glucose and ketones. If there is not sufficient glucose, then the liver takes fat and certain amino acids (called fatty-acid metabolism) and turns them into ketones, first to feed the brain, then the rest of the body. This is called keto-adaptation, or nutritional ketosis, and is thought to be an evolutionary adaptation.

## How are ketones measured?

Ketones are normally produced by the liver. They will be completely metabolized so there will be few, if any, that appear in a person's urine. Normally, 3 to 15 milligrams of ketones (a very small amount) are excreted in the urine daily. Increased amounts of ketones, usually determined from a ketone urine test, can mean several conditions, many of which resemble other health problems. These conditions can include:

- Poorly controlled diabetes
- Diabetic ketoacidosis (see below)
- Starvation (for example, not eating for long periods, usually 12 to 18 hours, or anorexia nervosa, bulimia nervosa, alcoholism, or fasting)
- Some metabolic disorders
- A too-high protein or low-carbohydrate diet
- Vomiting over a long period
- A hyperactive thyroid gland (meaning too much thyroid hormone)
- Some types of toxic poisoning

## How are ketone levels interpreted by physicians?

Physicians interpret ketone levels mainly on the basis of ketone urine tests. These may include test kits purchased at a drug store (they contain "dipsticks" coated with chemicals that react to ketone bodies by changing color) or sending a urine sample to a laboratory to be analyzed, usually a physician's choice to obtain a more accurate reading. (There are also blood glucose meters that can measure blood ketones; for more information about meters, see the chapter "Taking Charge of Diabetes.") The results are interpreted as follows (most often, abnormal results mean more tests must be made to determine the cause of the excess in ketones):

- A negative test result is normal, with a small amount of ketones in the urine.
- An abnormal result means there are ketones in the urine; results are broken down this way:
    1. small—less than 20 milligrams per deciliter
    2. moderate—30 to 40 milligrams per deciliter
    3. large—greater than 80 milligrams per deciliter

53

Ketone tests can produce false results. For example, there may be a false-positive test result but no indication of ketones upon further testing. This may indicate certain conditions, mainly dehydration or the result of taking particular medications (for example, phenazopyrazine or vitamin C). There can also be false-negative ketone results, usually with urine-testing kits.

## Is there a treatment if a person with diabetes tests positive for ketones?

Yes, if a person with diabetes tests positive for ketones when using a meter that detects ketone bodies, he or she should contact their diabetes educator or physician. The elevated numbers may mean the person needs additional insulin. According to the Joslin Diabetes Center, the person should also drink plenty of water and other fluids (that contain no calories) in order to flush out the ketones from the blood. The person is also advised to continue checking blood glucose levels for three to four hours, testing for ketones if the blood glucose level is over 250 mg/dl (milligrams per deciliter). In addition, a person with a blood glucose level over 250 mg/dl and ketones present should not exercise. There is a good reason: If both blood glucose and ketone levels are high, it can lead to a life-threatening condition called diabetic ketoacidosis (see below).

## What is diabetic ketoacidosis, also known as DKA?

Diabetic ketoacidosis can occur when a person with diabetes has an episode of extremely high blood glucose and elevated levels of ketone (called positive ketones). It is not common and is most often associated with type 1 diabetes. (People with type 2 diabetes can also experience DKA, especially if they have very late-stage, insulin-dependent diabetes. But DKA is rarer in people with type 2 diabetes than in those with type 1.) It is most often detected with a urine test, as the ketones spill out into the urine. It is also often identified with a ketone test if the physician suspects an overabundance of ketones in the blood.

## What happens if a person with diabetes develops diabetic ketoacidosis?

Diabetic ketoacidosis (DKA) occurs when a person with diabetes does not receive enough insulin. Without the insulin to help get the glucose into the body's cells, the person essentially goes into what can be called a "starvation mode." This triggers the liver to start making ketones out of fat and proteins to give the body's cells energy, especially in the brain. But because there is no insulin, the cycle continues, and more ketones are produced. Both glucose and ketones are then transferred to the urine. The kidneys begin emptying the bloodstream of excess glucose and ketones with water, causing the person to urinate more and become dehydrated. By the time ketones—especially beta-hydroxybutyrate (75 percent) and to a lesser extent aceto-acetate—reach around 15 to 25 mM (millimolars), the body's resulting pH balance (for more about pH, see this chapter) leads to metabolic problems, and the person becomes very ill. The metabolic disturbance usually causes low blood pressure and shock, and if not treated, the process can lead to a coma and eventual death.

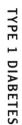
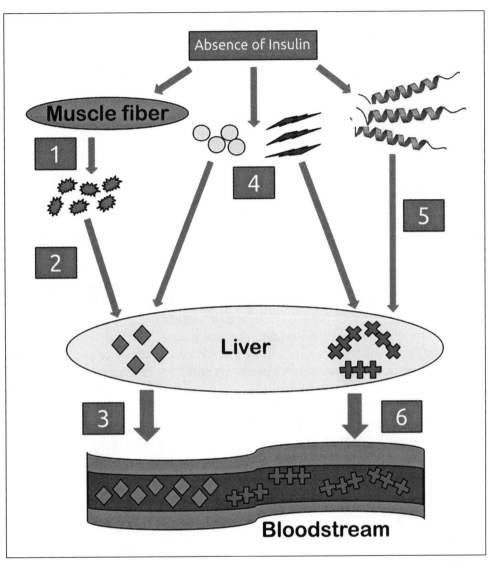

The diagram above outlines the process leading to diabetic ketoacidosis as follows: 1) amino acids escape from muscle fibers due to low insulin levels; 2) the amino acids are converted to glucose in the liver; 3) glucose enters the bloodstream; 4) lack of insulin also causes adipose tissue to release fatty acids and glycerol, which are then turned into ketones inside the liver; 5) glucose from lack of insulin is also converted by the liver into ketones; and 6) ketones build up even more in the bloodstream.

## Why are diabetic ketoacidosis and nutritional ketosis often confused?

The body normally produces some small amount of ketones every day. In nutritional ketosis, the body produces ketones when it burns fat for energy or fuel, occurring, for example, when a person loses weight or fasts. This is when the liver metabolizes fatty acids, turning them into ketones that are used as energy in various parts of the body. But

55

diabetics must be careful not to confuse normal ketosis with diabetic ketoacidosis—the first is usually something to be watched, while diabetic ketoacidosis is most often a medical emergency. In a person with diabetes, diabetic ketoacidosis means the blood glucose levels are high (hyperglycemia), the person has low insulin levels, and there are moderate to large amounts of ketones in the blood.

## Historically, was it often recorded how diabetes affected a person?

Yes, before the reasons and treatments for diabetes were better known, doctors watched their patients with diabetes go through a great deal of suffering. And although they did not know the details about diabetes—or even how ketones worked in a person with diabetes—many physicians' reports detailed the stages toward death. In the early twentieth century that meant most often people with type 1 diabetes.

It is now known that often one of the major reasons that caused a person to die from diabetes (usually type 1) was the body's buildup of ketone bodies. As the diabetic person's body slowed down metabolizing food, it used fatty acids for its energy. This led to a buildup of ketones, and over time, the chemical clogged the person's bloodstream and passed out in the urine. The person with an overabundance of ketones in his or her system would breathe out what was often called a "sickly apple smell" and continued to decline in health. As the ketones continued to accumulate, the body's pH (see below) dropped to dangerous acidic levels—what we now know as diabetic ketoacidosis. As the person sank into a deep coma, death was usually only a few hours away.

## Who should be aware of developing diabetic ketoacidosis?

People with type 1 diabetes, and insulin-dependent type 2, should be aware of their ketone levels (or symptoms of such a problem) so they do not develop diabetic ketoacidosis. Many physicians suggest monitoring ketones in all people with diabetes, especially in the following circumstances: if the person with diabetes misses an insulin injection or uses too little insulin during a period of illness or excessive or unusual stress; if the person's diet is low in carbohydrates, the person is exercising a great deal, or a combination of both; in pregnant women who have diabetes, or gestational diabetes; and when the person's blood glucose is high, or, if the person monitors ketones, if that level is very high.

## Is there a treatment for diabetic ketoacidosis?

For people who develop a more advanced case of diabetic ketoacidosis and get to a hospital for help, there are other more extensive treatments available. Commonly, the condition is treated with an intravenous infusion of fluids and insulin in order to rehydrate the person. This treatment also lowers the person's blood glucose levels and reverses the acidosis in the blood and body tissues. This is all done gradually to prevent the chance of hypoglycemia (low blood glucose levels) and hypokalemia (low potassium levels). Although measures are taken to help a person who develops diabetic ketoacidosis, it is estimated that almost 1,900 people with diabetes die each year from this condition.

## Can a person with diabetes keep track of ketones in his or her blood?

Yes, it is possible for a person with diabetes to keep track of the ketone levels in the blood. Along with being checked by a hospital or the person's physician, a person can use home blood tests and even some glucometers that detect the presence of ketones.

## What is pH?

The term pH is a chemical term taken from the French phrase *puissance d'hydrogen,* meaning "the power of hydrogen." The pH is based on a scale that ranges from 0 to 14, with a pH of 1 being very acidic, pH of 7 being neutral, and pH of 14 being very basic (alkaline). For example, battery acid has a pH of about 0; human stomach acid has a pH from 1 to 3; lemon juice has a pH of about 2.3; tomatoes, grapes, and bananas have a pH of 4.6; black coffee has a pH of about 5; urine has about a pH of 5 to 7; saliva has a pH between 6.2 and 7.4; blood has a pH of around 7.3–7.5 (a bit alkaline); seawater has a pH of 7.8 to 8.3; and oven cleaner has a pH of about 13.

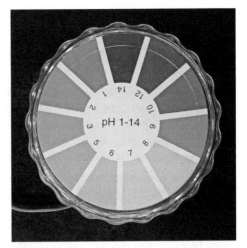

The pH scale measures how acidic or basic something is on a scale of 1 (very acidic) to 14 (very basic).

## Why is bicarbonate important to the body?

In general, bicarbonates in the body help to maintain the pH of the blood and other fluids, or the balance between acid and basic (for more about pH, acidity, and basic [alkaline] levels, see sidebar). The kidneys and lungs usually help the body to maintain the pH. For instance, the kidneys remove bicarbonate from the blood if the pH is too high. But sometimes the levels can be affected by certain foods or medications—or if a person has uncontrolled type 1 diabetes. Thus, a doctor will often measure bicarbonate levels to learn whether a patient has problems with acidity in the body.

## What is hypoglycemia?

Hypoglycemia occurs when a person has a very low blood glucose level. It is from *hypo,* or "low," and *glycemia,* or "sugar in the blood." It is often referred to as "a low" (mostly by people with diabetes), "insulin reaction," or "insulin shock." It is also the most common—and most dangerous—side effect that can often occur when a person has diabetes, especially if blood glucose levels are not monitored or the symptoms of hypoglycemia are ignored. (For more about hypoglycemia, see the chapter "Taking Charge of Diabetes.")

## What is severe hypoglycemia unawareness?

A certain condition often experienced by people with type 1 (and some with type 2) diabetes is called severe hypoglycemia unawareness, or the inability to sense that their blood glucose levels are dropping to an extremely low level. It is a dangerous condition and can lead to disorientation, unconsciousness, convulsions, and, if severe enough, even death. It is also considered a true emergency, as it makes people unable to help themselves.

One of the best ways to counteract a severe hypoglycemic episode is to give an injection of glucagon, the hormone that raises blood sugar, or intravenous glucose. The person with diabetes should always have an up-to-date glucagon kit at home and work for emergencies. (For more about what should go in a glucagon kit, see the chapter "Taking Charge of Diabetes.") In addition, they should explain to family members, friends, and co-workers what signs to watch out for and how to use the glucagon in case of an emergency. If the kit is not available, call a paramedic team immediately so they can administer an injection of glucagon. (Emergency personnel must always carry such a kit in case they have to treat a person with diabetes. Some also carry tubes with a special sugar mixture that is similar to cake icing in order to raise the person's blood glucose levels quickly.) Emergency medical technicians will also know whether the person having the hypoglycemic episode needs to be taken to the hospital.

## What is hyperglycemia?

Hyperglycemia is the opposite of hypoglycemia. It occurs when a person with type 1 or type 2 diabetes has too much glucose in his or her system.

## What is a hyperosmolar coma?

Although the condition is rare, if a person's blood glucose levels rise to extremely high levels—over 800 mg/dl—and there are no ketones present, it can lead to what is called a hyperosmolar coma, or diabetic hyperglycemic hyperosmolar syndrome. In this case, there will usually be severe dehydration, confusion, or a coma. This condition occurs mostly in elderly people with type 2 diabetes. In most cases, their blood glucose levels increase because of an impaired ability to recognize that they are thirsty, ill, or under great stress. If people don't drink more liquids at this stage (either because they are not thirsty or because of neurological damage from an event such as a stroke), then blood sugar levels can rise dangerously high. If it continues, the person will become sleepier and more confused and may have seizures following the dehydration, all of which can lead to a hyperosmolar coma. Such a condition most often requires hospitalization and can be fatal if not treated in a timely manner.

# PREDIABETES AND TYPE 2 DIABETES

## A PROPENSITY TOWARD TYPE 2 DIABETES

### What is prediabetes?

Prediabetes is a condition that often (but not always) occurs before a person develops type 2 diabetes. It is characterized by somewhat high blood glucose levels, which are caused by either a lack of insulin in the body or the body's inability to efficiently use insulin produced by the pancreas. In terms of measurement, prediabetes is considered to be present if blood glucose levels are higher than normal but not enough to be a diagnosis of diabetes.

### How does a person know if he or she has prediabetes?

For most people, there are no clear symptoms of prediabetes. In most cases, a person discovers he or she has prediabetes after a routine blood test or diabetes test. Because blood glucose levels rise slowly over time, a person may develop indicators of diabetes gradually or not at all, and thus, the symptoms may be overlooked. In addition, many of the symptoms experienced by a person who is prediabetic may be discounted, as they often represent several other conditions. This is also why prediabetes may go undiagnosed for years (and an often subsequent diagnosis of diabetes for many years, too).

### What are the major tests health care professionals use to diagnose prediabetes?

When a person has blood glucose levels—usually determined through a fasting plasma-glucose test—slightly above the normal range but not high enough to be diagnosable as diabetes, he or she is considered prediabetic. The following list, from Harvard Medical School and the American Diabetes Association, shows ranges of various tests that indicate whether a person is at high risk for developing diabetes (the random plasma-glucose test is not usually used to determine prediabetes; for more about the following tests, and the random plasma-glucose test, see the chapter "Taking Charge of Diabetes"). The symbols "mg/dl" represent milligrams per deciliter:

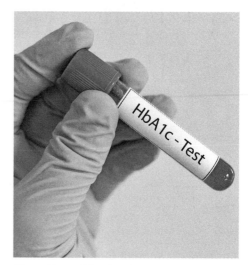

Glycated hemoglobin (or HbA1c or simply A1c) can be measured to determine plasma glucose levels.

- Fasting plasma glucose (or fasting blood glucose): 100 mg/dl to 125 mg/dl (if a person's number is in this range, it is often called impaired fasting glucose)

- Oral glucose tolerance (or OGTT 2-hour blood glucose): 140 mg/dl to 199 mg/dl (if a person's number is in this range, it is often called impaired glucose tolerance)

- HbA1c (also called A1C or A1c): 5.7 to 6.4 percent

## Are the terms impaired glucose tolerance (IGT) and impaired fasting glucose (IFG) both synonymous with prediabetes?

Many people have impaired glucose tolerance (IGT) or impaired fasting glucose (IFG), two ways of expressing what is commonly referred to as prediabetes. As the name "prediabetes" suggests, the condition occurs when a person has a higher blood glucose level than what is considered normal but one that is still below what is considered diabetes. These levels are usually measured by a blood glucose test. Doctors often refer to a person with prediabetes as having impaired glucose intolerance or impaired fasting glucose depending on the test that was used when the prediabetes was detected.

## Who is at most risk for prediabetes?

The people who seem to be most at risk for developing prediabetes are most often overweight or obese because the majority of people who develop type 2 diabetes carry extra weight. In addition, some people with prediabetes may already have some of the symptoms of type 2 diabetes or even the problems associated with the disease.

## Are there any symptoms if a person is prediabetic?

There are several signs that a person may be on the road toward developing diabetes. There are usually seven warning signs, and many of them mimic or seem to be symptoms of other ailments. For this reason, it is estimated that of the one in four people who has prediabetes, only about 4 percent know it. This means 96 percent of the population with prediabetes does not know it is at risk of developing type 2 diabetes. The "hidden" signs, as they are often called, are ones that increase a person's risk of developing diabetes and include the following:

*Red, swollen, and/or tender gums*—It is estimated that nine out of ten people with gum disease are at high risk for diabetes. This is compared to six out of ten without gum disease. Although some people have a predisposition to gum disease or have certain diseases that can affect their gums, it is often thought that people with gum disease who do not have diabetes check their blood glucose levels at least once a year.

*High blood pressure*—There are several statistics when it comes to high blood pressure, and especially involving women developing type 2 diabetes. It is estimated that women with high blood pressure are more than twice as likely to develop type 2 diabetes over a ten-year period as women with normal blood pressure. There is thought to be an elevated risk to women even if their blood pressure is a bit higher or when their blood pressure slowly rises over time.

*Gastrointestinal problems*—People who are prediabetic also have more upper-gastrointestinal problems. These include heartburn, acid reflux, some indigestion, and chest pain (not associated with heart disease). Also included are people who have ulcer-like pains that cause them to wake up at night but find that the pain goes away when they eat.

*Thirst*—Being thirsty much of the time is one of the classic symptoms not only of full-blown diabetes but also of prediabetes. This is because sugar tends to build up in the bloodstream when a person has the beginnings of diabetes (and with diabetes). This buildup causes the sugar to spill into the urine, and the kidneys begin to excrete more water in order to dilute the sugar. This process causes people to generate

## Why do some people seem to lose weight at the onset of diabetes—and sometimes after the diagnosis?

Many people with prediabetes—and even those with uncontrolled diabetes—seem to eat more during the day. This is because of insulin resistance (meaning their cells ignore insulin), which means it is difficult for glucose to get into the body's cells. This problem makes the muscles and organs want more energy, which means the person will burn fat and muscle to obtain that energy. Thus, they will lose weight, but in reality they are losing healthy muscle mass and not as much fat. This is because without a constant source of glucose in the body, the muscle tissues shrink over time. Such weight loss (or sometimes the inability to gain weight) is most notable in people with type 1 diabetes. It also occurs in people with type 2 diabetes, but because they are often overweight or obese to begin with, such weight loss goes virtually unnoticed.

a great deal of urine, making them go to the bathroom more often—and making them thirstier as they lose fluids.

*Numbness, burning pain, or tingling sensations*—This is especially true in the extremities, namely the hands and feet.

*Wounds that heal slowly*—This is also a sign of prediabetes, especially as the person's blood glucose levels begin to rise.

*Confusion and fatigue*—This is a more difficult symptom to connect to prediabetes. But for people who are developing diabetes, there are often signs of confusion and general fatigue.

### At what age should a person who may be at risk for diabetes be tested for prediabetes?

There are some indications that a person may be prediabetic, but the most common way it is detected is through a fasting blood glucose test. Many health care professionals suggest a person undergo a fasting blood glucose test after age 45, with some even suggesting their younger patients be tested after age 20, especially if there is a history of type 2 diabetes in the patient's family.

### What are some of the risks of being prediabetic?

Most people with prediabetes have a higher risk of becoming a type 2 diabetic, which is why health care professionals suggest that people who are diagnosed as prediabetic should have their glucose levels checked once a year (or more, if the doctor prescribes such tests). In fact, some statistics estimate that about half of people with prediabetes will go on to develop type 2 diabetes. In addition, this condition puts a person at a higher risk for developing cardiovascular and other related diseases. (For more information about cardiovascular disease, see the chapter "How Diabetes Affects the Circulatory System.")

But many people who are diagnosed with prediabetes never develop type 2 diabetes. In the majority of cases, this is because they change their lifestyle habits, including eating more healthfully, exercising more, and lowering their stress.

## LOWERING THE RISK OF PREDIABETES

### How can most people lower their risk of developing prediabetes and eventually type 2 diabetes?

For many people, there are ways to lower the risk of developing type 2 diabetes. In fact, according to the American Diabetes Association, a person can often lower his or her risk by about 58 percent by losing 7 percent of their body weight (for example, if a person weighs 200 pounds [90.7 kilograms], losing about 15 pounds [6.8 kilograms]) and by exercising moderately (for example, brisk walking) for 30 minutes a day, five days a week. In the same example as above, if a person weighs 200 pounds, even losing 10 pounds (4.5 kilograms) will make a big difference and lower the risk of developing type 2 diabetes. (It should be noted that for some people such measures may only slow the disease down. For example, those who have a genetic predisposition to diabetes or have other medical problems may still have an increased risk for developing type 2 diabetes.)

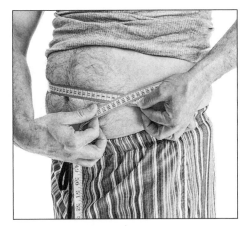

For many people who are prediabetic, losing a few pounds and getting regular exercise can stave off full-blown diabetes.

### What are some foods to avoid in order to lower the risk of developing type 2 diabetes?

Not all foods lead to diabetes, but some are more likely than others to increase the risk of diabetes. For example, foods high in saturated fats, trans-fatty acids, and fructose, along with highly processed foods, can contribute to a person's chances of getting type 2 diabetes. This is because many of those foods cause excess weight gain—especially if the person does not get much exercise—and additional weight sometimes increases a person's risk of developing type 2 diabetes. (For more about foods and type 2 diabetes, see the chapters "Diabetes and Nutrition" and "Diabetes and Eating.")

### If a person is prediabetic, will he or she always become diabetic?

According to Harvard Medical School, having prediabetes is no guarantee that a person will develop full-blown diabetes. What a prediabetes diagnosis means is that the person has a risk of developing type 2 diabetes. There are some often-debated averages concerning whether a person with prediabetes will develop full-blown type 2 diabetes. Some research indicates that half of the people with prediabetes will develop type 2. Other research suggests that about a quarter of people with prediabetes will develop type 2 and around half will stay in the prediabetic stage. The rest (the last quarter) will not develop type 2 diabetes and will revert to having normal blood glucose levels, mostly through lifestyle changes. Either way, most experts agree that being diagnosed with prediabetes should be a wake-up call for people to pay attention to their lifestyle in order to avoid developing type 2 diabetes.

# TYPE 2 DIABETES

### What percentage of people with type 2 diabetes are said to be obese?

In general, it is thought that about 90 to 95 percent of people with diabetes have type 2 diabetes, with almost 80 percent of those people said to be obese. Some research also indicates that the number of people who are obese and have type 2 diabetes are on the rise, not only in the United States but all over the world.

### How fast does type 2 diabetes develop?

There is truly no set "timetable" for when a person develops type 2 diabetes. Some studies indicate that if a person does not make changes to diet or exercise—or lifestyle changes—after being diagnosed with prediabetes, they have about a 50 percent chance of developing type 2 diabetes within ten years. This is not true for everyone who develops type 2 diabetes, as genetics or other conditions can lead to the disease, but on the average most people can stop or slow down the progression with lifestyle changes.

### What is thought to be a major risk factor in developing type 2 diabetes?

Although there can be several reasons for developing type 2 diabetes, research has shown that excess body fat is a major risk factor. In fact, people who are obese—those with a body mass index (BMI) of over 30—apparently have 100 times more risk of developing type 2 diabetes than people who have a lower BMI. (For more about body mass index, see the chapter "Diabetes and Obesity.")

### Is there a "standard" type of person who has type 2 diabetes?

In treating type 2 diabetes one must remember that people differ in size, shape, health risks, and medical problems. Thus, there is not a "standard" person with type 2 diabetes.

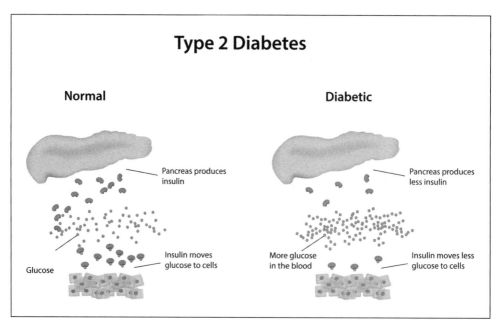

Type 2 diabetes results when the pancreas does not make enough insulin to carry sufficient amounts of glucose to the blood.

But doctors do mention common characteristics of a person with type 2 diabetes, including a lack of exercise, obesity, high blood pressure, and even a group of conditions called the metabolic syndrome. (For more about metabolic syndrome, see this chapter.)

## What are the warning signs of type 2 diabetes?

There are several warning signs of type 2 diabetes, although some people don't have such obvious signs. The following lists some of the general, traditional type 2 diabetes symptoms, which are similar to the type 1 warning signs:

- The onset is apparently sudden, although for many people (especially children) it may seem to occur slowly as some of the symptoms mimic other conditions.
- The person urinates frequently, as the body tries to rid itself of the excessive amounts of blood glucose.
- The person has excessive thirst as he or she urinates more frequently.
- The person may also find that cuts and bruises are slow to heal; the person may also have frequent infections.
- As the disease develops, the person may become progressively hungry, as the body burns its own fat for energy.
- Even though the person may be hungry and eat more, there may also be some sudden weight loss as the body continues to burn its own fat.
- Because the cells are not able to receive the sugar they need (due to poor insulin function), the person can become ill-tempered because of fatigue.
- The person may have tingling or numbness in the hands and/or feet.
- The person may also have vision problems; this is caused because as the blood glucose increases, fluid may be pulled from the lenses of the person's eyes, causing blurred vision.
- Some people with type 2 diabetes may have areas of dark skin in the folds or creases of their body (the neck and armpits are the most common sites), which is often considered a sign of being resistant to insulin.
- Although not as much of a sign as the others mentioned above, nausea and vomiting can accompany the disease in some people.

## Why are health care professionals so concerned that people are having type 2 diabetes at younger ages?

Health care professionals have several concerns about young people developing type 2 diabetes. One reason is the management of the disease, especially for those who are trying to maintain a balanced blood sugar throughout the day while in school (for more about diabetes and school, see the chapter "Who Gets Diabetes"). But one of the major reasons for concern is the risk of complications: the risk of heart attack, stroke, blindness, kidney failure, and amputations becomes greater the longer a person has diabetes.

## What gene was recently studied in connection with type 2 diabetes?

In 2016, it was announced that an international team of researchers had identified a gene that may be responsible for the development of type 2 diabetes. The scientists, led by a team from Flinders University in Australia, found a single gene called RCAN1 that may hold a key to the future of type 2 diabetes prevention. The researchers cross-referenced genes from people with Down syndrome, a genetic condition in which a person has an extra copy of chromosome 21 (the extra genetic material is called overexpression of particular genes). People with Down are also more likely to develop type 2 diabetes, as many have lower insulin secretion. The researchers looked at over 5,000 genes in four mouse models of Down syndrome (two exhibited high blood sugar, two did not). They then found 38 possible genes that were crossovers of Down and type 2 diabetes. Researchers noticed that when one gene called RCAN1 was overexpressed in mice, the mice secreted less insulin in the presence of high glucose. Thus, they extrapolated that RCAN1 may be responsible for type 2 diabetes in humans. Although it is unknown what types of changes occur in the pancreas to make the transition to type 2 diabetes, this discovery may lead to uncovering a primary cause of the disease. More research needs to be done, of course, with the next steps including using drugs to target RCAN1 and to see whether any of those drugs improves insulin secretion. Diabetes researchers hope that targeting this gene will eventually lead to possible prevention or reversal of type 2 diabetes. (For more about the future of genetics and diabetes, see the chapter "The Future and Diabetes.")

### At what age can a person develop type 2 diabetes?

A person can develop type 2 diabetes at almost any age. Even young children can develop type 2 diabetes, and in the past decade, the number of youngsters with the disease has grown. In fact, the youngest person on record to be diagnosed with type 2 diabetes was around three years old. (For more about young people and type 2 diabetes, see the chapter "Who Gets Diabetes?")

### What other diseases (besides diabetes) are associated with insulin resistance?

Insulin resistance is a condition in which the body's natural hormone insulin is less effective in reducing a person's blood glucose (sugar) levels. This causes blood glucose levels to rise, and if the increase becomes more severe, it can lead to type 2 diabetes and potential adverse health effects. But other diseases are also associated with insulin resistance, including metabolic syndrome, hypertension, and nonalcoholic fatty liver disease.

### Why do people often develop insulin resistance with type 2 diabetes?

The body's fat and muscle cells (and all other cells in the body) require insulin in order to absorb the glucose from certain foods. That glucose, in turn, gives the cells energy.

For a person with type 2 diabetes, there are three causes of insulin resistance: the person's muscles are not taking up glucose as they should, so there is an excess amount of glucose in the blood; the liver is taking up too little glucose and is even over-secreting glucose into the bloodstream; and the insulin production in the pancreas is not keeping up with the high levels of glucose in the bloodstream. As this system breaks down, the primary problem seems to be insulin resistance in the liver and the muscles. The person's blood glucose levels rise, but the body's cells cannot take in the glucose because of the lack of insulin.

Beta cells in the pancreas are in charge of storing and releasing insulin. If they malfunction, diabetes can result.

## Why do beta cells in the pancreas play a role in insulin resistance?

In most cases, people with type 2 diabetes have insulin resistance caused by a problem with the beta cells in the pancreas, specifically if the cells do not make enough insulin to keep up with resistance and/or if the beta cells become depleted. (For more about the pancreas and insulin, see the chapter "How Diabetes Affects the Endocrine System.")

## How is insulin resistance measured?

Insulin resistance is measured by taking a person's fasting insulin level or giving a glucose-tolerance test. There is also a test called the hyperinsulinemic euglycemic clamp to measure insulin resistance, which many consider one of the best indicators of insulin resistance. In addition, there are several other tests, such as the homeostatic model assessment (HOMA), the quantitative insulin sensitivity check index (QUICKI), and the modified insulin-suppression test.

## What are some risk factors linked to insulin resistance in a person with type 2 diabetes?

Several factors may contribute to a person's developing insulin resistance. These include a genetic risk (especially if a family member has type 2 diabetes); having insulin receptor mutations (called Donohue syndrome); and being African American, Hispanic, American Indian, or Asian. Other risk factors include being between the ages of 40 and 45, being obese, having a sedentary lifestyle, high triglyceride levels, hypertension, prediabetes, having had gestational diabetes (and having a baby who was more than nine pounds [four kilograms] at birth), and where a person stores fat (especially if the fat is mostly in the abdomen rather than in the hips and thighs).

**What is one way that may help lower the risk of developing insulin resistance that could lead to type 2 diabetes?**

Similar to what most doctors recommend for any type of diabetes, two of the best ways to lower the risk of developing insulin resistance are exercise and weight loss.

# TYPE 2 DIABETES AND THE METABOLIC SYNDROME

## What is metabolic syndrome and its connection to diabetes?

Metabolic syndrome (once called Syndrome X) is a cluster of metabolic risk factors that a person has, all putting the person at risk for various diseases. One of the major traits of metabolic syndrome is obesity, or being overweight, either through poor eating habits, not enough exercise, or other factors. Found mostly in adults (many with prediabetes), obesity includes too much fat around the waist (in other words, a large waist measurement), high blood pressure, high triglycerides, and abnormal blood fats (especially certain cholesterol levels).

In terms of diabetes, metabolic syndrome also includes high blood glucose levels, which go hand-in-hand with glucose intolerance. Not only does metabolic syndrome predict an increased risk of diabetes, it also predicts cardiovascular disease. (For more about cardiovascular disease, see the chapter "How Diabetes Affects the Circulatory System.")

## How many people are estimated to have metabolic syndrome in the United States?

It is estimated that about 34 percent of adults in the United States have metabolic syndrome. It is found to be higher in non-Hispanic white males than Mexican American and non-Hispanic black men. But in contrast, it is more common in Mexican American women than in non-Hispanic black or non-Hispanic white women.

## What are the numbers behind metabolic-syndrome traits?

According to many organizations, such as the National Heart, Lung, and Blood Institute (NHLBI), the American Diabetes Association, the American Heart Association (AHA), and the Diabetes Prevention Support Center, any three of the following five traits in the same person meet the criteria for metabolic syndrome. Many of these traits are related to the foods we eat (note: the term "mg/dl," also seen as "mg/dL," means milligrams per deciliter, a unit of measure):

> *Abdominal obesity*—One metabolic syndrome trait is a high waist circumference, often called an "apple-shaped" body (as opposed to what is called a "pear-shaped" body). This means a waist circumference of 40 inches (102 centimeters) or more in men and 35 inches (88 centimeters) or more in women (there are also different cri-

teria for various ethnic groups, too; for example, for Asian Americans, the values are greater than or equal to 35 inches [90 centimeters] in men and greater than or equal to 32 inches [80 centimeters] in women). (For more about abdominal obesity, see this chapter.)

*Serum triglycerides (or triglycerides)*—This reading is included in the test for metabolic syndrome if a person has a triglyceride reading of 150 mg/dl or above and is taking medicine for high triglycerides. (For more about triglycerides, see the chapter "How Diabetes Affects the Circulatory System.")

*Cholesterol*—The cholesterol in the body has "good" and "bad" types. The "bad" cholesterol is LDL (low-density lipoprotein), but that reading is not used in determining metabolic syndrome. The "good" cholesterol, HDL (high-density lipoprotein), is used: If the HDL cholesterol reads 40 mg/dl or lower in men and 50 mg/dl or lower in women, then it is part of the list for metabolic syndrome. In addition, taking medicine for low HDL cholesterol is included in the metabolic-syndrome list. (For more about cholesterol—good and bad—see the chapter "How Diabetes Affects the Circulatory System.")

*Blood pressure*—For blood pressure to be added to the list of metabolic-syndrome traits, there must be a reading of 130/85 or more (systolic over diastolic numbers), although this reading is often debated, usually in favor of a bit higher reading. Another trait of metabolic syndrome is taking medicine for high blood pressure. (For more about blood pressure, see the chapter "How Diabetes Affects the Circulatory System.")

*Blood glucose*—Another metabolic-syndrome trait is high blood glucose levels. Levels of fasting blood glucose would measure 100 mg/dl or above (although this number is also debated, with several researchers suggesting it should be even lower). Taking medicine for high blood glucose is also included in metabolic syndrome.

## How is metabolic syndrome treated?

According to almost every health-related organization, such as the American Heart Association and the American Diabetes Association, there are several things a person with metabolic syndrome can do to help

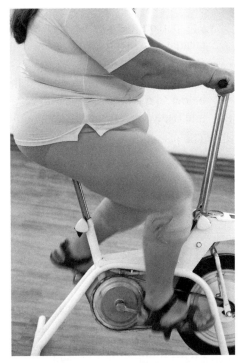

A common sense treatment for obesity and related diseases such as metabolic syndrome is weight loss through exercise.

lower the risk of developing cardiovascular disease and/or diabetes. The major ways are for a person to lose weight, eat a healthy diet, and increase physical activity.

# RISKS OF TYPE 2 DIABETES

### For adults between 18 and 45, what are some risk factors for developing type 2 diabetes?

People between the ages 18 and 45, and with a body mass index of 25 or higher (for more about body mass index, or BMI, see the chapter "Diabetes and Obesity") should be tested if they have one of the following risk factors for developing type 2 diabetes:

- The person has a mother, father, brother, or sister with diabetes.
- The person is physically inactive.
- The person is of African American, Asian American, Hispanic American, Native American, or Pacific Islander decent.
- The person has given birth to a baby weighing more than 9 pounds (4 kilograms) or has had gestational diabetes during pregnancy (for more about gestational diabetes, see the chapter, "Other Types of Diabetes").
- The person has a blood pressure of around 140/90 mm Hg or higher or is being treated with blood pressure-lowering medications (for more about high blood pressure, see the chapter "How Diabetes Affects the Circulatory System").
- The person has abnormal blood lipid (fat) levels, such as HDL cholesterol levels below 35 mg/dl or triglyceride levels over 250 mg/dl. (For more about cholesterol and triglycerides, see the chapter "How Diabetes Affects the Circulatory System.")
- The person has measured levels that indicate impaired glucose tolerance or impaired fasting glucose after being tested for diabetes.
- A female has polycystic ovary syndrome or (males and females) a history of vascular problems.
- The person has an HbA1c level that is greater than 5.7 percent. (A reading of 5.7 percent means a person is not yet considered to have diabetes but has a higher chance of developing diabetes; health care professionals consider a person to be diabetic if the HbA1c number is greater than 6.5 percent.)

If one or more of these items fits a person, and he or she is found not to have diabetes, then the test should be repeated in three years or as the health care professional suggests—or repeated, of course, if the person starts to develop symptoms.

### For a person older than 45, what are risk factors for developing type 2 diabetes?

There are several risk factors for type 2 diabetes for adults age 45 years or older. They include:

- A family history of diabetes, especially in the immediate family.
- Being overweight, and especially if a person is obese (generally a body mass index, or BMI, over 30; for more about BMI, see the chapter "Diabetes and Obesity").
- A lack of regular exercise (often connected with a sedentary lifestyle in older people).
- Being from an ethnic or racial group that is more inclined to type 2 diabetes, including African Americans, American Indians, Hispanic Americans, Asian Americans, and Pacific Islanders.

## Do people with type 2 diabetes ever need insulin injections instead of oral medication?

When people with type 2 diabetes have the disease for a long time, their use of oral medications may not work as well. Thus, one of the only ways to keep the blood glucose levels in balance is to begin using insulin. In combination with eating well, physical activity, and often other medications (including oral diabetes medicines), insulin becomes an additional help in controlling blood glucose levels. (For more about diabetes medications, see the chapter "Taking Charge of Diabetes.")

## What are some long-term complications of diabetes, especially type 2?

There are possible complications if a person has diabetes in the long term—in other words, the longer a person has diabetes, the more the possible risk of complications increases. These complications include heart attack, stroke, blindness, kidney failure, and amputations. But many of these risks can be mitigated or at least lessened by rigorous blood-sugar control and also by treating a diabetic for high blood pressure and/or high cholesterol if necessary.

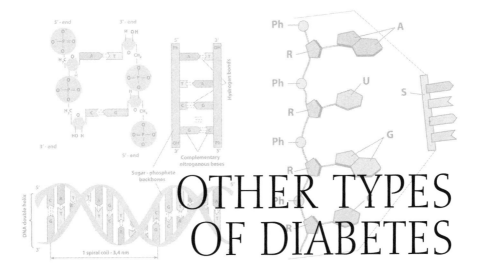

# OTHER TYPES OF DIABETES

## GESTATIONAL AND PREGESTATIONAL DIABETES

### What are some connections between diabetes and pregnancy?

One connection between diabetes and pregnancy is pregestational diabetes. This is when a woman already has insulin-dependent diabetes and becomes pregnant (see below). The most well-known connection between diabetes and pregnancy is a condition called gestational diabetes. In the United States, it occurs in about 4 to 9 percent of pregnant women (the percentage varies depending on the study). Worldwide, it has been reported by some studies to occur in about 19 percent of pregnant women.

### What is gestational diabetes?

Gestational diabetes occurs when a pregnant woman develops high blood glucose levels, even if she did not have diabetes before pregnancy. This type of diabetes generally develops during the woman's second trimester and usually disappears after the baby is born. According to the American Diabetes Association, this condition is also thought to raise the mother's and child's risk for developing type 2 diabetes later in life.

### Why do some pregnant women develop gestational diabetes?

Although not all studies agree, most research seems to indicate gestational diabetes may be caused by the hormones in the fetus's placenta. This connection between the mother and fetus, which supplies the nutrients the baby needs, may block the action of the mother's insulin throughout the body. If left untreated, gestational diabetes can result in very large babies and possibly the need for a caesarean delivery.

## What is the O'Sullivan test?

The O'Sullivan test is a one-hour glucose-tolerance test (GTT) that is given to pregnant women to screen for gestational diabetes. It is most often performed between the 24th and 28th weeks of pregnancy.

## What is pregestational diabetes?

Pregestational diabetes is used to describe the condition of a woman who already has insulin-dependent diabetes and becomes pregnant. Like gestational diabetes, pregestational diabetes can have consequences for the woman's infant, especially if the mother's blood glucose levels are not controlled during pregnancy.

## What percentage of pregnant women develop pregestational or gestational diabetes?

Although studies vary, it is estimated that gestational diabetes affects around 4 to 9 percent of pregnant women, or 4 to 9 of every 100 women who become pregnant in the United States. It is also estimated that gestational diabetes is 100 times more common than pregestational diabetes. There are also ethnic and racial groups that are at higher risk for gestational diabetes. It is thought that the Pima Indians of Arizona have 40 percent chance of having gestational diabetes, or a tenfold higher risk than the general population. Other groups are also at an increased risk, including African Americans, obese women, women who are at an older maternal age at pregnancy, women with a family history of diabetes, women whose babies are large for their gestational age, and women with a prior history of gestational diabetes during other pregnancies.

## Do any groups have a lower risk of developing gestational diabetes?

Yes, it has been estimated that teenage pregnant women have a lower risk—about one-fourth lower—of developing gestational diabetes than pregnant women age 35 or older. In addition, certain studies have indicated that Asian, Asian American, and Filipino women seem to have a lower risk of developing gestational diabetes, but more studies are needed to confirm the results.

## How can having pregestational diabetes affect a woman's unborn child?

If a mother who has insulin-dependent diabetes has uncontrolled blood glucose, excess glucose is often transferred to the fetus. Because of this, the baby's system se-

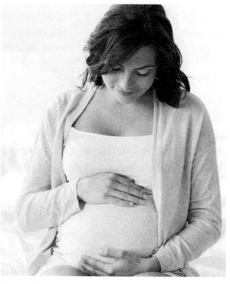

About 5 to 10 percent of women in the United States will be affected by gestational diabetes.

## Can a woman develop diabetes by becoming pregnant?

No, there is no research that supports the idea that pregnancy causes a woman to develop diabetes, but there is the possibility of developing gestational diabetes. However, some research indicates that if a woman has had gestational diabetes, she may be at a higher risk for developing type 2 diabetes later in life. Other research seems to indicate that breastfeeding a child will lower the mother's risk of developing type 2 diabetes. But overall, no true connection between becoming pregnant and developing diabetes has been shown.

cretes an increased amount of insulin, which can cause an increase in tissue and fat deposits in the baby. According to Stanford Children's Health, these deposits can increase the risk of birth defects, especially during the development of the fetus's heart, brain, spinal cord, and gastrointestinal system. In many cases, too, the infant of a mother with pregestational diabetes is often larger than expected for the gestational age.

## In what way does gestational diabetes differ from pregestational diabetes in terms of the fetus?

According to Stanford Children's Health, pregestational diabetes (if the mother has uncontrolled blood glucose levels) has been associated with birth defects in certain organs of the fetus as they form. Gestational diabetes generally does not cause birth defects. This may be because women who develop gestational diabetes develop it later in their pregnancy. Thus, most women will have normal blood glucose levels during the first trimester when the fetus's organs are forming.

## What is the White Classification?

The White Classification of Diabetic Pregnancies classifies the risks associated with a woman who is pregnant and has diabetes. It was presented by American physician and researcher Priscilla White (1900–1989), who, in 1924, joined the practice of Elliot Joslin and began caring for pregnant women who had diabetes. (She was also one of the founders of the Joslin Diabetes Center in Boston; for more information about Joslin, see the chapter "Introduction to Diabetes," and for more about the center, see the chapter "Resources, Websites, and Apps.") White's system was based on a pregnant woman's age at the onset of diabetes, the duration of the disease, and whether the woman had any vascular complications. The class system White presented in 1949 included Class A, meaning the diagnosis of the diabetes is based on a glucose-tolerance test and deviates slightly from the normal levels. Class B means the pregnant woman has had diabetes less than ten years, with the onset at age 20 or older, and no vascular disease. The diabetes and associated diseases increases as the classes continued down the alphabet. For example, class F means the pregnant woman with diabetes has nephritis, or inflammation of the kidneys.

## How has the White classification changed— and how does it often cause confusion?

As research uncovered information about diabetes, the White Classification of Diabetic Pregnancies listing changed accordingly. Other more complex revisions were made in the classification, based on differences in research and new discoveries of how diabetes affects other parts of the body. For example, one later classification listed class A as involving a pregnant woman having diabetes that can be controlled by diet alone, at any duration or onset age. Class B means the onset age is older than 20, with the duration less than ten years (same as with the White classification). But such listings also become more complicated. For instance, also in this listing, the classes are even farther down the alphabet, such as class H, in which arteriosclerotic heart disease is clinically evident, and class T, which is listed as "prior renal transplantation," or excessive kidney disease that led to a kidney transplant. Still other classifications list not only other symptoms in each class but add different and/or more classes. Thus, many researchers are now calling for a more standardized classification to simplify—yet explain the complexities of—the list of types of diabetes in pregnant women.

### Is there a classification based on just gestational diabetes?

As with many diseases, there are often several classifications. Gestational diabetes also has its own classification that differs from the White and subsequent listings (see above). One of the simplest states that if a pregnant woman can control her diabetes through diet, then it is called class A1; if a pregnant woman needs insulin or oral medication to control her diabetes, then it is called class A2.

### Are multiple pregnancies connected to diabetes?

Multiple pregnancies, or pregnancies with more than one fetus, often pose special risks because of the extra demands on the mother's system. For example, the need for oxygen and other nutrients for each fetus is multiplied. In addition, two common health conditions often affect the mother in multiple pregnancies. One is called preeclampsia, or having high blood pressure and protein in the urine. The other condition is gestational diabetes, or high blood sugar levels during the pregnancy (see above).

### Why is breast milk so nutritious for a baby, and how is it connected to diabetes?

After a baby is born, the mother's breast milk becomes extremely important for the baby's nutrition. The milk has an amazingly consistent composition, and in most mothers, it is almost a "perfect food" for the child (although it is usually low in vitamin D and fluoride). Certain studies indicate that breastfeeding a baby decreases the risk of respiratory infections, high blood pressure, asthma, and a tendency to develop certain allergies. In some studies, it has been found that when a baby is breastfed, he or she will have a lower incidence of diabetes in later years. But realistically, such benefits also depend on the mother's lifestyle habits. In other words, the nutrition of the breast milk is directly related to the nutrition of the mother. And if a nursing mother has poor nutrition, then it is often the amount of milk more than the quality that suffers.

## Can breastfeeding protect a mother from type 2 diabetes?

Although several studies seem to indicate that breastfeeding can cause certain changes in a mother's body that may help protect against type 2 diabetes, the connection has not been proven. But there are

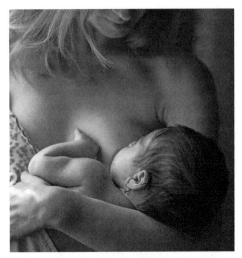

Breastfeeding is thought to be much healthier for infants than bottle feeding. One benefit is that breastfed babies have a lower incidence of developing diabetes later in life.

some indications that this may be true. For example, one recent study looked at 1,000 ethnically diverse women who had been diagnosed with gestational diabetes. The researchers examined each woman in terms of, for example, lactation intensity and duration. They then tested the women's blood glucose six to nine weeks after delivery and annually for two years after. By that time, almost 12 percent of the women developed type 2 diabetes, and after accounting for several factors (such as age or other risk factors), the researchers found that women who exclusively breastfed or mostly breastfed were about half as likely to develop type 2 diabetes as those who did not breastfeed. In addition, the researchers found that the length of time a woman breastfed affected her chances of developing type 2 diabetes. Women who breastfed longer than two months lowered the risk of type 2 diabetes by almost half and beyond five months lowered the risk by more than half. But again, more research needs to be done.

## Should a mother take diabetes medication while breastfeeding?

If a mother with diabetes decides to breastfeed her baby and takes either insulin or oral medication, it is important to understand certain safety factors while breastfeeding—not only for the baby's health but for the mother's sake, too. According to the American Diabetes Association, most diabetes medications can be taken safely as a woman breastfeeds her baby, but the ADA strongly advocates that the woman check with her doctor just to be sure.

## What are some tips for mothers who have diabetes and wish to breastfeed their infant?

According to the American Diabetes Association, breastfeeding can be a challenge for mothers who have diabetes, especially because it often makes it harder to stabilize blood glucose levels. The organization suggests that to prevent lower blood glucose levels, the mother should plan to have a snack before or during nursing, drink plenty of fluids (such as water or a caffeine-free beverage) while nursing, and have something nearby to eat in case of low blood glucose so the child's feeding will not be interrupted. And as always when breastfeeding, it is best to get the right amount of fluids, nutrients, and proteins. Such a nutritional plan can be worked out between a health care professional or dietitian and the breastfeeding mother.

# GENES AND VARIOUS TYPES OF DIABETES

## What are chromosomes and genes?

A chromosome is the threadlike part of a cell that contains DNA, or deoxyribonucleic acid. It also contains the genetic material of a cell. In some cells, the chromosomes consist entirely of DNA and are not enclosed in a membrane (called a nuclear membrane). In other cells, the chromosomes are found within the central nucleus of the

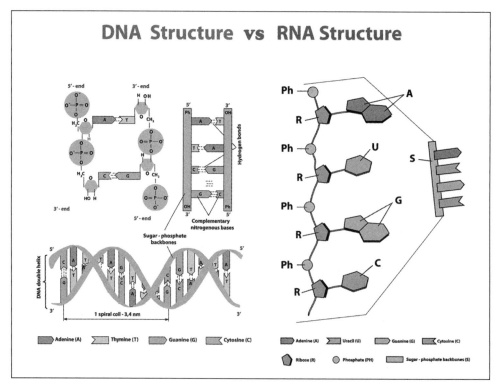

The chemical structures of DNA (left) and RNA. These are the molecules so important to maintaining life processes and genes.

cell and contain both DNA and RNA (ribonucleic acid). Overall, the human genome contains 24 of these distinct, physically separate units. (For more about DNA and RNA, see sidebar.) Arranged linearly along the chromosomes are tens of thousands of genes (from the Greek term *genos,* meaning "to give birth to"). They are complex protein molecules and are responsible—as a unit or in biochemical combinations—for the transmission of certain inherited characteristics from the parent to the offspring, such as eye color.

## What are DNA and RNA?

DNA, or deoxyribonucleic acid, is a nucleic acid found in the body. DNA forms from the repetition of the simple "building blocks of life" called nucleotides. These nucleotides are made of a phosphate, sugar (deoxyribose), and a nitrogen base. There are five types of bases—called adenine (A), thymine (T), guanine (G), cytosine (C), and uracil (U). In a DNA molecule, this basic unit is repeated in a double-helix structure made from two chains of nucleotides linked between the bases. These are linked either between A and T or between G and C. (There are no other links because these particular base structures do not allow any other combinations.) DNA molecules in a single human cell are extremely long. In fact, if one were stretched out and laid end to end, it would measure approximately 6.5 feet (2 meters) in length. The average human body contains 10 billion to 20 billion miles (16 billion to 32 billion kilometers) of DNA distributed among trillions of its cells. In fact, if the total DNA in all the cells from one human were unraveled, it would stretch to the sun and back more than 500 times.

RNA, or ribonucleic acid, is also a nucleic acid found in the body. But unlike DNA, it consists of a single chain instead of a double, and the sugar is ribose rather than deoxyribose. The bases are the same as in DNA, except that the thymine (T) is replaced by another base, uracil (U), which, like the thymine in DNA, links to adenine (A). All RNA exists in three different forms and depending on the cell is formed either in the central nucleus or in the nucleoid region (an irregularly shaped region within certain types of cells).

## What is a mutation?

A mutation is a change (or alteration) in the DNA sequence of a gene. Although people often use the term "mutant" in a disparaging manner, mutations are important because of the variation they contribute to a population's gene pool. Without mutations, there would be no variations and no natural selection within the population—human or otherwise. But mutations can also create harmful effects that cause diseases and disorders. One example of a mutation and resulting disease is sickle-cell disease (also called sickle-cell disorder or anemia). It occurs when a person inherits two abnormal copies of the hemoglobin (the oxygen-carrying protein) gene, one from each parent. The disease causes red blood cells to become rigid and sickle-like in shape and, thus, unable to carry as much oxygen throughout the body.

### Have any genes been found in connection with type 1 diabetes?

To date, researchers have identified several different genes that are believed to make a person more likely to develop type 1 diabetes. But they have not found any one single gene that makes all people who inherit it develop the disease (which is why some family members never develop type 1 diabetes, whereas other siblings do develop the disease). Overall, scientists call the genes they have found "diabetes susceptibility" genes.

### What is polygenic diabetes?

Polygenic diabetes is actually what doctors most often refer to when discussing type 1 and type 2 diabetes. This means that there are multiple genes—more than one and often several—that can increase the risk of developing type 1 and type 2 diabetes.

### What is monogenic diabetes?

Monogenic diabetes is when a person has one gene mutation that causes diabetes. It is estimated that of the human body's 25,000 genes, more than 20 are associated with monogenic diabetes. An error in one of these single genes can cause an adult or child to develop monogenic diabetes. It accounts for an estimated 1 to 5 percent of all cases of diabetes, depending on the study. According to the American Diabetes Association, it is most common in infants, children, and young adults. Monogenic diabetes includes maturity-onset diabetes in the young (MODY) and neonatal diabetes mellitus (NDM). Not everyone knows that he or she has this single gene and diabetes, with estimates as high as 80 percent of all cases of monogenic diabetes going undiagnosed. In fact, if this form of diabetes is not treated correctly, goes undiagnosed, or is confused with type 1 diabetes, it can lead to problems. (See also MODY and NDM, below.)

### Is there genetic testing for monogenic diabetes?

Yes, genetic testing can be used to detect monogenic diabetes, but as of this writing, it is often expensive, and some insurance companies do not pay for the screening. Many health care specialists will test babies who seem to have routine high blood glucose levels. But not all children who have any type of monogenic diabetes will be diagnosed unless they show classic symptoms that lead the health care professional to test for diabetes. This is why it is estimated that almost half of all infants who have or will develop a form of monogenic diabetes go undiagnosed.

### Who gets neonatal diabetes mellitus (NDM)?

A rare condition called neonatal diabetes mellitus (NDM) appears in neonates, or babies in the first six months of their life. It is caused by a mutation in a single gene and is considered a form of monogenic diabetes. The number of infants born with neonatal diabetes is not precisely known, but it is thought that one in every 100,000 to 500,000 live births, and about one in 400,000 infants, are diagnosed with neonatal diabetes in the first six months of life.

## What is polyglandular autoimmune syndrome, type II?

Polyglandular autoimmune syndrome, type II (it is sometimes used interchangeably with Schmidt syndrome) is a rare autoimmune disorder. It most often occurs when there is an extreme lowering of the levels of several hormones from the glands that secrete the hormones. It usually refers to a combination of many diseases, such as Addison's disease (an autoimmune adrenal [kidney] insufficiency), autoimmune hypothyroidism or hyperthyroidism, type 1 diabetes mellitus, and/or others.

## Is there a difference between neonatal diabetes mellitus and type 1 diabetes?

There is a definite difference between neonatal diabetes mellitus (NDM) and type 1 diabetes (the type most associated with children, although it can occur later in life, too). In particular, type 1 diabetes normally appears after the infant's first six months of life, whereas NDM can affect the health and development of a child beginning at conception.

## Why does neonatal diabetes mellitus occur?

The reason for neonatal diabetes mellitus (NDM) has to do with genes. In fact, to date, more than a dozen different genes (some research suggests more than 20) have been found to cause neonatal diabetes, with some causing both temporary and permanent NDM. For example, according to the American Diabetes Association, if an infant is born with such a defective gene, he or she may have neonatal diabetes throughout adult life. Two of the most common single mutated genes are labeled KCNJ11, which represents 30 percent of all cases of permanent neonatal diabetes, and ABCC8, representing about 20 percent.

## How are some children affected by neonatal diabetes mellitus (NDM)?

According to the National Institutes of Health, a child's health can be affected from birth onward if he or she has neonatal diabetes mellitus. For example, some fetuses with NDM may show signs of slow growth, high blood sugar, dehydration, and even difficulty growing after they are born. Children with NDM may also continue to grow more slowly than other children their age, and if the NDM is severe enough, the child may also experience developmental problems.

## Can infants outgrow neonatal diabetes mellitus (NDM)?

Yes, some infants will eventually outgrow neonatal diabetes (in that case it's called transient neonatal diabetes mellitus), while others will have it all their lives (permanent neonatal diabetes mellitus). Nearly 50 percent of the babies born with neonatal diabetes will see the disease disappear by age 18, but the rest will have permanent neonatal diabetes.

81

## What is autoimmunity?

**A**utoimmunity occurs when the immune system of a person's body attacks cells that are considered good for the body, mistaking them for foreign cells. This is one reason that scientists believe type 1 diabetes occurs as the autoimmune system attacks the beta cells (the insulin-producing cells) in the pancreas, and the body can no longer make insulin. (For more about beta cells and the pancreas, see the chapter "How Diabetes Affects the Endocrine System"; for more about autoimmunity and the immune system, see the chapter "Diabetes and Body Connections.")

## What are HLAs?

HLAs, or a set of proteins known as human leukocyte antigens, may predispose a person to diabetes. The HLAs are actually a set of proteins formed by a set of genes. These genes code for certain proteins called antigens that usually identify a person's cells as their own cells—in other words, they tell the immune cells not to destroy the cells that are part of the person's body. Researchers suggest that some of the HLAs incorrectly tag a person's own beta cells as "unfriendly," causing the immune-system cells to attack the beta cells in a form of autoimmunity that can easily affect blood glucose levels.

## What is the MODY form of diabetes?

A genetic form of diabetes, caused by a single gene mutation, is called maturity-onset monogenic diabetes of the young, or MODY. It most often occurs as a child approaches puberty or young adulthood, with most people diagnosed by age 25. It is thought that 3 to 5 percent of all patients with diabetes have MODY (the numbers vary depending on the study). It is also estimated that every child born to a parent with MODY has a 50 percent chance of developing the condition. As for symptoms, the child may or may not show any at all.

Genetically speaking, at least 11 different genes are responsible for the different forms of MODY, and each appears to have different symptoms attached, thus demanding different treatments. For example, according to the Diabetes Genes group in the United Kingdom, people who have a defect in the GCK gene may have hyperglycemia, with an A1c ranging from 5 to 7 percent—with little effect by diet and exercise modification on their blood glucose levels.

## Is there a difference between MODY and MODY1?

Yes. In particular, MODY is "maturity-onset diabetes of the young" and due to mutations in the HNF1A gene, while MODY1 is "maturity-onset diabetes of the young, type 1," caused by mutations in the gene HNF4A on chromosome 20. There are also other MODYs, such as MODY2, due to mutations in the GCK gene on chromosome 7, and depending on the mutation, MODY3, MODY4, and so on. A person with a certain type of

## Why are some treatments given to people with MODY1 often questioned?

**M**ODY1 occurs when the beta cells in a person's pancreas—the cells that secrete insulin—are under stress. Most health care professionals provide the standard therapies given to people with type 2 diabetes in order to make the beta cells secrete more insulin, but a study in 2016 questioned this practice. Most health care professionals treat MODY1 patients with the standard type 2 diabetes drug therapies, including oral medications that make the pancreas's insulin-secreting beta cells more active. But the researchers believe that the type 2 medications given to a person with MODY1 to increase the activity of the beta cells actually increases stress on those cells. This, in turn, may cause the destruction of the cells, causing even more problems with blood glucose levels. Thus, many researchers caution professionals who diagnose diabetes in patients to determine whether or not the patient has type 2 or MODY1 diabetes before initiating treatments.

MODY will have complications based on the mutation, and in general, these conditions disrupt insulin production. The most common forms are MODY2 and MODY3.

## What is congenital hyperinsulinism?

Congenital hyperinsulinism is not common, but it occurs when a person has abnormally high levels of insulin. Because of this, the person may experience frequent episodes of hypoglycemia, or low blood glucose levels. It is caused by mutations in the genes that regulate the release of insulin, leading to an oversecretion of the hormone by the pancreas's beta cells.

# OTHER LESSER-KNOWN FORMS OF DIABETES

## What diabetic condition is often associated with iron?

"Bronze diabetes" (also called the "Celtic Curse") is when the body is unable to eliminate excess iron properly, and some of the overabundance of iron collects in the pancreas. As the name implies, a person who has bronze diabetes takes on a bronze skin hue because of the accumulation of iron. This form of diabetes is actually caused by an underlying condition called hemochromatosis, an autoimmune disease that causes the body to store excess iron not only in the liver and pancreas but also in the heart, sexual organs, skin, and joint tissues. If or when the overabundance of iron eventually collects in the pancreas, it can "overload" the organ, creating this type of diabetes.

## What is hemochromatosis?

Hemochromatosis is often classified with other "iron-overload" diseases, or those caused by an excessive amount of iron in the body. Normally, a person's body extracts the correct amount of iron from foods in the intestines. If a person has hemochromatosis, this mechanism fails. As more and more iron is absorbed, the body cannot excrete the excess. It eventually accumulates the excess iron in specific tissues in the body, especially the pancreas, liver, and heart.

## How is hereditary hemochromatosis connected to genetics?

Hereditary hemochromatosis (HH) is a genetic form of hemochromatosis caused by a single gene defect. According to the National Human Genome Research Institute, the main gene, called HFE, was first identified on chromosome 6 in 1996. Most cases of HH result from a common mutation in this gene, known as C282Y. But other mutations have been identified that cause this disease, including one known as H63D. Hemochromatosis is most often inherited from both parents. If only one parent has the gene, then he or she becomes a carrier for the disease but usually does not develop it (although he or she may have a slightly elevated amount of iron in the system).

## Who is likely to develop bronze diabetes in the United States?

According to the American Diabetes Association, it is thought that one in every 200 (some studies say 300) people in the United States may have both copies of the gene for hemochromatosis. Of this number, it is estimated that about half of them will eventually develop complications, including bronze diabetes. According to the Centers for Disease Control and Prevention, as many as 75 percent of patients with hemochromatosis eventually develop bronze diabetes. In the United States, it is estimated that 1 million people have hemochromatosis.

Some more recent studies also indicate that bronze diabetes may be age- and/or even gender-driven. This is because bronze diabetes is rare in children, young adults, and pre-

---

### Was there a single ancestor who began the genetic mutation for hereditary hemochromatosis?

Yes, according to many studies, the origin of hereditary hemochromatosis was most likely from a single individual in Europe around 60 to 70 generations ago. The mutation in the HFE gene in this person was passed on to subsequent generations. And because this mutant gene does not cause problems early in life—especially through the child-bearing years in women—there was no reason for the mutation to be "stopped" by natural selection as with other mutations. Thus, hemochromatosis often affects Caucasians of Northern European decent and, to a lesser extent, other ethnic groups that develop other "iron-overload" diseases.

## Did writer Ernest Hemingway suffer from hemochromatosis?

Many researchers believe that American writer Ernest Hemingway (1899–1961) suffered from undiagnosed hemochromatosis, or bronze diabetes. It is thought that the disease often has a family history; for Hemingway, that appeared to be the case, as many members of his family reportedly committed suicide. (The iron accumulation plays a role in affecting mood and brain function.) Because depression and suicide are closely associated with hemochromatosis, as is the diabetes that afflicted Hemingway (along with his liver problems, heavy drinking, and high blood pressure), the disease could have been the cause of his suicide at age 61 (just weeks short of his 62nd birthday).

menopausal women under 50, while men between the ages of 40 and 60 are more likely to be diagnosed. There may be an understandable reason that women under 50 do not develop the disease as readily as men. Women regularly lose a significant amount of blood each month through menstruation until menopause, as well as during childbirth. Because of this, they lose a significant amount of iron. For most women with the defective gene that causes hemochromatosis, the blood loss before age 50 is often enough to keep the disease—and thus possibly bronze diabetes—at bay until well after menopause.

## How do health care professionals diagnose hemochromatosis?

Diagnosing hemochromatosis purely from symptoms is difficult, as it often mimics other conditions. In addition, a person may not show any signs or symptoms until the illness has progressed to the later stages. In the early stages, the symptoms seem nonspecific, including joint pain, lack of energy, weight loss, and abdominal pain. As more iron accumulates, people may develop arthritis, problems with sexual activity, and thyroid problems, often hypothyroidism (an underactive thyroid). In the later stages, the iron accumulates first in the liver, possibly causing liver diseases such as cirrhosis. From there, it can affect the heart and pancreas, eventually often leading to heart disease and/or diabetes.

If hemochromatosis is suspected, there are several ways to diagnose the disease. One way is through a blood test to learn whether there is too much iron in the body. This is done using a transferrin saturation test or a serum ferritin test. Another way is to test for the defective gene HFE (see above for more information about this gene).

## What could happen to a person with hemochromatosis if it is not treated?

According to the American Diabetes Association, if a person with hemochromatosis is not treated for the condition, it can affect the pancreas (leading to diabetes), liver (leading to cirrhosis), and heart (leading to heart disease). As with many conditions, because the symptoms for hemochromatosis resemble so many other diseases, it is thought to be severely underdiagnosed.

## How is hemochromatosis treated?

The good news is that, once diagnosed, hemochromatosis is relatively simple to treat (as long as it hasn't progressed too far). The treatments include phlebotomy, in which blood is removed from the body through a vein over multiple sessions. (On average, it is usually once or twice a week for several months, up to a year or more.) According to the National Institutes of Health, a newer treatment that includes fewer treatments than a phlebotomy is called erythrocytapheresis, in which red blood cells are separated from the whole blood, and the iron is removed.

In addition, the person's diet can help slow down iron overload. This means avoiding iron-containing supplements and limiting intake of such iron-rich foods as red meat and especially organ meats, such as liver. Some health care professionals also suggest avoiding supplements that contain vitamin C, as that vitamin is known to increase iron absorption in the body.

## What is the history behind the term "brittle diabetes"?

Brittle diabetes has often been used to describe a type of diabetes characterized by large and sudden swings in blood glucose levels. The true meaning of brittle diabetes is often debated. Some health care professionals believe it is a myth, while others believe it is a distinct condition. The concept was first mentioned in the literature in the 1940s to describe type 1 diabetics that did not respond well to insulin treatment. The biggest challenge of defining brittle diabetes was obvious. There were few ways that diabetics could easily measure their blood sugar levels, as there were no blood glucose meters or continuous blood glucose monitors. Thus, brittle diabetes became known as sudden episodes of low glucose levels (severe hypoglycemia) and recurrent, extremely high blood glucose levels (or recurrent diabetic ketoacidosis, or DKA; for more about DKA, see the chapter "Type 1 Diabetes"). Many experts believe this term was once used when a doctor did not know how to treat such extreme highs and lows of blood glucose. Today, the term is sometimes used to describe the unexplained variability of glucose levels.

In fact, with modern technology—in the form of glucose monitors and meters—it is much easier for a person with diabetes to control blood glucose levels. Thus, the number of people with so-called brittle diabetes has gone down significantly. According to some recent studies (in particular, those that included people with type 1 diabetes), life-interfering glucose fluctuations are rare, and some experts believe it is becoming even less common. The main reasons are the advancement of glucose metering and monitoring technology, better medications, and the advances in treating an individual diabetic—not only the physical but also the emotional conditions that can cause such extreme blood glucose levels.

# NOT TRULY DIABETES

## What has been called "type 3 diabetes"?

The term "type 3 diabetes" was introduced around 2005 as another name proposed for Alzheimer's disease. This was suggested because of the possible connection between insulin resistance in the brain and the eventual onset of Alzheimer's. Other recent studies indicate that Alzheimer's is accompanied by inflammation, or the body's response to an invading microbe (in fact, postmortem studies commonly reveal microbes in the brains of the elderly). Perhaps one day researchers will discover that inflammation and diabetes may be two of the major conditions that lead to the development of Alzheimer's, especially since a person with type 1 or type 2 diabetes often has difficulty fighting off inflammation. But at this writing, the true reason(s) for Alzheimer's is still highly debated.

## What is Alzheimer's disease?

Alzheimer's disease occurs when there are nerve-cell changes in certain parts of the brain. These changes result in the death of a large number of cells, causing several symptoms that range from mild forgetfulness to serious impairments in thinking, judgment, and the ability to perform daily activities.

## What is diabetes insipidus?

Diabetes insipidus (DI) is not a true form of diabetes but rather a rare disease linked to the body's hypothalamus and pituitary gland. Similar in some symptoms to diabetes mellitus (DM), DI causes frequent urination and excessive thirst, but that is where the similarities end. Diabetes mellitus is associated with the body's pancreas and is caused by insulin deficiency or resistance, thus leading to an imbalance in blood glucose (sugar) levels. On the other hand, DI occurs when the system that regulates the kidney's handling of fluids is upset by certain circumstances, such as disease or trauma.

## What steps lead to developing diabetes insipidus?

Diabetes insipidus occurs when the body's fluids become unbalanced. Normally, the body balances fluid volume and composition, with the fluid intake governed by thirst and the rate of excreting urine by the production of vasopressin, also called antidiuretic hormone (ADH). This hormone is made in a small gland in the brain called the hypothalamus. The ADH is then stored in the nearby pituitary gland and released when needed into the bloodstream. When the ADH reaches the kidneys, it concentrates urine by reabsorbing some of the filtered water into the bloodstream, therefore making less urine. When this system is not working properly—in other words, when the kidneys' ability to regulate fluids does not work well—the result is often DI.

## How does a doctor test for diabetes insipidus?

Because diabetes insipidus and diabetes mellitus have a crossover of symptoms—chiefly frequent urination and excessive thirst—a health care provider may suspect that a person with DI actually has diabetes mellitus. Therefore, testing is needed to distinguish the difference, including urinalysis (to determine the concentration of a person's urine) and a fluid-deprivation test (which will change body weight, urine output, and urine concentration when fluids are withheld, all of which can be used to learn whether there is any defect in ADH production or the kidneys' response to ADH).

## What are the various forms of diabetes insipidus (DI)?

There are several different forms of diabetes insipidus. The following lists some of these forms and the factors that explain the differences:

- *Central DI*—This is the most common form of DI. It is caused by damage to the pituitary gland, which stops the normal storage and release of ADH (antidiuretic hormone). Damages to the pituitary gland can be caused by a variety of diseases, head injuries, neurosurgery, or even genetic disorders.

- *Nephrogenic DI*—This is caused by a disruption in the kidneys' ability to respond to ADH. The disruption can be caused by various drugs (lithium, for example) or by several types of chronic diseases, such as sickle-cell disease, inherited genetic disorders, kidney failure, or partial blockage of the ureters. It is often treated with several drugs, including hydrochlorothiazide.

- *Dipsogenic DI*—This is caused by an actual defect in or damage to the body's thirst mechanism, which is located in the brain's hypothalamus. Abnormal increase in thirst and fluid intake are seen in a person with this problem, and those, in turn, suppress ADH secretion—and increase the urine output. So far, there is no real treatment for dipsogenic DI. (For more about ureters and the urinary system, see the chapter "How Diabetes Affects the Urinary System.")

- *Gestational DI*—Similar to gestational diabetes, gestational DI occurs only during pregnancy, but that is where the similarity ends. Gestational DI results when a specific enzyme made by the placenta destroys the ADH in the mother. (The placenta is the system of tissues and blood vessels that develop with the fetus; it is attached to the mother, supplying nutrients and eliminating waste products between the fetus and mother.) It is most often treated with desmopressin (although there is a rare form of gestational DI, in which the thirst mechanism is abnormal, which is not treated with desmopressin).

## What is "uric acid diabetes"?

According to a recent study, there may be a connection between uric acid and how the body metabolizes carbohydrates and fats (lipids). The researchers suggested the phrase "uric acid diabetes" after discovering a statistically high incidence of diabetes in people with hyperuricemia (an abnormally high amount of uric acid in the blood), gout, or both. But more studies need to be conducted to verify whether there truly is a uric acid–diabetes connection. (For more about uric acid, see the chapter "How Diabetes Affects the Urinary System.")

# DIABETES AND BODY CONNECTIONS

## SOME HUMAN MOLECULES AND DIABETES

### What are the major organic molecules in humans?

The major organic (also called bioorganic) molecules in the human body are carbohydrates, lipids (or fats), proteins, and nucleic acids. These molecules are characteristic of all life—from the smallest to largest cells. They all have basic roles in the body's cells, such as storing and producing energy, providing structural materials within a cell, and storing hereditary information. (For more information about carbohydrates, lipids, and fats, see the chapter "Diabetes and Food.")

### Are glucose levels affected by carbohydrates, fats, and proteins?

Yes, glucose levels in the body are affected by what a person eats, whether the foods contain carbohydrates, fats, or proteins (along with vitamins, minerals, and other nutrients). All of these bioorganic molecules can affect people's glucose levels whether they have diabetes or not—albeit in different ways.

### What is an enzyme?

An enzyme is a protein that acts as a biological catalyst. It decreases the amount of energy needed (activation energy) to start a metabolic reaction. Different enzymes work in different environments, owing to changes in temperature and acidity. For example, the amylase enzyme that is active in the mouth cannot function in the acidic environment of the stomach; pepsin, which breaks down proteins in the stomach, cannot function in the mouth. In fact, without enzymes, the stomach would not be able to obtain energy and nutrients from food. In the human body, there are thousands (ranging from

1,000 to 5,000 depending on the source of information) of enzymes that help with cellular reactions.

## What are proteins, and what is their purpose?

Proteins are large, complex molecules composed of smaller subunits called amino acids. Human life could not exist without proteins, as these complex molecules help build, maintain, and repair the body and especially the body's cells.

## What are some important enzymes—or proteins—in the human body?

The enzymes that are required for all metabolic reactions are proteins. These proteins also are important to structures such as muscles, and they act as both transporters and signal receptors. The following lists the types of proteins and examples of their functions, including those associated with blood glucose:

| Type of Enzyme/Protein | Examples of Functions |
| --- | --- |
| Defensive | Antibodies that respond to invasion |
| Enzymatic | Increase the rate of reactions; build and break down molecules |
| Hormonal | Insulin and glucagon, which control blood glucose levels |
| Receptor | Cell-surface molecules that cause cells to respond to signals |
| Storage | Store amino acids for use in metabolic processes |
| Structural | Major components of muscles, skin, hair |
| Transport | Hemoglobin carries oxygen from lungs to cells |

# THE IMMUNE SYSTEM, INFECTION, AND INFLAMMATION

## What is an autoimmune disease?

An autoimmune disease is one in which the body triggers an immune response against its own cells and tissues. Autoimmune diseases can affect almost every organ and system in the body. The cause or causes of most autoimmune diseases is unknown. They may be systematic (meaning they affect and damage many organs) or localized (affecting only a single organ or tissue). The following lists only a few autoimmune diseases that affect certain body systems (those associated with diabetes are italicized):

| Autoimmune Diseases and Their Effects | |
| --- | --- |
| Body System | Autoimmune Diseases |
| Blood and blood vessels | Autoimmune hemolytic anemia; pernicious anemia; systemic lupus; Wegener's granulomatosis |
| Digestive tract | Autoimmune hepatitis; Crohn's disease; scleroderma; ulcerative (including the mouth) colitis |

| Body System | Autoimmune Diseases |
| --- | --- |
| Eyes | Sjögren's syndrome; *type 1 diabetes mellitus* |
| Glands | Graves' disease; thyroiditis; *type 1 diabetes mellitus* |
| Heart | Myocarditis; rheumatic fever; scleroderma; systemic lupus |
| Joints | Rheumatoid arthritis; systemic lupus erythematosus |
| Kidneys | Systemic lupus erythematosus; *type 1 diabetes mellitus* |
| Lungs | Rheumatoid arthritis; scleroderma; systemic lupus erythematosus |
| Muscles | Myasthenia gravis; polymyositis |
| Nerves and brain | Guillain-Barré syndrome; multiple sclerosis; systemic lupus erythematosus |
| Skin | Psoriasis; scleroderma; systemic lupus erythematosus |

## Besides diabetes, what other illnesses are often caused by the body's own immune system's "attacking" itself?

One explanation for the development of type 1 diabetes is thought to be the immune system's antibodies attacking the insulin-producing cells in the pancreas. But this is not the only way the body's immune system "mutinies" against itself—attacking the organs it is supposed to defend. For example, autoimmune diseases include rheumatoid arthritis, in which antibodies attack the tissues of the joints. Another is multiple sclerosis, which is thought to be caused when antibodies attack the myelin sheath surrounding nerves. (For more about arthritis and diabetes, see the chapter "How Diabetes Affects Bones, Joints, Muscles, Teeth, and Skin.")

## What is the difference between inflammation and infection?

Inflammation does not mean infection, even when the infection causes the inflammation. An infection is caused by a bacteria, fungus, or virus, while an inflammation is the body's response to the infection.

## Do people with diabetes often have more infections?

Yes. Because high blood glucose levels can weaken a person's immune system—along with damaging nerves and reducing blood flow—people with diabetes are more apt to have infections. These include infections

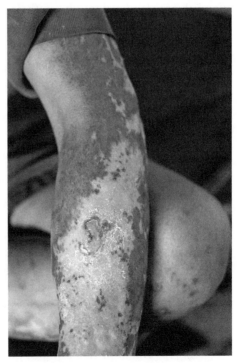

Scleroderma is an autoimmune disease affecting the skin, in many cases, but it can also afflict internal organs such as the lungs and kidneys.

91

of the skin (in particular the feet), bladder, kidney, and mouth, and for women, often vaginal infections.

## Do older people with diabetes seem to have more infections?

Yes, according to some studies, older people with diabetes seem to get more infections. In particular, common sites of such infections include the urinary tract, along with the skin (mostly areas that remain moist; for instance, the groin and armpits), and the soft structures (for example, between the toes) and bony structures (such as with bunions) of the feet. There are several reasons for more of these infections in the elderly, especially a less-efficient immune system, traumas, neuropathies, and infections that go unnoticed or are ignored by the person.

## Which skin cells are involved with the immune system and deterring infections?

Keratinocytes, found in the top layer of skin called the epidermis, assist the immune system. They produce hormone-like substances that stimulate the development of certain white blood cells called T lymphocytes. In turn, the T lymphocytes defend against infection caused by disease-causing pathogens—mainly bacteria and viruses. (For more about the skin, see the chapter "How Diabetes Affects Bones, Joints, Muscles, Teeth, and Skin.") For people with diabetes, defense against infections is often less efficient, as high blood glucose levels often weaken their immune system.

## What are the types of immune responses in the body?

The body has two major forms of ridding the body of disease or invading microbes that result in inflammation. Natural (or innate) immunity operates against microorganisms and dead cells and cell parts and is usually present when a person is born. The body's acquired immunity responds to the presence of specific antigens (toxins, often) and is usu-

### What is the role of fever in infection?

The normal body temperature for humans is 98.6°F (37.2°C), although this can vary up or down by a few degrees. A fever is defined as a higher-than-normal body temperature, and it most often occurs when certain pathogens (a bacterium, virus, or other microorganism that causes disease) invade the body. For example, bacteria often release certain toxins when they invade the body, many of which cause an infection. These toxins (or antigens) cause the body's immune system to respond by releasing special proteins that regulate body temperature. The increase in body temperature also causes a person's metabolic rate to rise and speeds up the body's reactions that aid in getting rid of infection. One of these includes a fever, which seems to inhibit the growth of certain microbes. It also stimulates the liver to hoard certain substances that bacteria seem to require, which helps to stop the microbes from growing.

ally acquired after birth as the body is exposed to certain antigens as the person ages. For example, if a person gets a splinter, the tissue around the entry wound becomes irritated, hot, painful, red, and swollen. This is the result of the body's immune response to fight off the microorganisms that are on the splinter. In this case, the body's immune system sends out what are called phagocytes, or cells in the blood that (if working properly) approach their prey, engulf it, and destroy it with special enzymes.

## What is inflammation in the human body?

Inflammation (from the Latin *inflammo* or "ignite") is the body's natural way of fighting off microbes that enter the body; it is also referred to as part of the body's immune response. It is a positive feature, as it is the body's attempt to protect itself against harmful stimuli and to begin healing. But it can also cause more inflammation, becoming almost self-perpetuating.

Most people are familiar with inflammation. For example, the body responds to a bug bite, rash, or skin infection—all of which cause inflammation in the infected area. Inflammation can be acute, meaning it starts rapidly and quickly becomes severe, such as when a person accidentally cuts a finger with a knife. Inflammation can be chronic, meaning long-term inflammation that can last months or several years. This type of inflammation can cause several diseases and conditions, including atherosclerosis, periodontitis, hay fever, and rheumatoid arthritis. And although scientists know that inflammation can play a role in, for example, heart disease and possibly diabetes, it is still unknown what drives inflammation in the first place.

## What is the connection between inflammation and diabetes?

There seems to be a connection between inflammation and, in particular, type 2 diabetes. Recent studies seem to indicate that inflammation inside the body may actually play a role in the development of type 2 diabetes. Some research indicates that fat may be the problem, especially in people who are obese and have fat around the belly. It is thought that these fat cells produce chemicals that lead to inflammation, which some researchers believe contributes to the development of chronic diseases such as type 2 diabetes.

In fact, it is known that people who have type 2 diabetes have higher levels of inflammation in their bodies, including higher cytokines, or inflammatory chemicals in the body. It is also known that they also have elevated cytokine levels inside their fat tissues. Thus, excess body fat probably causes chronic, low levels of inflammation in a person with type 2 diabetes, altering the insulin's ability to do its normal task and further contributing to the disease. This does not mean that inflammation causes type 2 diabetes, but it appears to be involved in the development of the disease.

## Why is exercise good to fight inflammation and type 2 diabetes?

It is thought that physical exercise—even 30 minutes of walking a day—may not only help prevent type 2 diabetes in those who are at risk of developing the disease but may also help increase insulin sensitivity. This is because exercise releases several anti-inflammatory chemicals into the body. It also helps the body's muscle (and other) cells increase their sensitivity to insulin and, in turn, helps reduce chronic inflammation.

### What is the inflammatory factor (IF)?

The inflammatory factor (IF), described almost a decade ago, is a way of rating foods based on their potential ability to increase or decrease inflammation in the body. The numbers in the range vary widely (there are no upper or lower limits), and each rating is considered to be dependent on serving size. Most studies on the IF have shown a mixed result, and the topic is highly debated. Some people say there is

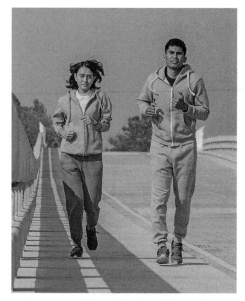

Walking 30 minutes a day is a good way to help stave off the possibility of contracting type 2 diabetes.

no way to control inflammation in our systems using this method, while others believe eating foods with the IF in mind will help decrease inflammation in the body.

### What is an anti-inflammatory diet, and can it help a person with type 2 diabetes?

An anti-inflammatory diet is just as the phrase implies: Some foods have natural anti-inflammatory properties and attributes. Eating such a diet does not prevent type 2 diabetes, but it does help with weight loss—a contributor to the disease for people at high risk for developing type 2 diabetes. The foods often mentioned include fats such as omega-3 fatty acids (olive, flaxseed, and canola oils), avocados, walnuts, and most fruits and vegetables (oranges, tomatoes, leafy greens, blueberries, etc.). Foods that can *cause* inflammation are those that contain trans-fatty acids, vegetable shortening, red meat (especially beef and pork), and margarine. (For more about foods and diabetes, see the chapter "Diabetes and Food.")

# DIABETES, HIV, AND AIDS

### What is the difference between human immunodeficiency virus (HIV) and acquired immunodeficiency syndrome (AIDS)?

The term AIDS (acquired immunodeficiency syndrome) applies to the most advanced stages of HIV (human immunodeficiency virus) infection. According to the Centers for

Disease Control and Prevention, AIDS includes all HIV-infected people who have fewer than 200 CD4+ T cells per cubic millimeter of blood. (Healthy adults usually have CD4+ T cell counts of 1,000 or more.) The HIV definition also includes 26 clinical conditions (including many infections that occur as complications of the disease) that affect people with advanced HIV.

## How is HIV diagnosed?

The only accurate way to diagnose HIV is through antibody testing. The immune system of an individual infected with HIV will begin to produce HIV antibodies to fight the infection. Although these antibodies are ineffective in destroying the HIV virus, their presence is a positive indication of the presence of HIV.

## How is the HIV virus transmitted from one person to another?

HIV is transmitted via unprotected sexual contact with an infected partner or through contact with infected blood. Over the past few decades, rigorous screening of the blood

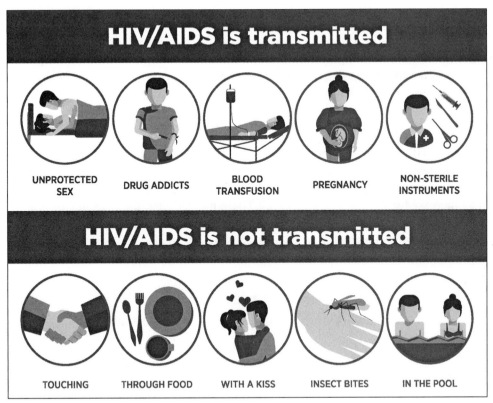

HIV is not transmitted through casual contact such as kissing or hand holding. Instead, there needs to be direct contact with another person's blood, such as through a needle or as can happen through unprotected sexual intercourse.

supply and heat-treating techniques for donated blood have reduced the rate of transmission via blood transfusions to a very small percentage. However, sharing needles and/or syringes with someone who is infected is still a mode of transmission of the HIV virus. In the past, HIV was frequently passed from a mother to her baby during pregnancy and/or birth. Treatments are now available that reduce the chances of a mother's passing the virus to her child to 1 percent.

### Why should people with diabetes and AIDS be aware of infections?

The immune system of individuals with AIDS is severely compromised and weak, so the body cannot fight off certain bacteria, viruses, fungi, parasites, and other microbes. Because such infections can easily establish themselves, it is usually more difficult to fight off an infection for a person with HIV/AIDS who also has diabetes.

### Why should a person taking metformin for diabetes, along with certain HIV medications, be aware?

According to the National Institutes of Health, people taking metformin for diabetes, plus getting certain HIV treatments, may be at higher risk of lactic acidosis (for more about lactic acidoses, see the chapter "Taking Charge of Diabetes"). They also warn that if a person has liver or kidney problems, or they binge drink or drink alcohol regularly, they are also at higher risk of lactic acidosis. As always, it is best for a person with diabetes and HIV to discuss medications, alcohol habits, and general health with their doctor.

### Do HIV medications increase the risk of type 2 diabetes?

No, not all HIV medications increase the risk of type 2 diabetes, but according to the National Institutes of Health, some do. In particular, NIH says HIV medicines in the nucleoside reverse transcriptase inhibitor (NRTI) and protease inhibitor (PI) drug classes may increase the risk of type 2 diabetes. These include such drugs as didanosine (an NRTI) and indinavir (a PI) that seem to make it more difficult for the body to respond to and use insulin. This insulin resistance causes a rise in blood glucose levels that can

---

**What should a pregnant woman with HIV
be aware of in terms of gestational diabetes?**

The American Diabetes Association suggests that women who are pregnant and are being treated for HIV be screened early in their pregnancy by their doctor for gestational diabetes. This means around 24 to 28 weeks' gestation or even earlier if the woman is taking certain HIV medications and/or if she has any other risk factors for developing diabetes.

eventually lead to type 2 diabetes. Thus, it is important to have blood glucose tests after starting these (and to be safe, other) HIV medications.

# DIABETES AND SLEEP

## Are women who have difficulty sleeping at risk for type 2 diabetes?

Yes, according to a study in 2016, women who have sleeping difficulties—both in quantity and quality of sleep—may be at an increased risk for type 2 diabetes. The study followed more than 133,000 women for ten years. Examining the women who developed type 2 diabetes, the researchers defined difficulty sleeping as: (1) trouble falling asleep or staying asleep; (2) sleeping less than six hours a night; (3) frequent snoring; and (4) either shift work disrupting sleep or sleep apnea. In most cases, these problems resulted in several conditions, including a higher body mass index (BMI; for more about BMI, see the chapter "Diabetes and Obesity") that would indicate being overweight or obese, more hypertension (for more about hypertension, see the chapter "Diabetes and the Circulatory System"), less exercise, and depression.

Even without these conditions, the researchers showed, sleeping difficulties were still tied to a 22 percent increased risk for type 2 diabetes in the female participants.

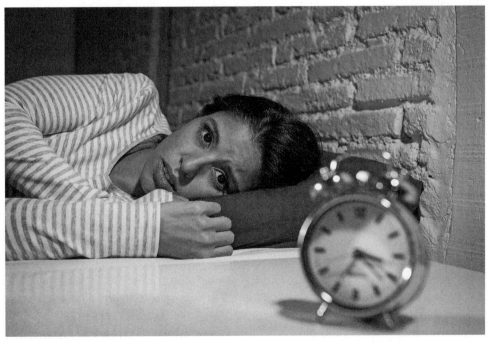

Studies have shown that women who have trouble sleeping have an increased risk of getting type 2 diabetes. This may be because lack of sleep is the result of increased levels in the hormones ghrelin or cortisol, which are related to hunger and stress, respectively; and these, in turn, are related to diabetes risk.

And if four of the above problems were prevalent, it meant the woman had almost four times the risk of developing type 2 diabetes. In this case, the explanation for the lack of sleep may be mostly hormonal. Sleep problems are often associated with the excess secretion of ghrelin (resulting in a boost in appetite) and cortisol (resulting in an increase in stress and insulin resistance), both of which increase the risk of type 2 diabetes.

### What did a recent study show about A1c blood glucose levels and sleep duration?

According to a recent study, sleep and A1c blood glucose levels may definitely be linked. The researchers found that people with type 1 diabetes who slept less than an average of 6.5 hours a night had higher A1cs than those who slept longer (for more about A1c measurements, see the chapter "Taking Charge of Diabetes"). In addition to the finding of sleep length and A1cs, the researchers found that these shorter-term sleepers were "non-dippers," or people who also have blood pressure levels that do not get lower at night—a definite indicator of health problems.

### What is nocturnal hypoglycemia?

Nocturnal hypoglycemia is as the words indicate: a low blood glucose level during night-time sleep. Often an episode of nocturnal hypoglycemia wakes a person, but sometimes it does not. If it does, it is often treated by the eating of fast-acting carbohydrates, such as glucose tablets or gel, to boost glucose levels back to normal. Thus, for safety reasons, most health care professionals suggest that a person with diabetes check his or her blood sugar at bedtime—and consider it one of the most important checks of the day.

### What did a recent study find about insulin sensitivity and sleep duration in men?

In yet another recent study from the Netherlands, researchers found that there was a connection between insulin sensitivity and how long a male slept. Insulin sensitivity in this study was based on how sensitive a person is to the effects of insulin. High insulin sensitivity means less insulin is needed to lower blood glucose levels, whereas low insulin sensitivity means more insulin is needed to lower them. High or low sensitivity depends on how well the pancreas is producing or the body is using insulin. The researchers found that men who sleep for less than or more than seven or eight hours of sleep had lower insulin sensitivity. In addition, men who slept for shorter periods had lower beta cell function (beta cells produce and release insulin) in the pancreas. More research is needed because no one knows the real cause and effect.

## What can occur if a person with diabetes has high or low blood glucose levels at night?

If a person with diabetes experiences high or low blood glucose levels at night, most of the time the episode has no effect, especially if the highs or lows are not too extreme. But if the levels become extreme, there may be certain problems if they are too high or low. For example, if people with diabetes have high blood sugar levels at night, it may be harder for them to sleep because they may feel too warm, irritable, and unsettled. If the levels are very low, it may cause problems within the person's central nervous system, including nightmares, sleepwalking, restlessness, and confusion.

## Why should a person with type 2 diabetes be aware of the "dawn phenomenon"?

Most people have a rise in hormones—for example, cortisol and glucagon—during the early hours of the morning, usually from about 2 A.M. to 8 A.M. Called the dawn phenomenon, it occurs as various organs attempt to keep a person's blood glucose levels from going too low at night. This hormonal activity helps to tell the liver to produce more glucose. In response, there is an increase in insulin to handle the extra glucose. And this, in turn, allows a person to wake and start the day after fasting all night. But for a person with diabetes, such a rise in insulin may cause fasting glucose levels to be dramatically elevated as the system cannot handle the extra glucose.

## Could daytime sleepiness be associated with lower blood glucose levels in type 2 diabetics?

Yes, some people with type 2 diabetes who have excessive sleepiness during the day could be at a higher-than-normal risk for hypoglycemia (low blood glucose levels). In a recent study, researchers speculated that when the blood glucose level dips low during nighttime sleep, it disrupts the diabetic person's sleep, creating daytime sleepiness. In fact, that daytime sleepiness can make a person less aware of a hypoglycemia event during the day, thinking instead that he or she is just tired, and thus, a person who has not been diagnosed with diabetes may ignore the early warning signs of disease.

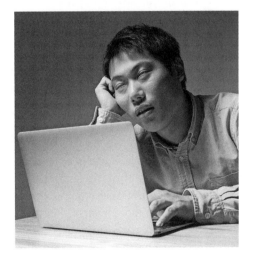

## What is sleep apnea?

Sleep apnea, clinically called obstructive sleep apnea (or OSA, the most common form of sleep apnea), is a condition in which a person's windpipe is temporarily closed as he or she sleeps, usually causing

One symptom of type 2 diabetes can be a chronic feeling of being sleepy and tired.

the person to pause his or her breathing. This commonly occurs when the upper respiratory airway is blocked, either because the throat muscles collapse, the tongue falls back into the airway, or the tonsils and/or adenoids are enlarged, impeding the air flow. The lapses in breathing also cause the individuals to wake up briefly because their breathing has been interrupted and may even stop for a brief period. Sleep apnea is often further described as a condition in which a person frequently stops breathing for ten seconds or more during sleep, with some experiencing a lack of breathing sometimes hundreds of times a night. A person who has apnea awakens frequently during the night gasping for breath. It is thought to be a medical problem for many reasons. For example, this pause in breathing can reduce the blood oxygen in the body, putting a strain on the cardiovascular system (especially the heart), which is why many people with sleep apnea are considered at risk for cardiovascular disease. It can also have an effect on a person with diabetes, causing a fluctuation in blood glucose levels during sleep (see below).

### Is there a connection between type 1 diabetes and sleep apnea?

Although it has not been investigated as much as sleep apnea in people with type 2 diabetes, recent studies have shown that people with type 1 diabetes may have more sleep apnea (and associated problems) than previously thought. For example, in 2015, a study showed that 67 people with type 1 diabetes had a high prevalence of obstructive sleep apnea. Sleep apnea was also associated with kidney complications and retinopathy (for more about the eyes and retinopathy, see the chapter "Diabetes and Inside the Human Body"). One interesting result of the study was that it was uncommon for people with

---

### Who gets sleep apnea?

Sleep apnea (OSA) most often occurs when air cannot flow into or out of the person's nose or mouth as he or she breathes. According to the National Sleep Foundation, sleep apnea often occurs in conjunction with snoring. And although snoring may be harmless for most people, it can be an indication of sleep apnea, especially if it is accompanied by mild to severe daytime sleepiness, which is why it is also often responsible for people's having auto accidents owing to daytime grogginess.

Of course, most people who have sleep apnea may not know it as they are asleep when snoring or not breathing. Men seem to have apnea more than women, as do people who are obese, but it can occur in anyone at any age for various other reasons. For example, it can happen to people with a large neck, people with small airways (the nose, throat, or mouth), people who sleep on their backs, and people who have a misaligned jaw. Another cause can be that, as an individual ages, the muscles around the back of the throat become relaxed. One of the telltale signs of this condition is snoring. Another sign can be complaints of lack of sleep by the person's bed partner.

type 1 diabetes and sleep apnea to be obese or have daytime sleepiness, which may be why a sleep apnea diagnosis was overlooked.

Although there were few people in this study, other more recent studies are indicating the same results. For example, one study indicated that sleep apnea was higher in people who have been affected by type 1 diabetes the longest. Also, people with poorly controlled type 1 diabetes have more sleep apnea problems than those who have more control over their blood glucose levels. And, like people with type 2 diabetes and sleep apnea, people with type 1 often are fatigued and depressed, not only from lack of sleep but also from difficulty controlling their blood sugar levels both day and night.

### Is there a connection between type 2 diabetes and sleep apnea?

Yes. Overall, it is estimated that up to 80 percent of people with diabetes—at this writing, mostly people with type 2 diabetes—have the condition. In particular, heavier people who have sleep apnea appear to have more health problems, including an increased risk for diabetes (no doubt because of being heavier or obese, which is connected to the risk of type 2 diabetes). If they already have type 2 diabetes, sleep apnea sufferers have difficulty controlling their blood sugar levels. For people with type 2 diabetes, sleep apnea also increases the risk of developing other diseases and conditions, including heart disease, high blood pressure, acid reflux, dementia, and depression.

### What device may help stabilize blood sugar levels in people with sleep apnea (OSA) and type 2 diabetes?

In a preliminary study conducted in 2016, researchers found that people with diabetes who used a device called a continuous positive airway pressure (CPAP) device had improved blood glucose levels. The researchers evaluated the effects of a CPAP machine on people with both OSA and poorly controlled type 2 diabetes. They found that people using the CPAP experienced statistically significant improvements in insulin sensitivity at three to six months after using the device. There was also a decrease in insulin resistance and HbA1c levels at six months (for more about HbA1c, or A1c, testing, see the chapter "Taking Charge of Diabetes"). Another positive result was that the participants had lower levels of certain inflammatory molecules and LDL cholesterol (considered the "bad" cholesterol; for more about LDL, see the chapter "How Diabetes Affects the Circulatory System"), along with

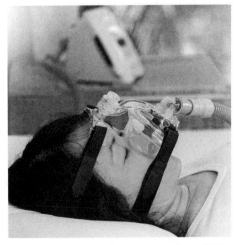

Sleep apnea can be greatly eased by wearing a CPAP mask at night to assist with breathing. A good night's rest has health benefits, including reducing the risk of diabetes.

higher levels of adiponectin, a hormone involved in regulating blood glucose levels. But there are a few caveats: the number of people tested was small, and there was no placebo testing. Thus, more research is necessary to see whether the CPAP can truly help many people with type 2 diabetes.

### Is there a connection between gestational diabetes and sleep apnea?

Yes, some studies indicate that sleep apnea may be more common than previously believed in women with gestational diabetes. (For more about gestational diabetes, see the chapter "Other Types of Diabetes.") One study in particular looked at a group of pregnant Asian women who were obese and had gestational diabetes. The researchers found that the majority of women in this group also had sleep apnea, which also caused their blood glucose levels to rise. The study did not determine causality—whether the sleep apnea led to the high blood sugar or high blood glucose levels led to the sleep apnea—but other studies seem to indicate that gestational diabetes is associated with the increased risk for obstructive sleep apnea.

# DIABETES AND SMOKING

### Is diabetes caused by smoking?

No, there is no evidence that smoking causes diabetes, but smoking can aggravate health conditions associated with diabetes. In fact, tobacco use—from cigarettes to cigars—increases the risk of developing type 2 diabetes and even makes managing the condition much harder if a person develops the disease.

### What recent research indicated a connection between seniors who smoke and diabetes?

In a study conducted in Germany, the data showed that seniors who smoked were almost three times more likely to develop type 2 diabetes than those who never smoked. (In this study, seniors were people age 60 or over.) If a senior also had prediabetes and was a smoker, the number rose to eight times more likely to end up with type 2 diabetes.

## What are some health problems associated with smoking that are exacerbated by diabetes—and vice versa?

Although diabetes is not caused by smoking, the disease can exacerbate some conditions associated with smoking. The Canadian Diabetes Association says recent studies indicate that smoking is an independent risk factor for type 2 diabetes—with those who smoke 25 or more cigarettes a day having double the diabetes risk than nonsmokers. Diabetes can cause damage to a person's heart and larger blood vessels, and smoking compounds the risk of this damage. Smoking is also thought to contribute to hardening of the

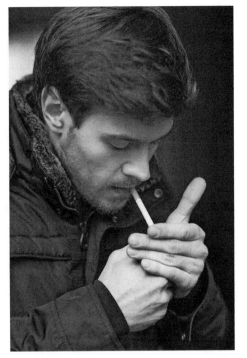

Recent studies indicate that smokers have a greatly increased risk of diabetes than nonsmokers.

arteries, which, when combined with high blood glucose levels from diabetes, can accelerate the development of diabetic complications. Thus, it is estimated that a person with diabetes who also smokes has about three times the risk of a heart attack compared to someone who does not smoke.

There are other problems with diabetes and smoking. Smokers who have diabetes can also have higher risks for serious health complications, such as kidney disease, retinopathy (eye disease that can cause blindness), and peripheral neuropathy (damaged nerves in the arms and legs that cause weakness, numbness, pain, and sometimes poor coordination). In addition, smoking by a person with diabetes increases the chances of stroke, faster nerve damage, and poor blood flow, especially in the extremities (hands and feet). If there is poor blood flow in the legs and feet because of smoking and diabetes, it can lead to infections and ulcers that are often difficult to treat. And in terms of blood vessels and nerve damage in the extremities, there is added incentive to quit smoking if a person has diabetes: It is estimated that some 90 percent of people with diabetes who have a foot amputated are smokers.

## Is it true that diabetes can be harder to control after a person stops smoking?

Not necessarily. Some researchers believe that after a smoker quits smoking, he or she gains weight and finds diabetes control more difficult, especially if the person doesn't exercise and eat a healthy diet. But other research suggests that smoking, while it does lower the body mass index (BMI; for more about BMI, see chapter "Diabetes and Obesity"), may actually redistribute a person's body weight into a pattern that can lead to obesity, which in turn can lead to diabetes. Thus, most health care professionals advise patients that smoking does increase the risk of diabetes (and often other diseases), making cessation of smoking that much more advantageous to a person's present and future health.

### How much of an increased risk for type 2 diabetes is there for smokers?

According to a 2015 study published in the *Lancet Diabetes & Endocrinology,* compared with people who have never smoked, people who smoke have a 37 percent increased risk for type 2 diabetes. For people who formerly smoked, the number decreased to a 14 percent increased risk for type 2 diabetes. The researchers even broke down the amount a person smokes and diabetes risk: Compared with a person who never smoked, a light smoker had a 21 percent increased risk of type 2 diabetes, a moderate smoker a 34 percent increased risk, and heavy smokers a 57 percent increased risk. The research also indicated that a smoker who has either type 1 or type 2 diabetes increased the relative risk of total mortality and cardiovascular events (such as heart attacks and strokes) by about 50 percent.

### Can secondhand smoke affect a person with diabetes?

Yes, according to some studies, if a person with diabetes is exposed to secondhand smoke (in most cases, if a nonsmoker lives with a smoker), it does have an effect on the disease. In 2015, a mega-analysis of 88 studies (which included a total of around 6 million people) found that people exposed to secondhand smoke have a significantly increased risk of developing type 2 diabetes. According to the data, compared with people who never smoked, inhaling secondhand smoke raised the risk of type 2 diabetes by 22 percent. Thus, the researchers pointed out that past studies of passive smoking's effect on health showed an increased risk of cardiovascular disease and cancer (mostly lung)—and also the risk of developing type 2 diabetes.

### If a person with diabetes quits smoking, how does it affect his or her overall health?

There is good news if a person with diabetes (or even without the disease) quits smoking. According to Harvard Medical School, some of the health benefits occur right away, especially a better stabilization of a person's glucose levels. In addition, researchers have found that a person with diabetes who quits smoking will notice that insulin resistance begins to decrease as soon as eight weeks after that last cigarette.

# DIABETES AND CANCER

## What is a common definition of cancer?

Cancer is caused by the unrestrained growth of cells in the body. Cells that do not "follow the rules" of the normal cell life cycle may eventually become cancerous. This means that the cells reproduce more often than normal, creating cellular overgrowth commonly referred to as tumors. Usually this happens over an extended period of time and begins with changes at the molecular level. There are more than 100 distinct types of cancer, each of which behaves in a specific fashion and responds to treatments differently.

## What types of cancer are associated with diabetes?

Diabetes is often associated with several types of cancer, including a higher risk of developing pancreatic, hepatic (liver), endometrial (ovaries), breast, lung, bladder, and colorectal cancers. These cancers are all independently associated with insulin resistance and also hyperinsulinemia. The reason for this connection between so many cancers and diabetes is still being explored, but there are a few possible explanations. For example, according to Harvard Medical School, cancer and diabetes share several risk factors, including obesity, aging, and a sedentary lifestyle, along with a diet high in fat and refined carbohydrates. Another connection is that the changes in the body associated with diabetes, including insulin resistance, high blood glucose levels, and inflammation, may also help contribute to the risk of developing cancers. This is why most health care professionals suggest that a person with diabetes stick to a healthful lifestyle and schedule routine cancer screenings.

## Are there any treatments for diabetes that may lower the risk of cancer?

Yes, but some also may raise the risk. Metformin is often cited as reducing the risk of many types of cancer, and a class of oral medications called thiazolidinediones (for example, pioglitazone) have been noted to lower the risk of some cancers, while increasing the risk of others (often cited is bladder cancer and even other medical problems such as an increased risk of heart failure). In addition, GLP-1 therapies (or glucagon-like peptide 1 receptor agonists, which are often mentioned as a treatment for type 2 diabetes) have often been connected to an increased risk of pancreatic and thyroid cancers. But as usual, many of these connections have not been proven by extensive research.

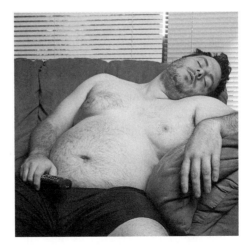

Having a sedentary lifestyle puts you at greater risk of not only diabetes but also some types of cancer.

### Does any type of cancer cause diabetes?

No, no research has found that any type of cancer causes diabetes, although, as seen above, diabetes is often associated with a higher risk of several cancers. This lack of association makes sense, as both diseases develop for different reasons.

# DIABETES AND ALLERGIES

### What is an allergic reaction?

An allergic reaction is a response to a substance that is often harmless to most other people. Allergens, the antigens (chemical substances, mostly in the form of proteins) that can cause an allergic reaction, are found in many foods and medications, along with responses to various plants, animals, chemicals, dust, or molds. The more common allergic reactions are allergic rhinitis (hay fever), allergic conjunctivitis (an eye reaction), asthma, atopic dermatitis (skin reactions), urticaria (hives), and what are called severe systemic allergic reactions (such as anaphylaxis).

### Do allergies cause diabetes?

No, there is no evidence that any allergies cause diabetes (although there have been some rare reports of allergies to insulin in people with type 2 diabetes). But that does not mean people with diabetes don't have allergies (such as allergies to certain foods and medications).

### How can certain medications for allergies affect a person with type 2 diabetes?

Several over-the-counter (OTC) and prescription allergy medications can affect a person with type 2 diabetes. For example, certain medicines, especially OTC decongestants

---

## What is anaphylactic shock?

Anaphylactic shock, or anaphylaxis, is a severe allergic reaction to certain allergens, usually within minutes after exposure. For example, many people who are severely allergic to the venom in bee stings can experience anaphylactic shock. Anaphylactic reactions usually involve one or several organs in the body, such as the skin (often as a rash), respiratory system (usually as breathing difficulties), and gastrointestinal tract (most often as vomiting and/or diarrhea).

Many people who may suffer severe reactions to bee stings or snake bites carry what is called an Epipen™ with them, a needle-and-syringe medical device that provides a premeasured, single dose of epinephrine. When delivered soon after exposure to the allergen, this self-delivered injection usually helps to stave off a potentially life-threatening reaction.

> ## What drug causes the most allergic reactions?
>
> Penicillin is a common cause of drug allergy. One research study found that approximately 7 percent of normal volunteers react to penicillin-allergy skin tests (IgE antibodies). Anaphylactic reactions to penicillin occur in 32 of every 100,000 exposed patients.

taken orally, can constrict blood vessels in the body and cause such effects as a rise in blood glucose. During allergy season, taking cough drops that are not sugar-free can often cause a rise in glucose levels. Some prescription nasal sprays for a stuffy nose may contain steroids, which can stimulate the liver to produce more glucose—raising blood glucose levels.

## What allergies can a person develop?

There are a large number of allergens that can affect humans and cause allergies. The most common allergens are dust and mites. People can also be allergic to various foods, pollen, chemicals in cosmetics, medications, fungal spores, insect venom, various microorganisms—even a person's own body cells can develop abnormally, causing an allergic reaction. If a person is sensitive to one of these allergens, allergies can develop. In people who are not sensitive, there will be no response.

## Can some allergy medications affect a person's diabetes?

Yes. Most people take allergy medications if they have reactions to tree, grass, and weed pollen, especially in the spring. Many of the allergy medications—for example, from the prescription name-brand Flonase to the over-the-counter Nasacort—contain corticosteroids. These drugs reduce the inflammation caused by seasonal allergies but can also cause a rise in blood glucose levels. Because of this, most health care professionals recommend that seasonal allergy-prone diabetics pay closer attention to their blood glucose levels. They may also want to discuss modifying their diabetes medicine or insulin with their health care provider or see whether there is another allergy medicine that does not contain corticosteroids.

# DIABETES AND INSIDE THE HUMAN BODY

## INSIDE THE HUMAN BODY

### What is an "organ" in the human body?

An organ is a group of several different tissues working together as a unit to perform a specific function or functions in the body. Each organ performs functions that none of the component tissues can perform alone. This cooperative interaction of different tissues is a basic feature of animals, including humans. For example, the heart is an organ that consists of cardiac muscle wrapped in connective tissue, with nerve tissues controlling the rhythmic contractions of the heart's muscles.

### How many organs are in the human body?

About 78 organs are in the human body, each one with a different size, shape, and function (or sometimes the same, as with two kidneys). The largest organ, with respect to its size and weight, is the skin. Not everyone has organs in the same place. For example, sometimes the kidney may be located closer to the pelvis, or only one kidney may be present. These differences can be due to genetics, differences in the organ's cell growth, or even disease.

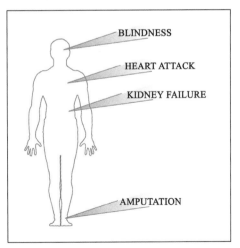

Several body systems are negatively affected by diabetes, which can damage everything from the heart and kidneys to causing blindness or damaging peripheral nerves, which could even necessitate amputations.

## What body systems are most affected by diabetes, especially when the disease is left untreated?

If a person's diabetes is left untreated, then many—often life-threatening—complications will arise in other parts of the body. In particular, major problems can develop with the heart, eyes, kidneys, nerves, and circulatory system. Often just as much of a problem, the muscular, reproductive, immune, and integumentary (skin) systems can be affected by untreated diabetes. (For more information about how diabetes affects these systems, see their respective chapters.)

## What are the major organ systems in the human body?

An organ system is a group of organs working together to perform a vital body function. There are 12 major organ systems in the human body. The following lists those organ systems, along with their components and functions:

### Major Organ Systems

| Organ System | Components | Functions |
| --- | --- | --- |
| Cardiovascular | Heart, blood, and blood vessels | Transports blood throughout the body, supplying nutrients and carrying oxygen to the lungs and wastes to the kidneys |
| Digestive | Mouth, esophagus, stomach, intestines, liver, and pancreas | Allows the ingestion of food and breaks it down into smaller (chemical) units |
| Endocrine | Pituitary, adrenal, thyroid, and other ductless glands | Coordinates and regulates the activities of the body, including metabolism |
| Excretory | Kidneys, bladder, and urethra | Helps to remove wastes from the bloodstream |
| Immune | Lymphocytes, macrophages, and antibodies | Removes foreign substances from the bloodstream |
| Integumentary | Skin, hair, nails, and sweat glands | Protects the body; the skin holds in the organs |
| Lymphatic | Lymph nodes, lymphatic capillaries, lymphatic vessels, spleen, and thymus | Captures body fluids and returns them to the cardiovascular system |
| Muscular | Skeletal muscle, cardiac muscle, and smooth muscle | Allows the body to move |
| Nervous | Nerves, sense organs, brain, and spinal cord | Receives external stimuli, processes information, and directs activities |
| Reproductive | Testes, ovaries, and related organs | Carries out reproduction |
| Respiratory | Lungs, trachea, and other air passageways | Exchanges gases (captures oxygen [$O_2$] and disposes of carbon dioxide [$CO_2$]) |
| Skeletal | Bones, cartilage, and ligaments | Protects and provides support for the body's motions and movements |

# DIABETES AND THE SENSES: TOUCH, HEARING, SMELL, AND TASTE

## What is diabetic neuropathy, and how does it affect a person who has diabetes?

In general, diabetic neuropathy is the loss of sensation—including touch—because of diabetes. This occurs because over time, diabetes can cause nerve damage as high blood glucose levels damage the body's nerve fibers. This damage often causes several symptoms, including loss of feeling, especially on the skin and in the extremities. (For more about nerve damage and diabetes, see the chapter "How Diabetes Affects the Nervous System.")

## Can diabetes cause hearing loss?

No one truly knows whether diabetes can cause hearing loss, but it is known that many people with diabetes have some hearing loss. Some researchers believe that, as with nerve damage in the eyes, high blood glucose levels in a person with diabetes may damage the small vessels and/or nerves in the inner ear, causing hearing loss. Other reasons can add to the hearing loss, including exposure to toxins, injury (loud noises such as heavily amplified music through headphones), or genetic disorders.

## What is tinnitus?

Tinnitus is the perception of sound in the ears or head where no external source is present. In almost all cases, tinnitus is a subjective noise, meaning that only the person who has tinnitus can hear it. It is often referred to as "ringing in the ears." Persistent tinnitus usually indicates the presence of hearing loss. The exact cause of tinnitus is not known, but there are several likely sources, all of which are known to trigger or worsen the condition. They include noise-induced hearing loss, wax buildup in the ear canal, medicines that are toxic to the ear, ear or sinus infections, head or neck trauma, jaw misalignment (often associated with the temporal mandibular joint), and Meniere's disease.

## How are tinnitus and diabetes connected?

According to many studies, there may be a connection between tinnitus and diabetes. This is because those who experience tinnitus often have elevated blood glucose levels, which can lead to diabetes, or they already have diabetes with uncontrolled blood glucose levels. Because the inner ears depend on oxygen and glucose from the bloodstream for their energy (as in the brain, there are no fat reserves to use for energy in the ears), when a person's glucose is interrupted, the parts of the ear called the cochlea and vestibular (inner ear) system cannot function well, resulting in tinnitus. In fact, one study indicated that close to 90 percent of the participants who had inner ear problems (called peripheral vestibular disorder) had higher glucose levels and problems metabolizing insulin. This is why many health care professionals suggest that people with diabetes who have "ringing in the ears" keep good control over their blood glucose levels to lessen the effects of—or even help stop the development of—tinnitus.

## How does a person taste and smell?

A person's ability to taste comes from certain cells located in clusters (taste buds) on the tongue, roof of the mouth (palate), and within the lining of the throat. A person tastes thanks to the thousands of nerve endings associated with the taste buds (everyone is born with about 10,000, but lose many with age). In general, each taste bud strongly responds to a certain taste according to its position on the tongue. Sweet receptors are concentrated at the tip of the tongue, while sour receptors are more common at the sides of the tongue. Salt receptors occur most frequently at the tip and front edges of the tongue, and bitter receptors are most numerous at the back of the tongue. These nerve endings help a person to distinguish among spicy, sweet, and sour foods. The nerves also help a person to distinguish smells. Because the aroma of a particular food also contributes to its taste, most people can tell the difference between foods, such as an orange from an apple. This is also why, if a person has diabetes, the sense of smell and taste can also be affected, as the nerve endings can be damaged by high blood glucose levels (for more about neuropathy, see the chapter "How Diabetes Affects the Nervous System").

## Do many people have impaired taste and smell?

According to the National Institute on Deafness and Other Communication Disorders (NIDCD), around 15 percent of adults may have a problem with their ability to taste and/or smell. As with many other conditions, it is estimated that only around 200,000 seek medical help for either condition. In fact, the NIDCD estimates that almost 75 percent of all adults ages 57 to 85 have some type of taste impairment, which is why it is often difficult to persuade older people to eat healthful foods to stay well.

## Does type 1 or type 2 diabetes affect a person's ability to taste and smell?

For many people who have type 1 or type 2 diabetes, the disease will not affect taste or smell. But there are some indications that taste in some people with diabetes can change. For example, one study (although the number of participants was small) indicated that of the people who had type 1 diabetes, around 70 percent had impaired taste, compared with 16 percent who did not have diabetes. In yet another study, participants who were newly diagnosed with type 2 diabetes seemed to have more trouble tasting sweet foods. In addition, some medications can affect a person's taste (and often smell), including metformin, one of the most common medications to treat type 2 diabetes.

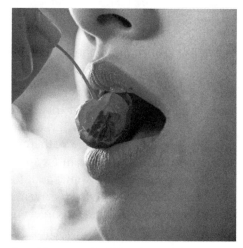

About 70 percent of people with type 1 diabetes have an impaired ability to taste foods.

# DIABETES AND THE EYES

## What are the parts of the eye and their functions?

The major parts of the eye and their functions are summarized in the following chart:

**Parts of the Eye**

| Structure | Function |
| --- | --- |
| Sclera | Maintains shape of eye; protects eyeball; site of eye muscle attachment; it is also referred to as "the white of the eye" |
| Cornea | Refracts incoming light; focuses light on the retina |
| Pupil | Admits light |
| Iris | Regulates amount of incoming light |
| Lens | Refracts and focuses light rays |
| Aqueous humor | Helps maintain shape of eye; maintains intraocular pressure; nourishes and cushions cornea and lens |
| Ciliary body | Holds lens in place; changes shape of lens |
| Vitreous humor | Maintains intraocular pressure; transmits light to retina; keeps retina firmly pressed against choroids |
| Retina | Absorbs light; stores vitamin A; forms impulses which are transmitted to brain; the macula of the retina is responsible for clear, sharp central vision |
| Optic nerve | Transmits impulses to the brain |
| Choroid | Absorbs stray light; nourishes retina |

The extra (accessory) structures of the eye include the eyebrows, eyelids, eyelashes, conjunctiva (mucus membrane that covers the front of the eye and inside the eyelids), and tear duct areas (called the lachrymal apparatus). These structures have several functions, including protecting the front portion of the eye, preventing the entry of foreign particles, and keeping the eyeball moist.

## Can there be a connection between eye diseases and diabetes?

There is often a connection between diabetes and eye diseases. According to the American College of Family Physicians, almost all people who have had diabetes for 15 years or more—they estimate 98 percent—have some sort of eye disease that is connected with their diabetes. Some studies also suggest that male and female hormonal changes during puberty, along with diabetes, can increase a child's odds of developing eye problems. One study notes that children who develop type 1 diabetes before age ten have a higher risk of developing diabetic retinopathy as they get older (for more about diabetic retinopathy, see below).

## What are cataracts?

According to the American Academy of Ophthalmology, a cataract is a cloudy or opaque lens in a person's eye. Because the incoming light is not properly reflected onto the light-sensitive tissue lining the back of the eye (the retina), the person's vision becomes blurred, distorted, or cloudy.

### Why do people develop cataracts?

Although cataracts are often associated with people who have diabetes (see below), there are other reasons for them. Cataracts mainly occur in older people and are more common in smokers. Development of cataracts also runs in families. They can also occur in people who take high doses of steroids and/or steroids for a long time; if they take certain other medications; if they have had certain surgeries that contribute to cataract development; or if they have other types of eye diseases and/or eye in-

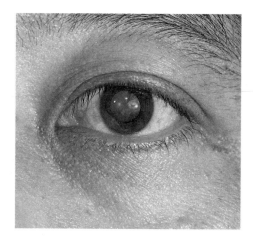

When the lens of an eye becomes cloudy or opaque, a cataract has formed, compromising one's vision. Diabetes increases the chance for cataracts to develop.

juries that lead to the clouding of the lens. In addition, it is thought that eye exposure to the sun also can contribute to cataract development, which is why so many health care professionals recommend wearing sunglasses outside in the sunshine (or on snow or water) and/or having special ultraviolet coating added to eyeglasses.

### Do people with diabetes develop more cataracts than those without diabetes?

Yes, according to the American Diabetes Association. In fact, it is estimated that people with diabetes are 60 percent more likely to develop cataracts. It is also estimated that around 20 percent of people who have cataract operations have diabetes. People with diabetes also seem to develop cataracts earlier in life and more quickly than people who do not have the disease.

### Why does diabetes often lead to the development of cataracts?

The main reason for the development of cataracts in people with diabetes has to do with blood glucose levels. The eye's lens—the object that becomes cloudy when a person has cataracts—gets its nutrients from the aqueous humor (the fluid in the front of the eye). When a person's blood glucose levels are not in control, the sugar levels rise in the aqueous humor and lens. When this occurs, the lens swells, causing the person's vision to blur. This is why many people with diabetes often mention blurred vision, an increased problem with glare (especially during nighttime driving), and yellowish or faded views around them. As with most problems encountered by people with diabetes, one of the best ways to keep cataracts at bay is to maintain healthy blood glucose levels.

### What is diabetic retinopathy?

Diabetic retinopathy is a phrase commonly used to describe many different eye disorders caused mainly by diabetes. It is also the major cause of blindness in the United

## Why does diabetes often cause blindness?

According to Harvard Medical School, diabetes is the leading cause of new cases of blindness in people ages 20 to 74. The high blood-sugar level in diabetes weakens blood vessel walls in the retina and choroids of the eye. This weakening, in turn, increases the eye's susceptibility to hemorrhaging, scarring, and retinal detachment, all of which can contribute to blindness.

States among adults ages 20 to 65, and is most associated with people who have diabetes—both types 1 and 2. According to Harvard Medical School, diabetic retinopathy is considered a degenerative eye disorder; it occurs when chronic high blood sugar causes the tiny blood vessels in the retina (capillaries) to break down and leak fluid into the surrounding tissue. Not only can the leakage leave what are called hard exudates, or deposits of fat and protein, but if it is near the macula, it will impair the person's sight—a condition called macular edema.

These vessels also nourish the eyes, and if the capillaries are damaged, it is more difficult for them to supply nutrients and eliminate wastes from the surrounding tissues. The vessels can also eventually become blocked, and although new vessels form to compensate in the later stages of retinopathy, the newer vessels are more fragile. This fragility can often lead to bleeding into the vitreous humor (the gel-like substance in the inner eye); the bleeding, in turn, temporarily blocks light and causes a sudden change in vision. Although the blood is often reabsorbed, scar tissue forms. This tissue can pull at the retina, often causing retinal detachment. If this condition is not caught in time, it can lead to permanent vision loss or blindness.

## What are the major types of diabetic retinopathy?

According to the American Diabetes Association, there are commonly two major types of diabetic retinopathy—proliferative and nonproliferative. In proliferative retinopathy, new blood vessels form as others become blocked. The growth of these new vessels often leads to scar tissue, severe bleeding, and even retinal detachment. The more common type, nonproliferative retinopathy, forms as capillaries in the back of the eye form pockets. This type of retinopathy is also caused when blood vessels become blocked but usually does not require treatment.

## How do eye specialists detect diabetic retinopathy?

According to the National Eye Institute, there are certain ways in which an ophthalmologist (eye specialist) can detect diabetic retinopathy in a person with diabetes. During a dilated-eye exam, in which the doctor dilates, or widens, a person's pupil to better see the retina and optic nerve, the tests include a visual acuity test (using an eye chart to measure a person's ability to see at various distances), a tonometry test (to measure

115

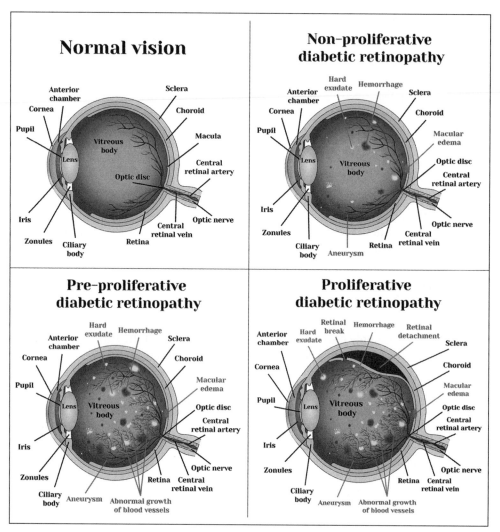

## Normal vision

Anterior chamber
Cornea
Pupil
Iris
Zonules
Ciliary body
Lens
Vitreous body
Optic disc
Central retinal vein
Retina
Sclera
Choroid
Macula
Central retinal artery
Optic nerve

## Non-proliferative diabetic retinopathy

Anterior chamber
Cornea
Pupil
Iris
Zonules
Ciliary body
Lens
Vitreous body
Aneurysm
Hard exudate
Hemorrhage
Retina
Sclera
Choroid
Macular edema
Optic disc
Central retinal artery
Optic nerve
Central retinal vein

## Pre-proliferative diabetic retinopathy

Anterior chamber
Cornea
Pupil
Iris
Zonules
Ciliary body
Lens
Vitreous body
Aneurysm
Abnormal growth of blood vessels
Hard exudate
Hemorrhage
Retina
Central retinal vein
Sclera
Choroid
Macular edema
Optic disc
Central retinal artery
Optic nerve

## Proliferative diabetic retinopathy

Anterior chamber
Cornea
Pupil
Iris
Zonules
Ciliary body
Lens
Vitreous body
Aneurysm
Abnormal growth of blood vessels
Hard exudate
Retinal break
Hemorrhage
Retinal detachment
Retina
Central retinal vein
Sclera
Choroid
Macular edema
Optic disc
Central retinal artery
Optic nerve

Normal vision compared to pre-proliferative retinopathy, non-proliferative retinopathy, and proliferative retinopathy.

the pressure inside the eye), and an optical coherence tomography or OCT (similar to an ultrasound but using light waves, not sound waves, to produce an image of the tissues inside the eye).

## How does an ophthalmologist treat diabetic retinopathy?

In reality, it is the person with diabetes who can "treat" diabetic retinopathy by keeping his or her blood glucose levels under control. If an ophthalmologist suspects that the patient has diabetic retinopathy, then the doctor may suggest a test called a fluorescein angiogram, in which a fluorescent dye is injected (most often into an arm vein). As the dye reaches the eyes, images of the retinal blood vessels are taken and examined for possible retinopathy. If diabetic retinopathy is confirmed, there are usually two major ways of helping the person's eyesight. According to the American Academy of Ophthalmology, one procedure uses lasers and is usually performed in a doctor's office. The laser treatment causes abnormal new vessels to shrink and often prevents them from growing. Another procedure is vitrectomy, which is usually performed in a hospital or surgery center operating room (usually on an outpatient basis). The procedure removes blood and scar tissue that often accompany abnormal blood vessels (that cause the bleeding) in the eye. When such hemorrhaging is eliminated, light rays are able to focus on the retina again.

## What is diabetic macular edema?

Diabetic macular edema (DME) is most often associated with diabetic retinopathy. With retinopathy, chronic high blood sugar can cause the blood vessels in the retina to break down and leak fluid. If the leakage is near the center of the macula, it can cause the macula to swell. This condition is called diabetic macular edema. Because the macula is the part of the eye responsible for sharp, straight-ahead vision, the person's vision will blur. DME is the most common cause of diminished vision in people with diabetes.

## Are there ways to prevent macular degeneration?

According to Harvard Medical School, there are several ways to prevent macular degeneration in many people. These include the following: don't smoke; wear sunglasses (especially in reflective places, such as around the ocean or snow); eat dark, leafy greens (kale and spinach are two of the best sources); exercise (choose a type that fits your lifestyle); if not allergic, eat nuts and oily fish (they both have omega-3, which some research indicates helps prevent macular degeneration); and especially avoid developing diabetes, mainly by eating healthfully and keeping weight in a normal range for your age and height.

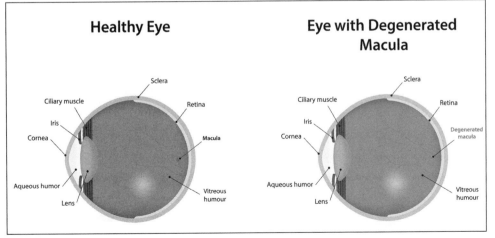

Macular degeneration occurs when the center of the retina deteriorates. It affects about 10 million Americans.

## What is macular degeneration?

Macular degeneration occurs when a small central portion of the retina called the macula deteriorates. The most common symptoms are slightly blurred vision, difficulty recognizing faces, and the need for brighter light with which to see. According to the American Diabetes Association, age-related macular degeneration is the most common cause of vision loss in people over age 55 (in the United States). Macular degeneration cases are expected to grow as the population ages.

## Can a person with diabetes develop eye aneurysms?

Yes, if people with diabetes have damaged blood vessels in the retina from chronic high blood sugar, they can eventually develop what are called microaneurysms, or small sac-like pouches that affect the smaller blood vessels, or capillaries. (The pouches have been associated with diabetic retinopathy since 1879; the microaneurysms of the eye from diabetes were first described in 1943.) The recognition of eye microaneurysms is often used to predict the development of diabetic retinopathy. In some studies, the microaneurysms have been found to be directly correlated with HbA1c values. For example, in one study, the researchers found that every 10 percent increase in HbA1c value (for instance, from 8.1 percent to 9.0 percent) was associated with an increase of 0.7 microaneurysms. This is not a huge amount, but it does indicate that a person's overall blood glucose level can have an effect on the formation of eye microaneurysms.

# HOW DIABETES AFFECTS BONES, JOINTS, MUSCLES, TEETH, AND SKIN

## DIABETES, BONES, AND JOINTS

### What is arthritis?

The word arthritis is derived from the Latin via Greek word *arthron* ("joint") and *itis* ("inflammation"). Arthritis is a disease in which a person's joints become inflamed, most often resulting in joint pain and stiffness. There are more than 100 types of arthritis, some affecting the skin, muscles, bones, and internal organs, as well as the joints. For example, one type of arthritis is rheumatoid arthritis, in which the joint pain is caused by the immune system's attack on the membrane lining the joints. Together, these types of arthritis are called rheumatic diseases and are considered to be one of the most common chronic health problems. (For more about immune system and inflammation, see the chapter "Diabetes and Body Connections.")

### Are people with diabetes more prone to arthritis?

According to the Arthritis Foundation, as of this writing, 47 percent of adults with arthritis also have another chronic condition. And of the 52.5 million American adults with arthritis, 16 percent (around 7.3 million) have type 2 diabetes, and 47 percent of adults with diabetes (both type 1 and type 2) have arthritis.

### Are people with type 1 diabetes more prone to rheumatoid arthritis?

Many studies seem to indicate an association between rheumatoid arthritis and type 1 diabetes. According to the Arthritis Foundation, both conditions are autoimmune diseases, with inflammation as the common condition in both. In a person with type 1 diabetes, the insulin-producing pancreas is attacked, which means the person does not produce insulin. In a person with rheumatoid arthritis, the body attacks the tissues lining the joints.

**119**

In addition, people who have rheumatoid arthritis have high levels of what are called inflammatory markers in their systems. For example, C-reactive protein, or CRP, is a marker that is also found in increased levels in people with type 1 diabetes.

### Is there a connection between type 2 diabetes and osteoarthritis?

Some researchers believe there is a connection between people with type 2 diabetes and osteoarthritis, but it is not because of inflammation, as with type 1 diabetes and rheumatoid arthritis. Because it is estimated that up to 80 percent of people with type 2 diabetes are overweight or obese, the additional weight puts stress on the joints, especially those of the lower body. In addition, the pancreas has to produce more insulin to compensate for the excess glucose in people with type 2 diabetes. This means the heart and blood vessels are stressed, causing problems with blood flow to joints. Because of these added stressors on the joints, osteoarthritis of the knee and hip are often found in people with type 2 diabetes.

### How are musculoskeletal problems in the body connected to glucose?

The term musculoskeletal means something that is connected to both muscles and bones in the body. It usually implies the range of motion in the hands, wrists, shoulders, and other joint areas and concentrates on the connective tissues surrounding the joints. According to Harvard Medical School and the American Diabetes Association, many musculoskeletal complications stem from changes in these connective tissues, including in people who have diabetes. These complications should not be confused with osteoarthritis (see above) but mostly appear to result from the attachment of glucose to the connective tissues. This often results in the stiffening of joints all over the body.

### What hand problems do people with diabetes sometimes face?

Many people with diabetes face musculoskeletal problems, especially of the hands. For example, diabetic stiff hand syndrome (or diabetic cheiroarthropathy) is a disorder that causes the skin on the fingers to become thick, tight, and waxy, thus causing the fingers—and often the entire hand—to become limited in movement. Usually, the first sign is a problem keeping the fingers together without leaving a gap (it is often called a "prayer sign"). It is thought to be caused by several reasons, including consistently high blood glucose levels that cause excess collagen (a structural protein that literally holds

### Why is arthritis often connected to foods a person eats?

Arthritis appears to be an ailment that is affected by what a person eats. Many studies indicate that some foods, such as processed or fried foods, cause more inflammation in our bodies. Foods such as fresh vegetables and fruits, along with nuts and teas, can cut back on the inflammation that affects a person's arthritic joints.

the body together) in the skin. At this writing, there is no cure for the syndrome.

Another problem with the hands—again in the fingers—is called trigger finger, or flexor tenosynovitis. This occurs when the tendon (and the sheath around it) that extends into the finger or thumb becomes inflamed. Lumps (nodules) can form on the tendon, causing it to stop moving correctly through the sheath and stopping the finger from moving. This causes the finger to become locked in a bent or straight position, thus the term trigger finger.

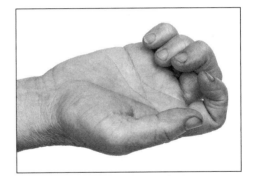

Flexor tenosynovitis—also called trigger finger—is an inflammation of the finger tendons that makes them hard to move.

Yet another hand problem for many people with diabetes has to do with the tissue under the skin of one or both palms. Dupuytren's contracture is when the palm's skin becomes thicker and tightens. If left to thicken over several years, it can lead to pain, stiffness, and the inability to straighten the finger joints, especially affecting the middle and ring fingers. Certain treatments are often suggested, including surgery to break apart the thick tissues or injections of steroids into the palm.

## Do people with diabetes have more problems with carpal tunnel syndrome?

One of the more well-known musculoskeletal wrist problems for people with diabetes—and those who do not have diabetes—is called carpal tunnel syndrome. It is caused by the thickening or swelling of the tendons found in the wrist, which compress the nerve that runs from the forearm into the hand. The most common symptoms include burning, shooting pains, and numbness in the hand and/or the wrist. It is mostly caused by repetitive movement (and thus called a repetitive injury) for most people. It is estimated that up to 20 percent of people with diabetes experience carpal tunnel problems, primarily because their nerves are more sensitive to compression from a repeated motion. (For more about nerve damage and diabetes, see the chapter "How Diabetes Affects the Nervous System.") For many people, the treatment can include steroid injections to reduce inflammation and physical therapy. But for more severe cases, surgery is often suggested to cut the connective tissue that is putting pressure on the nerve.

## What shoulder problems do people with diabetes sometimes face?

People with diabetes often face a musculoskeletal problem with their shoulders called adhesive capsulitis, or frozen shoulder. This occurs when the shoulder gradually stiffens, causing pain and decreasing the joint's range of motion. Although it is not fully understood what causes a frozen shoulder, it is usually found in association with other musculoskeletal problems, such as in people with diabetes (especially those who have such diabetic-related conditions such as retinopathy and neuropathy), thyroid disease, or certain autoimmune diseases. Frozen shoulder can be difficult to treat. The most common treatments range from administering medications for pain (such as nonsteroidal anti-inflammatory drugs [NSAIDs] or corticosteroid oral medications [for example, prednisolone] or corticosteroid injections in the joint), physical therapy for stretching the joint, and/or arthroscopic surgery to cut the adhesions that are usually involved in restricting the joint's mobility.

## What recent study indicated that diabetes may be linked to tendon pain?

It is known that chronically high blood glucose levels can increase the risk of developing tendinopathy, a condition that commonly causes the tendons to thicken. If a person has tendinopathy, then he or she usually has painful and inflamed tendons when exercising or with movement and, in particular, in response to overuse. A recent study showed there may be a link between type 2 diabetes and tendon pain. The researchers discovered that people with diabetes are more than 3.5 times as likely as those without diabetes to have tendon pain (and if severe, tendinopathy) in any tendon of the body. They also found that those with tendinopathy were 1.3 times more likely to have type 2 diabetes. The study also showed that the risk of tendinopathy also increases with the number of years a person has diabetes.

## Is there a connection between diabetes and bone fractures?

There is evidence that people with both type 1 and type 2 diabetes have a higher incidence of bone fractures than the general population. In fact, although people with type 2 diabetes usually have above-average bone density (carrying around extra weight helps maintain bone density, as does weight-bearing exercise), they still have more bone fractures. For example, two recent studies showed that people with type 1 diabetes had a risk of hip fracture 6.3 to 6.9 times higher, and those with type 2 diabetes 1.4 to 1.7 times higher, compared with people without diabetes. The reasons for these bone fracture and diabetes connections are unknown.

### Why is osteoporosis associated with bone fractures?

Osteoporosis is a bone disease that causes an increase in the risk of fractures and breaks, usually in older adults. Osteoporosis occurs when the person's bone mineral density decreases, causing the bones to deteriorate. This deterioration causes a loss of bone strength, lower bone mass, and a higher risk of fracturing the bones of the hip, spine, and wrist. In advanced osteoporosis, the bone is literally porous, with small holes altering the bone structure, which allows the bones to break more easily. (For more about osteoporosis, see the chapter "Who Gets Diabetes?") According to the most recent data, it is estimated that around 10 million Americans have osteoporosis. It is considered to be the most common type of bone disorder in both females and males, although more females experience the disease.

But there are several theories. One suggestion is that most people with type 2 diabetes are overweight or obese, making balance and coordination more difficult. Thus, people with diabetes and larger body size (and high bone mass) may have higher fracture rates because of balance problems. In addition, many people with diabetes (type 1 and type 2) have peripheral neuropathy and/or vision problems, making them more likely to fall and fracture a bone. And if a person with diabetes (type 1 or 2) experiences a hypoglycemic (low blood glucose) episode, he or she may fall and fracture or break a bone, as low blood glucose causes the person to be confused or even pass out.

# DIABETES AND MUSCLES

## How many muscles are in the average human body?

Most research says there are about 650 muscles in the average human body, although the numbers vary from one person to another. But other scientists believe there may be as many as 850 muscles, depending on how you categorize and look at each muscle group.

## What are the three main types of muscle tissue?

The three main types of muscle tissue are as follows:

*Smooth muscles*—found in the walls of blood vessels, in the walls of major organs (digestive, respiratory, urinary, and reproductive tracts), and in the iris of the eye.

*Cardiac muscles*—as the name implies, found only in the heart; they are responsible for pumping blood throughout the body.

*Skeletal muscles*—attached to tendons, which, in turn, are attached to bones; they help with the movement of the body.

## Where are sources of energy stored for muscle cells?

The muscle cells that make up the body's muscles use various sources to power their contractions. For example, if they need quick energy, they can use stored molecules in the cells (called ATP and creatine phosphate), which are usually depleted after about 20 seconds of activity. Then the muscles switch to other sources, especially glycogen (a carbohydrate made up of a string of glucose molecules). It is glycogen that helps the body make it through work-

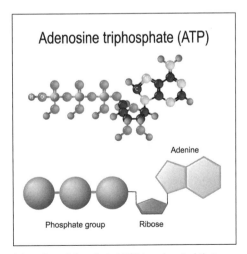

Adenosine triphosphate (ATP) is a chemical that helps store energy in cells, including muscle cells, which can use the energy to contract.

outs—whether a person is lifting weights or running—and glycogen originates with the foods a person eats. The following lists the major sources of energy for the body's systems and where the sources are stored in the body:

**Body System Sources of Energy**

| Source | Storage Site |
| --- | --- |
| Carbohydrates | Glycogen; there is an average of 500 grams stored most of the time in the average human, mainly in the liver and skeletal muscles. |
| Fats (lipids) | Adipose tissue (although it has several other tasks) stores energy in our system as fats (in the form of triglycerides); it is estimated that a healthy adult male has 12 to 18 percent body fat, while healthy adult females carry about 12 to 25 percent body fat. |
| Protein | Found throughout the body; usually the body's last choice as an energy source. |

### In general, what are the processes the body uses to maintain energy—especially glucose?

When a person is not eating or is exercising, the body must draw on its internal energy stored in various places. The major source is glucose, but the body follows several steps in order to obtain this energy:

*Glycogenolysis*—This is the process that occurs when the body breaks down carbohydrates, or glycogen, into simple glucose molecules.

*Lipolysis*—This is when the body breaks down fats into glycerol and fatty acids.

*Gluconeogenesis*—This is a multistage process in which amino acids are used to make glucose.

*Fatty acids*—If there is no gluconeogenesis, the body can break fatty acids down directly to get energy.

### What is muscle mass, and can it be affected by diabetes?

Muscle mass is usually interpreted as the amount of skeletal muscle in the human body. And yes, it can be affected by diabetes. In particular, people tend to lose muscle mass as they age. If an older person also has diabetes, he or she tends to lose muscle mass much faster than people without diabetes of the same age. Because of this, the American Diabetes Association recommends that people with diabetes partake not only in regular aerobic exercise but also in strength training at least twice a week if possible. In the majority of cases, this will not only help increase muscle mass but also improve the person's blood glucose levels.

### Does muscle mass affect glucose?

There appears to be a link between glucose and muscle mass. In general, in response to insulin, skeletal muscles use glucose in the bloodstream for energy. For some people, this is good news, as it balances the amount of insulin in their system. This is also why exercise is so important to lower the risk of developing diabetes. (For more about exercise and diabetes, see the chapter "Diabetes and Exercise.")

# DIABETES AND TEETH

## Can the gums be an indicator of diabetes?

Yes, in some people with diabetes, one of the more insidious and "hidden" signs of the disease is often red, tender, and/or swollen gums. It is estimated that nine out of ten people with gum disease are at high risk for diabetes, compared to six out of ten who do not have gum disease.

## What are some signs of gum disease?

One of the first possible signs is called gingivitis, or when the gums become inflamed and sensitive or tend to bleed, especially while a person is brushing the teeth. Gingivitis is usually caused by the buildup of plaque—or a combination of food, bacteria, and mucus, a mix that attaches to the gums and teeth (it is usually seen as an off-white soft layer, usually at the gum line). If the teeth are not properly cleaned and the plaque re-

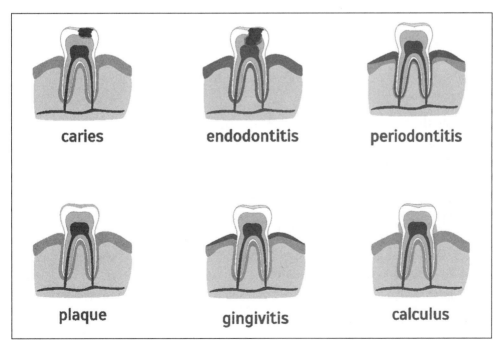

Dental problems are even more important to keep track of when one has diabetes because they can be precursors to even more serious health issues.

moved—which is why visiting the dentist regularly, especially for a person with diabetes, is necessary—then this plaque can harden into calculus, a hard substance resembling whitish plaster, that can form at and under the gum line. Calculus can irritate and infect the gums, eventually leading to periodontitis, an irreversible disease that is often thought to account for more tooth loss than dental cavities.

### Why is it important for a person with diabetes to be aware of tooth pain?

A person with a toothache from tooth decay is most often actually experiencing problems—including infection—with the tooth's pulp, or the inner structure in which the blood vessels and nerves reside. When the decaying tooth is exposed to hot or cold foods or drinks, the person usually feels a great deal of tooth pain. The solution is usually to remove the tooth pulp to stop the infection from reaching the bone that holds the tooth in place (in a procedure called a root canal). If not caught in time, tooth decay can lead to root decay and also destroy the bone. If the bone does become involved, then it can cause the tooth to loosen or even abscess (an internal infection usually below the gum line), with the affected tooth needing to be extracted.

For a person with diabetes, keeping track of tooth pain is even more important. Because diabetics often have higher blood sugar levels, the sugar keeps their immune system from fighting off infections the way it should. In addition, because high glucose levels tend to narrow blood vessels, the sugar can reduce blood flow, or circulation to the tooth, slowing down healing. Thus, once such a tooth infection starts, it is often harder for a person with diabetes to fight it off. (For more about diabetes and the immune system, see the chapter "Diabetes and Body Connections.")

# DIABETES AND THE SKIN

### What are the major functions of the skin?

The skin is considered the largest organ in the human body. It has several major functions, including:

*Hydration*—The skin provides protection from both injury (such as cuts or abrasions) and dehydration (water loss). Because the outer skin cells are dead, the skin is waterproof enough to prevent water loss and to prevent water from entering the body when a person is immersed.

*Barrier*—The skin is a barrier against invasion by bacteria and viruses and is involved in the regulation of body temperature.

*Vitamin D*—The skin is also the organ responsible for the synthesis of a form of vitamin D. A substance called 7-dehydrocholesterol forms from cholesterol in the wall of our intestines. When the sun's ultraviolet radiation strikes the surface of the human skin, it causes the 7-dehydrocholesterol that reaches the skin's surface to form cholecalciferol, or vitamin D-3.

## Does the average person's skin vary in thickness?

Yes, the thickness of a person's skin varies, depending on where it is found on the body. Skin averages 0.05 inches (1.3 millimeters) in thickness, and most of the body is covered by thin skin, which is 0.003 inches (0.08 millimeters) thick. The thinnest skin is found in the eyelids and is less than 0.002 inches (0.05 millimeters) thick, while the thickest skin is on the upper back (0.2 inches or 5 millimeters).

*Touch*—The skin contains receptors that receive the sensations of touch, vibration, pain, and temperature. In fact, for many people with diabetes, the skin's touch is most often affected, as high blood glucose levels can damage the nerves in the skin.

## Why should people with diabetes pay particular attention to their skin in the summer?

For a person with diabetes, the summer heat can cause certain problems with the skin. For anyone, heat can cause more sweating, and moisture can get trapped in the folds of skin or between a person's toes. This excessive moisture can cause more of a problem for a person with diabetes, as bacteria feed off the sugar-concentrated skin cells, and this bacteria growth, in turn, can lead to infections. In addition, dry skin is often a problem in the summer (and sometimes in the winter with dry, inside heat). If a person's diabetes is not under control and he or she has too much glucose in the bloodstream, then it is difficult for the body to retain moisture. When this happens, the skin can become dry and cracked, often leading to infection. Thus, health care professionals suggest that one of the best ways for a person with diabetes to help his or her skin in the summer (or in any season) is to keep the blood glucose under control. (For more about diabetes and being outdoors, see the chapter "Taking Charge of Diabetes.")

## What is diabetic dermopathy?

Much like age spots, diabetic dermopathy causes light-brown, scaly patches to form on a person's skin. They are also called "shin spots," as they most often form on the shins. These spots usually occur in people who have diabetes and are over 50 years old. They have also been associated with heart disease—which means a person with diabetes and such spots should mention the patches to a health care provider.

## Is there a connection among psoriasis, obesity, and diabetes?

According to a 2016 Danish twin study (in which all the participants were twins), there seems to be a link among psoriasis, obesity, and diabetes. Psoriasis is a chronic skin condition in which the skin is inflamed and breaks out in red-and-pink itchy patches. The researchers looked at the participants' psoriasis conditions, along with their body mass indexes (or BMI, which usually indicates whether a person is obese or not; for more about BMI, see the chapter "Diabetes and Obesity") and diagnosis of type 2 diabetes. The results indicated that there appears to be an association among the three conditions, but the cause of the connection is still unknown. Some researchers suggest that psoriasis could lead to a sedentary lifestyle (people with the skin condition are often afraid to go out into the public), which can lead to obesity and diabetes. Another suggestion is that diabetes and obesity could cause skin inflammation, eventually causing psoriasis.

### Should people with diabetes use antibacterial soap to clean their skin?

For most people, keeping their skin clean is necessary to fight dirt, grime, and certain bacteria. In the case of insulin-dependent diabetes (mainly people with type 1) diabetes, keeping the skin clean at an injection site is necessary. But all skin normally has some type of bacteria, and many of those bacteria help us fight off disease and infection. Thus, keeping skin clean is good, but not necessarily by using antibacterial soap. Most health care professionals suggest that using regular soap is enough and that thorough and consistent hand washing is truly what keeps away infection, not antibacterial soap.

Many experts believe the overuse of antibacterial soap may eventually help lead to a proliferation of antibiotic-resistant bacteria. In fact, in late 2016, the Food and Drug Administration (FDA) banned the use of certain chemicals found in antibacterial soap. They found data that suggested long-term exposure to certain active ingredients used in antibacterial products—for example, triclosan (liquid soaps) and triclocarban (bar soaps)—could pose health risks, such as bacterial resistance or hormonal effects. Thus, the FDA ruled that over-the-counter consumer antiseptic-wash products containing certain active ingredients can no longer be marketed.

### Do certain diabetic medications affect the skin?

Yes. For example, glipizide, a common diabetic medication classed as a sulfonylurea, can make the skin more sensitive to sunlight. Because of this, many dermatologists and other health care professionals suggest that a person with diabetes who is on certain medication similar to glipizide wear sunscreen with an SPF of 30 or higher. Some dermatologists suggest an even higher SPF number, especially if the person is fair skinned.

### What skin problems are often experienced by people with diabetes at injection sites?

People with diabetes who rely on insulin injections should watch their injection

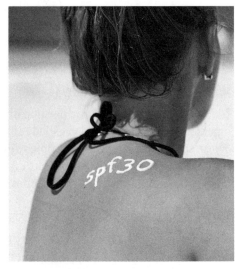

Because certain diabetes medications can make your skin more sensitive to sunlight, protecting skin from the sun is critical. Wear a strong sunscreen when planning to be outdoors during the day for an extended time.

sites for signs of infection. But two other common skin problems often accompany injections. Lipoatrophy and hypertrophy are two main skin problems at insulin-injection sites. Lipoatrophy occurs when the fatty tissue that lies under the skin essentially sinks, causing dents or dimples in the skin at injection sites (it somewhat resembles cellulite but on a smaller scale). It is thought that lipoatrophy may be caused by the body's immune reaction. In other words, the body believes the insulin is a "foreign" substance, and the immune system responds. In most cases, the problem does not occur if the person with diabetes is using highly purified insulin and preferably human insulin.

Hypertrophy occurs when the body's cells—most often fat cells—become overgrown, creating lumpy skin at the injection site that often resembles scar tissue. In this case, it is not the body's immune system responding to the insulin but a physical response to using the same injection site over and over. The condition is also called lipohypertrophy. When a site is used so many times, fat deposits accumulate in that area. Such a site may be more "comfortable" to use because hypertrophy can cause the area to become numb. However, the lumps that form are caused by abnormal cell growth and can diminish the absorption of insulin at that site. (For more about insulin, see the chapter "Taking Charge of Diabetes.")

## Can the two major skin problems around injection sites be prevented?

Many people with diabetes who inject insulin may prevent lipoatrophy and hypertrophy to some extent by rotating the location of the injection sites. Some researchers also believe that both skin problems may be caused by the type of insulin used. Thus, if a person with diabetes experiences either of these problems, then he or she may want to talk to the primary-care physician about the insulin used. (*Note*: It is also often recommended that a person with diabetes have his or her injection sites checked by a health care provider now and then for possible infection and these two skin problems.)

## What are diabetic foot ulcers?

Diabetic foot ulcers, or diabetic foot sores, are open sores or wounds that are most commonly located on the bottom of the foot. They develop for a number of reasons, including the lack of circulation and feeling in the foot from peripheral neuropathy (such that the wound often goes unnoticed); foot deformities; friction or pressure that irritates the foot; trauma to the foot; and having diabetes for a long time. With a lower blood flow in the feet and higher blood glucose levels (both due to diabetes), the body's ability to heal is reduced, increasing the possibility of infection and foot ulcers.

Foot ulcers are more prevalent in Native Americans, African Americans, Hispanics, and older men, especially those who have diabetes. People with diabetes who use insulin, and those with diabetes-related heart, kidney, and eye disease, are also at a higher risk to develop foot ulcers, as are those who are overweight and/or smoke. Thus, most health care professionals suggest that a person with diabetes check his or her feet every day for possible injury. If an ulcer is found, seek medical care immediately to reduce the risk of infection. (For more about diabetes and foot problems caused by nerve damage, see the chapter "How Diabetes Affects the Nervous System.")

## How are foot ulcers treated?

Health care professionals treat foot ulcers in several ways. When such an ulcer is found, the treatment includes taking pressure off the area of the foot that has the ulcer. It may also include gently removing some of the dead skin and tissue from the foot and applying a medication or dressing to the ulcer to help prevent infection. In addition, there will no doubt be a concentrated effort to manage the person's blood glucose levels and other health problems, all of which could ex-

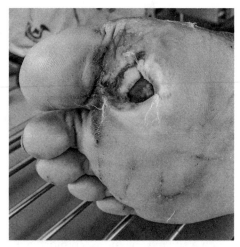

Diabetics are more prone to foot ulcers. If left untreated, they can become seriously infected and result in partial or full amputation of the foot.

acerbate the ulcer. And although not all ulcers will be infected (especially if noticed and treated right away), those that are infected may need a treatment of antibiotics, wound care (several hospitals have such wound-care facilities), and, if severe enough, hospitalization.

## How can a person with diabetes keep a foot ulcer from becoming infected?

There are several ways to try to keep a foot ulcer from becoming infected. The most important way is for people to keep their blood glucose levels stable. If they notice an ulcer, after consulting their health care professional to let them know about the ulcer, it is best to keep the wound clean and bandaged. They should also clean the wound daily and change the bandage or dressing—and avoid walking barefoot, especially outdoors or around the home (dust and dirt can enter and infect the ulcer). If the wound is on the bottom of the foot and being tended by a health care professional, the patient may be asked to wear special footwear to reduce the pressure and irritation to the ulcer area.

## What are the connections among diabetes, foot ulcers, and amputations?

According to the American Podiatric Medical Association, it is estimated that around 15 percent of people with diabetes experience some type of foot ulcer. Of these people, around 6 percent will be hospitalized because of infection and other ulcer-related complications. They also further estimate that around 14 to 24 percent of people with diabetes who develop a foot ulcer will eventually require an amputation and that foot ulceration precedes 85 percent of diabetes-related amputations.

## What should a person with diabetes do to keep track of potential foot problems?

Because people with diabetes often experience nerve damage in their feet from peripheral neuropathy and/or peripheral artery disease (for more about peripheral neuropathy, see the chapter "How Diabetes Affects the Nervous System") or from unnoticed injuries, it is important to check their feet daily (top and bottom, including between the toes) for possible injury. Besides the obvious other rules for maintaining foot health—especially keeping blood glucose levels balanced and maintaining a healthy weight—the American Podiatric Medical Association and other groups involved in helping people with diabetes suggest a daily foot exam that entails the following:

- Check feet for extremes in temperature, either very cold or hot. Keep feet clean by washing them each day. And keep them dry, especially between the toes, after showering, bathing, or swimming or on hot, humid days.

- Examine the skin on the feet (top and bottom) for ulcers, calluses, sores, blisters, dried or cracked skin that doesn't heal well, or any other unusual skin conditions, especially between the toes. If the person finds it difficult to see the bottom of his or her feet, it may help to use a mirror on the floor or ask a friend or family member for assistance.

- Do not try to remove calluses, corns, or warts on a foot, as over-the-counter products can burn the skin (most contain salicylic acid) and cause an infection, especially for people with diabetes. Ask a health care professional for help with any such skin problems on the feet.

- Do not wear tight socks or pantyhose. When socks, pantyhose, or sandals are removed, check them for blood, which indicates a cut or wound on the foot.

- Maintain footwear (shoes and socks) in good condition and, if possible, have new shoes properly measured so they fit well. There are also special types of socks (most are seamless) for people who have diabetes, usually found in drugstores, as well as some medical supply centers and hospital pharmacies.

- Exercise helps maintain weight and increases the circulation to the feet, but always wear the best-fit athletic shoes or sneakers when exercising. If there are other problems with a foot (or feet), such as bunions, hammertoes, or an internal structural injury, then consider orthotic insoles in shoes and sneakers that are made especially for people with diabetes.

- Be aware of improper fit, irritating seams, or tears in footwear that can irritate the skin. Before putting shoes or sneakers on, check for pebbles or other objects that may rub the skin, causing a wound.

- Try not to go barefoot, especially outside, where objects may injure a foot and lead to infection.

- Test water temperature with an elbow before entering a bath or hot-water soak to prevent burns. Also be aware of potential burns when putting feet near a fireplace, fire pit, grill, radiator, or any other heat source.

- Look for thin, fragile, or shinny skin, which may indicate a decrease in circulation in the feet, especially the toes.

- Check around the toenails for ingrown nails, splits or thickening of the nail, or fungal infection (such as athlete's foot—see below). Ask a health care professional for the best way to maintain nails on the hands and feet to prevent problems.

- Check for signs of neuropathy, meaning loss of sensation in any extremity—feet, toes, hands, or fingers.

- See a health care professional and discuss possible problems that a person with diabetes can have in terms of extremities. If possible for maintenance of the feet, see a podiatrist (the letters "DPM" after the name indicates a doctor of podiatric medicine) twice a year to help with foot care, as most are trained to treat foot conditions caused by diabetes, such as wounds, infections, peripheral neuropathy, and ulcers.

## Should a person with diabetes be aware of athlete's foot?

Yes, a person with diabetes should be aware of problems associated with athlete's foot, also called *tenea pedis*. It is considered to be a skin fungus, with the common name of ringworm (although it is not caused by a worm, and it does not involve a worm in any way). Many times it is associated with dogs and cats and can be very contagious, whether from human or animal. The symptoms of this skin fungus are scaling, itchy, flaky skin. It is usually associated with the toes, but it can extend to the bottoms of the feet. It thrives when the feet are hot and sweaty, especially if a person wears nonbreathable instead of breathable shoes and socks. It can also spread in public places; for example, it can be found on the floors of saunas, swimming pools, locker rooms, shower stalls, and washrooms—or places that are associated with humidity and people walking barefoot.

Athlete's foot is considered to be common in people with diabetes. It can usually be prevented by daily washing and drying of the feet, wearing sandals in public places such as swimming pools, and by wearing breathable shoes and socks. Although it is often diagnosed as just flaky skin, the problem for people with diabetes is not only the possibility of eventual infection in the area but also a secondary bacterial infection called cellulitis. This noncontagious infection occurs most often because of poor circulation in the extremities and weakened immune systems associated with diabetes, causing redness, swelling, and tenderness in the infected area. Antibiotics and anti-fungal creams or ointments are often prescribed, but if the cellulitis is not treated in time, it can lead to serious infections in the foot and lower limbs and, in the most extreme cases, to amputation.

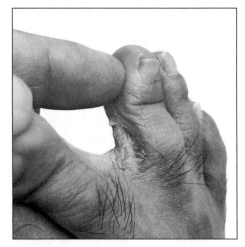

Even a common and relatively minor affliction such as athlete's foot can turn serious for a diabetic, who can develop serious infections.

# DIABETES, HAIR, AND NAILS

## How many hairs are on the human body, and where are most located?

On the average human body, there are approximately five million hairs. Males have a few hundred thousand more hairs than women. In males and females, hormones are responsible for the development of such hairy regions as the scalp, the axillary (armpit), and pubic areas, and, in addition in men, on the chest. Overall, the various types of hair grow all over the human body except for the soles of the feet, palms of the hand, eyelids, and lips.

## Does diabetes affect a person's hair?

In many cases, diabetes can affect a person's hairs—on the head, arms, legs, eyelashes, eyebrows, and other parts of the body—especially the loss of hairs. The hairs of an average adult without diabetes usually go through an active growth phase (two years or more, growing about 0.39 to 0.79 inch [1 to 2 centimeters] per month). Next is a resting phase (for a little over three months), and from there, some of the resting hairs fall out. But if a person has diabetes, these three phases are disrupted, with slower hair growth and/or more hair loss after the resting phase. This is most often caused by poor circulation to the person's scalp, which can cause hair loss and slow down hair growth.

Diabetes can also cause excess stress on a person's body, leading to hair loss. Hair loss can also be caused by medicines to treat diabetes, as well as by other chronic illnesses, such as thyroid disease.

## What is alopecia areata?

Alopecia areata often occurs if a person has diabetes ("alopecia" is the medical term for baldness). In this case, the immune system of the person attacks the hair follicles, causing the hairs all over the body or in specific spots to be lost in patches. This most often occurs in people with type 1 diabetes. Although type 2 diabetes is not thought of as an autoimmune disease like type 1, cases of alopecia areata have also been reported. Research also suggests a genetic component to this condition. In many cases, if a family member has alopecia areata, then others in the family have a higher risk of developing the condition. And if the family member also has an autoimmune disease, such as thyroid disease, lupus, or diabetes, then relatives may have an even higher risk of developing alopecia areata.

---

### How many hairs does the average person have on his or her head?

The amount of hair on the head varies from one individual to another. An average person has about 100,000 hairs on the scalp (blonds 140,000, brunettes 155,000, and redheads only 85,000). Most people shed between 50 to 100 hairs daily.

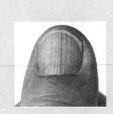
### Do people with diabetes have more toenail problems?

Most people with type 1 or type 2 diabetes have more problems than others with their toenails, including ingrown toenails, a fungus, or even foot ulcers. This is often due to the person's not noticing a problem with a toenail, mainly because diabetes causes nerve damage (he or she cannot feel the problem) and poorer circulation in the extremities. In addition, the person may also develop toenail fungus, meaning the nail becomes yellow and thick. If not treated, such a fungus can lead to a bacterial infection, which is often difficult for a person with diabetes to fight. This is why people with diabetes should check their feet and toenails regularly. And if a toenail problem is noticed, then a health care professional (including podiatrists, who are familiar with treating people with diabetes) should be consulted.

### Why do some people with diabetes have nails with bumps or ridges?

Bumps or ridges on a fingernail or toenail often indicate a previous injury to the nail, such as a blow (for example, accidentally hitting the fingernail with a hammer). They can also occur in the normal aging process or if a person is malnourished. If a person has diabetes, the nails may also have a profusion of bumps and ridges, mainly because of there is less blood flow to the extremities and/or poorly controlled blood glucose levels.

# HOW DIABETES AFFECTS THE ENDOCRINE SYSTEM

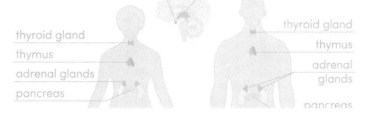

## ENDOCRINE SYSTEM AND DIABETES

### What is the endocrine system?

The endocrine system is one of two major regulatory systems that release chemicals in the body (the other one is the nervous system; for more, see the chapter "How Diabetes Affects the Nervous System"). The endocrine system, together with the nervous system, controls and coordinates the functions of all of the human body systems. It contains a group of glands that secrete hormones, all of which help maintain metabolic functions, allow the body to react to stress, and regulate growth, reproduction, and nutrient use by the body's cells.

### What are hormones and hormone receptors?

Hormones, or chemicals made and secreted by endocrine glands, are the main messengers of the endocrine system. Hormones are transported in the bloodstream to all parts of the body and interact with target cells (cells that contain hormone receptors and respond to a specific hormone in the body), which regulate metabolic rate (including glucose), growth, maturation, and reproduction. In most cases, hormones produce a specific effect on the activity of cells that are remotely located from the hormones' point of origin. Hormone receptors are located either on the surface of a cell's outer membrane or inside the cell itself (hormone receptors and hormones fit together much like a lock and key).

### What are the major endocrine glands and their respective hormones?

The major endocrine glands are the pituitary, thyroid, parathyroid, pineal, and adrenal glands. Other hormone-secreting organs are the central nervous system (hypothalamus), kidneys, heart, pancreas, thymus, ovaries, and testes. Some organs, such as the pancreas, secrete hormones as an endocrine function but also have other functions. The following lists some of the major glands, their target tissues, and their principal function in the body (those directly associated with diabetes are highlighted):

### Endocrine Glands and Their Functions

| Endocrine Gland/Hormone | Target Tissue | Principal Function |
|---|---|---|
| *Posterior pituitary* | | |
| Antidiuretic hormone (ADH) | Kidneys | Stimulates water reabsorption by kidneys |
| Oxytocin | Uterus, mammary glands | Stimulates uterine contractions and milk ejection |
| *Anterior pituitary* | | |
| Growth hormone (GH) | General | Stimulates growth, especially cell division and bone growth |
| Adrenocorticotropichormone (ACTH) | Adrenal cortex | Stimulates adrenal cortex |
| Thyroid-stimulating (TSH) | Thyroid gland | Stimulates thyroid hormone |
| Luteinizing (LH) | Gonads | Stimulates ovaries and testes hormone |
| Follicle-stimulating (FSH) | Gonads | Controls egg and sperm production |
| Prolactin (PRL) | Mammary | Stimulates milk production |
| Melanocyte-stimulating (MSH) | Skin | Regulates skin color in reptiles and hormone amphibians, but has an unknown function in humans |
| *Thyroid* | | |
| Calcitonin | Bone | Lowers blood-calcium level |
| *Parathyroid* | | |
| Parathyroid hormone (PTH) | Bone, kidneys, digestive tract | Raises blood-calcium level |
| *Adrenal medulla* | | |
| Epinephrine (adrenaline) and norepinephrine (noradrenaline) | Skeletal muscle, cardiac muscle blood vessels | Initiates stress responses; raises heart rate, blood pressure, metabolic rates; constricts certain blood vessels |
| *Adrenal cortex* | | |
| Aldosterone | Kidney tubules | Stimulates kidneys to reabsorb sodium and excrete potassium |
| Cortisol | General | Increases blood glucose |
| *Pancreas* | | |
| Insulin | Liver | Lowers blood glucose level; stimulates formation and storage of glycogen |
| Glucagon | Liver, adipose tissue | Raises blood glucose level |

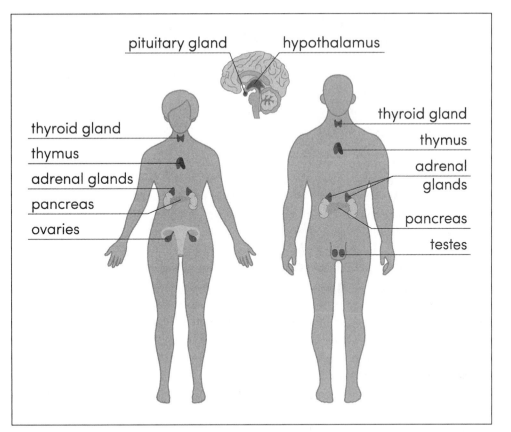

The endocrine glands excrete various hormones into the body that control various functions, such as water absorption, growth, and calcium levels in the blood.

| Endocrine Gland/Hormone | Target Tissue | Principal Function |
|---|---|---|
| *Ovary* | | |
| Estrogens | General; female reproductive structures | Stimulates development of secondary sex characteristics in females and uterine lining |
| Progesterone | Uterus, breasts | Promotes growth of uterine lining; stimulates breast development |
| *Testes* | | |
| Androgens (testosterone) | General; male reproductive organs | Stimulates development of male sex structures and spermatogenesis |
| *Pineal gland* | | |
| Melatonin | Gonads, pigment cells | Involved in daily and seasonal rhythmic activities (circadian cycles); influences pigmentation in some species |

137

## What is the hormonal response to stress and its connection to blood glucose?

The stress response has three basic phases: the alarm phase, the resistance phase, and the exhaustion phase. The alarm phase is an immediate reaction to stress, with epinephrine the dominant hormone. It is released along with activation of the sympathetic nervous system and produces the "fight or flight" response. Nonessential body functions such as digestive, urinary, and reproductive activities are inhibited. The resistance phase follows the alarm phase if the stress lasts more than several hours. Glucocorticoids (see below) are the dominant hormones of the resistance phase. Endocrine secretions maintain levels of glucose in the blood by moving fat and protein reserves, conserving glucose for nerve tissues, and synthesizing and releasing glucose by the liver. If the body does not overcome the stress during the resistance phase, the exhaustion phase begins. Prolonged exposure to high levels of hormones involved in the resistance phase can lead to the collapse of vital organ systems.

## How does the hormone adiponectin affect blood glucose?

Adiponectin is a hormone that is involved in regulating blood glucose levels. Medically, it is called a protein hormone that is produced and secreted exclusively by the fat cells (called adipocytes). These fat cells are responsible for regulating the metabolism of lipids (fats) and glucose. Thus, this hormone influences the body's response to insulin and also has an anti-inflammatory effect on the cells lining blood vessel walls. It is usually found in high levels in the bodies of people who are not obese. It can also be found in people who are obese and some who are overweight (but at much lower levels) and often in people with insulin resistance and type 2 diabetes.

# ADRENAL GLANDS AND DIABETES

## What are the physical characteristics of the adrenal glands?

The adrenal (from the Latin, meaning "upon the kidneys") glands sit on the upper tip of each kidney. Each adrenal gland weighs approximately 0.19 ounces (7.5 grams). The glands are yellow in color and have a pyramid shape. Each adrenal gland has two sections that may almost be considered as separate glands. The inner portion is the adrenal medulla (from the Latin, meaning "marrow"). The outer portion, which surrounds the adrenal medulla, is the adrenal cortex (from the Latin, meaning "bark," because its appearance is similar to the outer covering of a tree). The adrenal cortex is the larger part of the adrenal glands, accounting for nearly 90 percent of the gland by weight.

## What are the functions of corticosteroids?

The adrenal cortex secretes more than two dozen different steroid hormones called the adrenocortical steroids, or simply corticosteroids. The corticosteroids are vital for life and well-being, with each serving a unique purpose. The following lists the corticosteroids and their functions, including those associated with blood glucose and glycogen (which, in turn, are associated with diabetes):

## Corticosteroids and Their Functions

| Hormone | Target | Effects |
| --- | --- | --- |
| Mineralocorticoids | Kidneys | Increases reabsorption of sodium ions and water from the urine; stimulates loss of potassium ions through excretion of urine |
| Glucocorticoids | Most cells | Releases amino acids from skeletal muscles, lipids from adipose (fat) tissues; promotes liver glycogen and glucose formation; promotes peripheral utilization of lipids; anti-inflammatory effects |
| Androgens | | Promotes growth of pubic hair in boys and girls; in adult women, promotes muscle mass, blood cell formation, and supports the libido; in adult men, adrenal androgens are less significant because androgens are released primarily from the gonads |

## What are the major glucocorticoid hormones and their diabetes connections?

Cortisol, corticosterone, and cortisone are the three most important glucocorticoid hormones in the body. Cortisol, also called hydrocortisone, is the most abundant glucocorticoid produced, accounting for nearly 95 percent of the activity of the glucocorticoids. These hormones have many varying effects on the body. In terms of diabetes, effects include the stimulation of glucose synthesis and glycogen formation, especially within the liver. They also stimulate the release of fatty acids from adipose tissue, which can be used as an energy source; decrease the effects of physical and emotional stress (such as fright, bleeding, and infection, since the added glucose from the liver gives tissues a ready source of energy); suppress allergic and inflammatory reactions (which is important to a person with diabetes, as inflammation can lead to other problems); and decrease and suppress the activities of white blood cells and other components of the immune system.

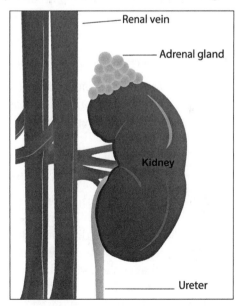

The adrenal glands rest on top of the kidneys; they produce hormones that affect such things as blood pressure and the body's response to stress.

# DIABETES AND THE THYROID AND PARATHYROID GLANDS

## What is the thyroid?

The thyroid is a butterfly-shaped gland in the neck. It is located just below the projection at the front of the neck (called the Adam's apple in men) and above the collarbone. Its major task is to regulate metabolism of the heart, liver, muscles, and other organs through the release of two hormones, thyroxine (T4) and triiodothyronine (T3). The gland also is part of a feedback mechanism that includes the pituitary gland (in the brain) and the hypothalamus (an area of the brain).

## What are T3, T4, and TSH and their functions in the body?

The thyroid itself has hormones and stimulates others to produce substances within certain areas of the body. These thyroid hormones have wide-ranging effects in regulating the function of virtually every organ, including how the body uses energy. Consequently, any changes in the thyroid hormone levels in the blood can affect many areas of the body and cause a wide range of symptoms if they are not balanced. In general, there is a sequence to the release of thyroid hormones. First, the thyroid-stimulating hormone (TSH) is produced when the brain's hypothalamus releases a substance called thyrotropin-releasing hormone (TRH). The TRH then triggers the pituitary gland to release the TSH. This release causes the thyroid to produce two hormones, triiodothyronine (T3) and thyroxine (T4), both of which help control the body's metabolism. From there, the brain's pituitary gland keeps track of the thyroid hormone levels in the blood, increasing or decreasing the amount of TSH released to keep the levels balanced.

## What are some statistics about people who have a thyroid disorder?

According to several thyroid organizations, millions of people have a thyroid disorder. Thyroid Federation International estimates that up to 300 million people worldwide have thyroid dysfunction, yet over half are unaware of their condition. According to the Amer-

---

### What is the most common cause of hypothyroidism?

The most common cause of hypothyroidism is dietary iodine deficiency, with an estimated 200 million people having the condition (although this number differs by a few tens of thousands depending on the report). In the United States, there is a lower incidence of hypothyroidism because iodine is usually added to salt and foods that contain salt. The most common reason for hypothyroidism in the United States is Hashimoto thyroiditis—an inherited autoimmune condition in which the immune system mistakenly attacks the thyroid and which affects more than 14 million Americans.

ican Thyroid Association, it is thought that around 20 million Americans, or 12 percent of the population, have a thyroid disorder (although some research indicates the number may be as high as 27 million). Gender-wise, it is estimated that women are five to eight times more likely to have a thyroid disorder than men. It is often said that thyroid disorders are second only to diabetes as the most common condition that affects the human endocrine system.

## What are hyperthyroidism and hypothyroidism?

If a person has an underactive thyroid gland, it is called hypothyroidism. ("Underactive"

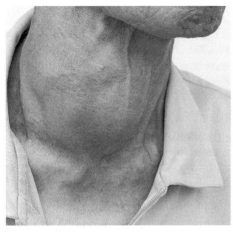

Hyperthyroidism can manifest as a goiter (the enlargement of the thyroid), which inhibits the gland's ability to process iodine.

means producing lower amounts of thyroxine than normal; a test would show too much TSH, or thyroid-stimulating hormone). If a person's thyroid gland is overactive (producing higher amounts of thyroxine than normal; a test would show too little TSH), it is called hyperthyroidism. This condition is less common than hypothyroidism. Neither condition is age related, but the conditions are often dependent on gender. For example, in the case of hyperthyroidism, it is often nine times more common in women than in men.

## Is there a connection between diabetes and thyroid disorders?

Yes, according to several studies, including those from the American Diabetes Association, many people who have diabetes are often affected by a thyroid disorder. In fact, people with diabetes have an increased risk for thyroid problems. In the general population, about 6 to 8 percent have some type of thyroid disorder, but this figure increases to 10 percent in people who have diabetes. There also seems to be an autoimmune connection. When a person has one autoimmune disorder, such as type 1 diabetes, he or she has an increased risk for developing another such disease. For example, statistics indicate that around 3 percent of women with type 1 diabetes have some form of autoimmune thyroid disease. Another example is postpartum thyroiditis, a form of autoimmune thyroid disease that causes thyroid dysfunction within a few months after delivery of a child. It is three times more common in women with diabetes. As for type 2 diabetes, although it is not an autoimmune disease, there is an unexplained higher occurrence of thyroid problems, especially hypothyroidism. Some studies suggest that this may be because type 2 diabetes and thyroid disorders often develop as a person ages.

## How are people with diabetes affected if they are hypothyroid or hyperthyroid?

Most studies indicate that, in general, if a person with diabetes has hypothyroidism, then there are few problems with blood glucose control, although the condition can reduce the removal of insulin from the bloodstream in people with type 1 diabetes (requiring that the dose of insulin be lower). If a person with diabetes has hyperthyroidism, he or she may have a more difficult time controlling blood glucose levels and may have to increase the insulin amount, as the condition causes an increase in glucose production in the liver, rapid absorption of glucose through the intestines, and increased insulin resistance. In addition, because diabetes can increase a person's risk for heart disease, and hyperthyroidism often increases the heart rate, the condition may exacerbate certain heart conditions, such as angina, or interfere with the treatment of a heart condition.

### What are the parathyroid glands?

There are four rice-grain-sized parathyroid glands located in the neck right behind the thyroid gland. Their main task is to keep calcium levels in the blood within a certain range by the release of the parathyroid hormone (PTH). The hormone not only helps muscles and nerves to work properly, but it is also connected to bone strength. In addition, if a person's blood calcium is too high, the parathyroid glands make less PTH, lowering the amount of calcium by filtering it out of the blood in the kidneys. If the person's blood calcium is low, the parathyroid glands make PTH, telling the body to increase the amount of the element in the blood. To do this, the body either absorbs more calcium from food in the intestines or it takes calcium from the bones.

### Do people with diabetes have more problems with hyperparathyroidism than other people?

Yes, according to several studies, hyperparathyroidism—or a high level of the parathyroid hormone in the blood (it can contribute to a loss of calcium and thus weaken bones)—is more prevalent in people with diabetes than in the general population. In addition, the prevalence of diabetes in patients with hyperparathyroidism is higher than in the general population. Studies have also shown that hyperparathyroidism—whether the person has or doesn't have diabetes—is almost three times more common in females than males and nearly seven times more common in postmenopausal women than in younger women.

# DIABETES, HORMONES, AND THE PANCREAS

### Where is the pancreas located?

The pancreas (from the Greek, meaning "all flesh") is located in what is called the abdominopelvic cavity, the area between and behind the stomach and the small intestine, and below the liver. It is an elongated organ that measures about 6 inches (12 to 15 centimeters) long.

## Why is the pancreas often called a "mixed gland"?

The pancreas is often called a "mixed gland" because it has both endocrine and exocrine functions. As an endocrine gland, it secretes hormones into the bloodstream, including insulin and glucagon for blood glucose regulation. But only 1 percent of the weight of the pancreas serves as an endocrine gland. The remaining 99 percent has exocrine functions, especially in its relation to the body's digestive system. (For more about the pancreas, including its functions as an exocrine gland, see the chapter "How Diabetes Affects the Digestive System.")

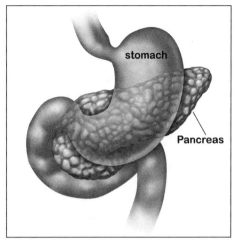

The pancreas is located behind the stomach.

## What are the pancreatic cells called the islets of Langerhans?

A cluster of cells in the pancreas is called the pancreatic islets (islets of Langerhans). They are also the cells that secrete hormones associated with blood glucose levels. In most adults, there can be between 200,000 and 2 million pancreatic islets scattered throughout the pancreas.

## How many different types of cells are found in the islets of Langerhans?

The types of cells in each of the islets of Langerhans include the alpha, beta, delta, and F cells. The two most important types of cells—especially in terms of diabetes—are the alpha cells that produce glucagon for the body and the beta cells that produce insulin (for more about using islets in the future, especially to help curb type 2 diabetes, see the chapter "The Future and Diabetes").

## Why are alpha and beta cells in the pancreas so important to a person with—or without—diabetes?

The pancreas contains two types of cells that help with insulin stability: alpha and beta cells. Within the islets of Langerhans, the beta cells secrete insulin in response to increased blood glucose levels. This secretion stimulates the cells to take up glucose, providing energy to the body. The alpha cells secrete the hormone glucagon in response to a decrease in blood glucose levels, with the hormone binding to glucagon receptors in the liver. This secretion helps stimulate the breakdown of glycogen and release glucose into the bloodstream. (There are also other cell types in islets, including those that secrete the hormones somatostatin, ghrelin, and pancreatic polypeptide Y, but the alpha and beta cells are the most important to controlling the blood glucose levels in the body.)

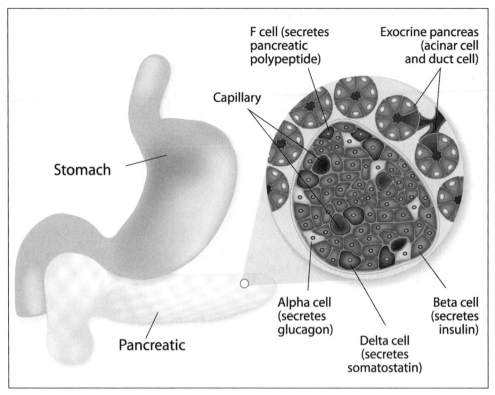

The islets of Langerhans contain three types of cells that secrete insulin: alpha, beta, and delta cells.

### Does any other chemical in the body stimulate the release of glucagon?

Yes. Although scientists know that glucose is the main factor in the release of glucagon, there are other factors including catecholamines (such as adrenaline) and amino acids (the "building blocks" of proteins) that also help stimulate glucagon release. In addition, insulin and fatty acids can inhibit the release of glucagon. There are many more factors, and scientists are currently trying to unravel the biology and hormone interactions in order to understand how cells respond (or don't respond) when a person has diabetes.

### How are the pancreas and insulin connected?

Insulin is made in the pancreas. As the blood glucose levels rise after a person eats a meal, the pancreas is triggered to release insulin. This hormone also enables the body's cells to take in sugar and other nutrients. It is necessary for energy and growth, which is why an imbalance of the hormone in the body (which most often means diabetes) can have a dramatic effect on a person's entire body system. When this system breaks down—in combination with other factors in the body—a person can develop insulin resistance, which is most often associated with type 2 diabetes. (For more about the pancreas, insulin resistance, and type 2 diabetes, see the chapter "Prediabetes and Type 2 Diabetes.")

## Who first described the pancreatic islets— and who discovered that the pancreas secreted insulin?

In the late 1860s, German pathologist and biologist Paul Langerhans (1847–1888) was the first to provide a detailed description of microscopic structures in the pancreas. What he found were uniquely shaped cells in the pancreas that were actually the islets. It was not until 1893 that French pathologist Gustave E. Laguesse (1861–1927) discovered that these polygon-shaped cells were actually the endocrine cells of the pancreas that secreted insulin.

## What is the function of insulin in the body?

Insulin is secreted when blood glucose levels rise above normal. One of the most important tasks of insulin is to help with the transport of glucose across a cell's membrane. In other words, insulin allows the glucose in the blood to diffuse into most body cells. It also stimulates the production of glycogen from glucose. The glucose is then stored in the liver to be released when blood glucose levels drop—for example, when the body needs energy during exercise. (For more about insulin, see the chapter "Taking Charge of Diabetes.")

## Does insulin just control the body's glucose levels?

No, insulin has other duties besides controlling the body's glucose levels. It also controls fat and helps the body store excess sugar as fat. Certain sugars and other carbohydrates with a high glycemic index are most likely to be stored as fat in the body. As the body's sugar goes up and down before, during, and after meals, the insulin follows along, keeping the glucose levels even and contributing to the body's fat stores. (For more about the glycemic index and how insulin and sugar are related to fat, see the chapter "Diabetes and Eating.")

# HOW DIABETES AFFECTS THE NERVOUS SYSTEM

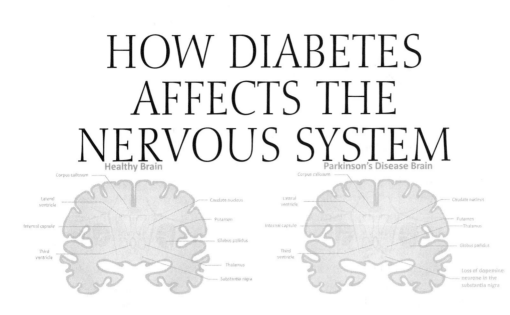

Healthy Brain

Corpus callosum

Lateral ventricle

Internal capsule

Third ventricle

Caudate nucleus

Putamen

Globus pallidus

Thalamus

Substantia nigra

Parkinson's Disease Brain

Corpus callosum

Lateral ventricle

Internal capsule

Third ventricle

Caudate nucleus

Putamen
Thalamus

Globus pallidus

Loss of dopamine neurone in the substantia nigra

## THE NERVOUS SYSTEM AND DIABETES

### What is the human nervous system?

The human nervous system is an intricately organized, interconnected system of nerve cells that relays messages to and from the brain and spinal cord (nervous systems are also found in organisms called vertebrates, or, literally, organisms with backbones, a group that includes humans). The human nervous system receives sensory input, processes the input, and then sends messages to the tissues and organs for the appropriate response. In humans (and other vertebrates), there are two parts to the nervous system. They are the central nervous system, consisting of the brain and spinal cord, and the peripheral system, consisting of peripheral nerves that carry signals to and from the central nervous system.

### Do some diseases that affect the nervous system have connections to diabetes?

Although there are several diseases of the nervous system, the more well-known ones are epilepsy, multiple sclerosis (MS), and Parkinson's disease. The two with the most possible connections to diabetes are epilepsy and Parkinson's disease (see below), but not multiple sclerosis. (MS is an autoimmune disease. It is a chronic, potentially debilitating disease that affects the sheaths surrounding the nerves [called myelin] in the central nervous system. In MS, the body directs antibodies and white blood cells against proteins in the sheaths, causing injury and inflammation to the sheaths, especially those surrounding nerves in the brain and spinal cord.) Overall, there is little evidence that diabetes—either type 1 or type 2—has any connection to MS, although people with either disease can develop the other one.

## How are seizures connected to diabetes?

Seizures, or a condition in which something interrupts the normal connections between the nerve cells and the brain, can under some circumstances be connected to diabetes. The definitions of seizures and shocks often differ depending on the research, but either way, a very low blood glucose reading can lead to a seizure. In particular, a hypoglycemic seizure from low blood glucose levels can cause clumsiness, weakness, trouble talking, confusion, loss of consciousness, seizures, or (rarely) death. Diabetic shock (severe hypoglycemia), also called insulin reaction, is a consequence of too much insulin. It can occur anytime there is an imbalance between the insulin in the person's system, the amount of food eaten, or the level of a person's physical activity. Hypoglycemic shock is similar (if not the same) as diabetic shock, caused by extremely low blood glucose levels, most often from an excessive amount of injected insulin, failure to eat after an insulin injection, or rarely by an insulin-secreting tumor of the pancreas. Whatever it is called, an extremely low blood glucose level can cause seizures and is considered to be a medical emergency.

## Is epilepsy connected to diabetes?

Epilepsy is a nervous system disorder in which clusters of nerve cells (neurons) in the brain sometimes send signals abnormally. When the normal pattern of nerve activity becomes disturbed, it causes strange sensations, emotions, and behavior or sometimes convulsions, muscle spasms, and loss of consciousness. There are thought to be many causes, including certain illnesses, brain damage, abnormal brain development and wiring, an imbalance of nerve-signaling chemicals (called neurotransmitters), or some combination of these factors. As for epilepsy's connection to diabetes, it is thought that there may be an increased risk—nearly three times more—of epileptic seizures in young people with type 1 diabetes as compared to others without type 1. One study also suggests that there may be an association between epilepsy and diabetic ketoacidosis in children with type 1 diabetes. (For more about diabetic ketoacidosis, see the chapter "Type 1 Diabetes.") As most researchers mention, more studies need to be conducted to determine whether there is a definite connection.

## Is there a relationship between Parkinson's disease and diabetes?

Several studies suggest a connection between Parkinson's disease and diabetes, including one report indicating that people with type 2 diabetes were 80 percent more likely to be diagnosed with Parkinson's disease. Parkinson's is a progressive neurological disorder (also called a neurodegenerative disease) that results from degeneration of neurons in a region of the brain that controls movement. This degeneration creates a shortage of the brain-signaling chemical (neurotransmitter) known as dopamine, causing changes in body movement—most often shaking of various parts of the body, including hands and head—that characterize the disease. No one knows whether there truly is a relationship, but one study suggests that many lifestyle factors, such as being overweight or obese, smoking, and being sedentary, seem to be associated with both disorders.

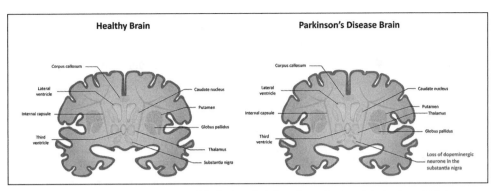

Parkinson's disease is caused when an area of the brain called the *substantia nigra* deteriorates, which lowers dopamine production, an essential chemical for muscle control. Patients with diabetes are more likely to get Parkinson's, but a direct connection has not yet been established.

## What recent research addresses why there may be a link between Parkinson's disease and type 2 diabetes?

In 2015, a study conducted at Ben Gurion University in Israel indicated that there may be a link between type 2 diabetes and Parkinson's based on certain proteins. The researchers were the first to discover the structure of a brain protein (alpha-synuclein) that can trigger Parkinson's by clumping and causing the death of nerve cells. There is also a protein (a short chain of amino acids) called amylin found in the pancreas in 95 percent of the people with type 2 diabetes—and it is also found in the brain. (In the pancreas, the amylin can harm insulin-producing beta cells, contributing to type 2 diabetes.) The researchers then studied a snippet of the brain protein alpha-synuclein (the snippet was called a non-amyloid-beta component, or NAC). Because of their research, they believe that the NAC and amylin may act together, causing the clumping in the brain and killing nerve cells—a possible link between both diseases. Researchers believe that if there is such a link, a drug may be developed that would prevent the interactions between the NAC component and the amylin. But as with many new discoveries, more research needs to be conducted on the possible link between the two diseases.

# DIABETES AND NEUROPATHY

## What is neuropathy?

Neuropathy is the general term that means nerve damage caused by various conditions that affect the body. It usually refers to the damage of a person's peripheral nerves (see below), as opposed to the nerves of the central nervous system (the brain and spinal cord). The nerves affected can be singular (mononeuropathy) or in sets (polyneuropathy). For example, in polyneuropathy, multiple nerves simultaneously malfunction, causing weak hands and feet, as well as the loss of sensation in those areas.

## What are the three types of nerves in the body that can be affected by neuropathy?

Overall, neuropathy for various reasons can occur if there is damage to three types of nerves (any number of these three types can affect a person at any one time):

*Autonomic*—The nerves that control the major systems of the body, such as the bladder; they can cause changes in a person's heart rate and blood pressure, along with sweating.

*Motor*—The nerves that allow the body to have power and movement; neuropathy of motor nerves can cause weakness in the hands and feet.

*Sensory*—These nerves control sensation; neuropathy of sensory nerves can cause pain, tingling, numbness, or weakness in the hands and feet.

## What are the common types of nerve damage often found in people with diabetes?

Not every person with diabetes will experience nerve damage, but for those who do, there are three different types of neuropathy:

*Peripheral neuropathy*—This is the most common type of neuropathy—and one of the major complications—in people with diabetes. It affects the long nerves that run from the spine to the arms, legs, and hands. Most researchers believe it is likely caused by damage to the delicate nerve fibers when the body experiences high blood glucose levels (see below). It is often called "diabetic peripheral neuropathy" (or "peripheral diabetic neuropathy") if these nerves are damaged from diabetes.

*Focal neuropathy*—This type of nerve damage affects a specific nerve or set of nerves and usually causes weakness in the face, arms, legs, or eye muscles. It often leads to weakness in the hands, double vision, or difficulty in raising the legs. If treated (most often by controlling the person's glucose levels), it typically disappears in two to six months.

*Autonomic neuropathy*—This nerve damage affects the autonomic nervous system, which controls such body functions as heart rate, digestion, blood pressure, sweating, and for men, erections. Autonomic neuropathy can cause a multitude of symptoms, including racing heartbeat, dizziness, or light-headedness. It can affect the digestive tract, causing vomiting, diarrhea, and/or constipation. It can also cause a person not to empty his or her bladder efficiently, which can predispose the individual to bladder infections. And for men, especially those who have had diabetes for many years, it may cause impotence (for more about impotence [also called erectile dysfunction] and diabetes, see the chapter "How Diabetes Affects the Reproductive System").

## Why do people with diabetes often develop certain types of neuropathy?

Most cases of chronic neuropathy are found in people who have diabetes. In fact, roughly 60 to 70 percent of people with diabetes have some type of neuropathy. Neuropathies in people with diabetes are thought to be caused by poorly controlled blood glucose levels. High levels of blood glucose can eventually damage delicate nerve fibers, interfering with nerve-signal transmission and damaging the nerves themselves. Although it is unknown why this happens, some researchers speculate that the damage is caused when glucose attaches to or affects the proteins found in nerve cells. This condition may either cause a chemical imbalance inside the nerves or restrict the blood flow to the nerves. Either way, once the network of nerves is damaged, the messages to and from different parts of the body are also affected. The nerve signals may slow down or send the wrong cues, or eventually, the nerves may stop working.

## What are some causes of peripheral neuropathy besides diabetes?

Numerous conditions can cause peripheral neuropathy. The most common cause of chronic peripheral neuropathy is diabetes, also called diabetic peripheral neuropathy. Other reasons for peripheral neuropathy include physical trauma (injuries such as broken bones can put pressure on nerves); infections (shingles, HIV infections, and Lyme disease often contribute to peripheral neuropathy); Guillain-Barré syndrome, a specific type of peripheral neuropathy triggered by infection; high consumption of alcohol; chronic liver and kidney diseases (both can cause peripheral nerve damage because of the imbalance in the body's overall chemistry); cancers (lymphoma can cause peripheral neuropathy); folate vitamin deficiencies (the lack of B2 in the diet can contribute to nerve damage); repetitive injuries (carpal tunnel syndrome); exposure to toxins (insecticides and certain solvents can cause peripheral neuropathy); and some drugs (some chemotherapy medication used to treat HIV often causes damage to the peripheral nerves). If the reason for the neuropathy is unknown—and it is estimated that the reasons for 30 percent of neuropathies are unknown—it is usually referred to as idiopathic peripheral neuropathy.

## Are there any treatments for a person who has diabetes and a certain type of neuropathy?

Yes, there are treatments for people with diabetes and neuropathy, depending on where the nerve damage is located. For example, if a person with diabetes has digestive problems because of nerve damage (a type of autonomic neuropathy), then he or she may need to eat more fiber. If a person with diabetes has bladder problems caused by autonomic neuropathy, then oral drugs, or even surgery, may help improve bladder function or reduce incontinence caused by the neuropathy.

## Can inflammation affect a person with peripheral neuropathy?

Yes, it is thought that peripheral neuropathy can be worsened by inflammation. This swelling of tissues—often accompanied by the area becoming hot—is the way the body fights off infection. But if there is too much inflammation along with neuropathy, these conditions can damage tissues and often cause pain.

## How can nerve damage affect the extremities of a person with diabetes?

Nerve damage can affect the extremities of a person with diabetes in several ways. These can include musculoskeletal complications in the hands, wrists, and shoulders, along with problems in the feet, toes, ankles, and legs. Most of this damage is caused by uncontrolled or high blood glucose levels that damage the delicate nerve endings in the extremities. (For more information about nerve damage and hands, wrists, and shoulders, see the chapter "How Diabetes Affects Bones, Joints, Muscles, Teeth, and Skin.")

### What are some of the dangers if a person with diabetes develops diabetic peripheral neuropathy?

There are some concerns if a person with diabetes develops diabetic peripheral neuropathy. For example, if a person has less sensitivity to vibrations, touch, and pain, owing to diabetic neuropathy (especially in the feet), then it could put him or her at a greater risk for foot injury. Such nerve damage could mean that conditions such as too tight shoes, high-impact exercise injuries, or even stepping on an object that punctures the bottom of the foot would go unnoticed. In extreme cases, a foot wound that goes overlooked for a long period could become infected, and if it does, the infection could lead to gangrene, eventually requiring amputation. In addition, with neuropathy, there may be more bladder and kidney infections or a decrease in muscle mass (or even muscle damage). If the person's digestive system is affected by neuropathy, along with frequent bouts of vomiting, it can result in poor blood glucose control.

### What are some of the symptoms of diabetic peripheral neuropathy?

Symptoms of peripheral neuropathy in people with diabetes include tingling, numbness, and reduced sensitivity to touch. It may also cause itching, weakness, and loss of balance, especially when it affects the legs and feet. In rare cases, it may also cause a burning or painful sensation in the extremities that continues up the arms or legs. People with diabetes and peripheral neuropathy commonly describe the sensation in various ways. For example, peripheral neuropathy in the feet has been described as "walking barefoot on cut glass."

### Why is it important for people with diabetes to care about their feet?

While everyone should practice good foot care, a person with diabetes should be extra vigilant. One of the more common side effects of diabetes is the loss of sensation because of diabetic peripheral neuropathy. Because of this, minor injuries to the feet could become a major problem. For example, if a person with diabetes gets a blister and has lost some of the sensation in the feet, he or she may not treat it properly or even know it exists. If the wound becomes infected, it may lead to ulcerations and, if severe enough, to amputation. (For more about diabetic foot problems, see the chapter "How Diabetes Affects Bones, Joints, Muscles, Teeth, and Skin.")

### Can diabetes cause a burning sensation on the soles of both feet?

Yes, a burning sensation on the soles of the feet is often reported by people who have diabetes. This can be caused by something as simple as ill-fitting shoes. But for a person with diabetes, it may be a sign of diabetic peripheral neuropathy, or damage to the peripheral nerves in the feet. It can also be caused by alcoholism and less commonly by vitamin deficiencies or lead poisoning. This burning sensation has even been attributed to a rare condition called erythromelalgia, a disorder that causes a burning feeling in the extremities brought about by an increase in blood flow to the hands and feet.

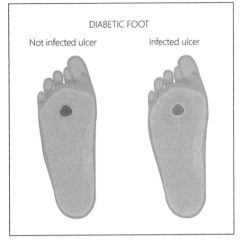

DIABETIC FOOT

Not infected ulcer          Infected ulcer

A sore on a foot for a diabetic person is much more prone to infection. If left untreated, the infection can get into the bones, even making amputation of toes, feet, or legs necessary.

## Why do some foot injuries go unnoticed by people with diabetes?

In most cases, the main reason that foot injuries go unnoticed is nerve damage from the diabetes and/or peripheral artery disease (PAD; for more about PAD, see the chapter "How Diabetes Affects the Circulatory System"). If a foot injury goes unnoticed, it is mostly because peripheral neuropathy often impairs pain sensations, and there is a decrease in the blood flow or complete blockage in the arteries feeding the foot. Thus, a cut, blister, bleeding wart, or even an ingrown toenail can cause an undetected infection to spread.

If the infection becomes severe, the foot's poor circulation from PAD or diabetic nerve damage exacerbates the problem by not allowing the body's natural infection fighters—such as white blood cells and antibodies—to attack the invading infection. If the infection remains uncontrolled, a foot ulcer can develop, which is a condition that needs immediate attention. If not treated, the infection can penetrate into the lower layers of the skin and reach the bone, causing a bone infection. If one or more toes, or another part of the foot, becomes involved, then the toes or even an entire foot often has be amputated. In extreme cases, a leg may have to be amputated. This is why it is often stressed that people with diabetes pay close attention to their extremities, especially the feet. (For more about foot ulcers, see the chapter "How Diabetes Affects Bones, Joints, Muscles, Teeth, and Skin.")

## What is Charcot's arthropathy (or Charcot's foot and ankle)?

Charcot's arthropathy, also called Charcot's foot and ankle or diabetic foot, is a syndrome that often affects a person with diabetes and who has severe diabetic peripheral neuropathy. (It can also affect other people who have loss of sensation in their feet for other medical reasons.) According to Harvard Medical School, this condition occurs when a person's foot and ankle joints and/or bones are destroyed, including such problems as bone disintegration, fractures, and dislocation of bones. These changes in the bones and joints can eventually cause deformities that interfere with walking. It is also one of the most serious foot problems that a person with diabetes faces.

Initially, there is minor trauma to a joint or bone in the foot from daily wear and tear. If this goes unnoticed—which often happens with severe diabetic peripheral neuropathy—then the damage often continues until the tissues are eventually destroyed. Again, this is why doctors stress that people with diabetes pay close attention to changes in their feet and ankles. If caught in time, the damage can potentially be minimized by changing the way a person walks (sometimes through physical therapy), modifying their footwear, or starting an exercise program.

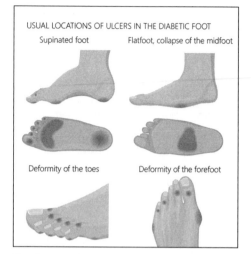

USUAL LOCATIONS OF ULCERS IN THE DIABETIC FOOT

Supinated foot      Flatfoot, collapse of the midfoot

Deformity of the toes      Deformity of the forefoot

The above graphic shows where dangerous ulcers most commonly develop on the feet of diabetics.

### How does a physician initially diagnose diabetic peripheral neuropathy?

The initial tests for diabetic peripheral neuropathy can usually be conducted during a physician's office exam. In fact, it is estimated that 60 to 70 percent of people with diabetes have some signs of neuropathy that can usually be detected with a physical exam or special tests. The best way to determine neuropathy is to test the reflexes and sensory perception of the patient. Other means of diagnosing will also be conducted, such as looking at the person's history (for example, any history of neuropathy in the family, exposure to toxins, medications taken, and alcohol consumption).

### What are some special tests to check a person with diabetes for peripheral neuropathy?

Sometimes a nerve conduction test may be needed to see whether certain nerves are affected, such as those in the arms or legs. This is done by attaching special electrodes to the skin over the nerve being tested. Another test is electromyography, which looks at the electrical activity of muscles. This is done by inserting a very thin needle with an electrode attached into the muscle being tested; the way the muscle responds is recorded on an oscilloscope. Not as common are nerve and skin biopsies, in which a small part of the suspect nerve is removed and examined under a microscope to detect damage.

### Is there a connection between food and peripheral neuropathy?

Yes, some studies indicate that there may be connections between food and the occurrence of peripheral neuropathy. The following are two of these possible connections (for more about food, see the chapter "Diabetes and Food"):

- Several studies indicate that high glucose levels after a meal are strongly associated with peripheral neuropathy. According to the Foundation for Peripheral Neuropathy, the best way to reduce after-meal glucose levels is to eat more foods that are slowly absorbed into the bloodstream. These include fruits, vegetables, beans, and nuts—and not refined starches and sugars. In addition, exercising after a meal will often cause blood glucose levels to decrease, and using fast-acting insulin can lower sugar. The best way to discover how to lower levels after meals is for a person to work with his or her health care professional to make certain medical and/or eating adjustments.

- Another culprit that connects food and peripheral neuropathy is inflammation. In fact, many foods are known to increase the amount of inflammation in the body. The greatest problem in determining how a food affects a person is just that—different foods cause different inflammations in different people. Some of the more well-known foods that can cause inflammation are trans fats, saturated fats, sugar, alcohol, and what are called omega-6 oils: corn, safflower, and soybean oils. (For more about omega-6, see the chapter "How Diabetes Affects the Digestive System.") Of course, other types of food, such as those that contain dairy, nuts, caffeine, and other foodstuffs, can also cause inflammation. To understand which foods may cause inflammation may take time. Again, the best way to uncover foods that cause inflammation is to work with an individual's health care professional.

## Why does having diabetes often increase the risk for amputations?

For some people with diabetes, there is an increased risk for amputation. This can be because of diabetic peripheral neuropathy but may also be from the complication of peripheral artery disease, or PAD. Both conditions raise the risk for nerve damage. If the damage is severe enough, it can eventually lead to amputation—especially if the tissue dies, and the extremity becomes infected. This often happens with the feet as foot injuries and ulcers may not be readily noticed because of nerve damage.

## What are some statistics concerning diabetes and amputations?

According to Harvard Medical School, diabetes is responsible for more than 60 percent of lower limb amputations that have not been caused by accidental injuries. The school also notes that a person with diabetes is ten times more likely to have an amputation than a person who does not have diabetes. But not everyone with diabetes will need amputation of extremities, especially if people keep their blood sugar levels under control and especially check their feet daily for possible cuts and wounds. If there is a wound, tend to it immediately so it does not become infected.

# THE BRAIN AND DIABETES

## Why do human brain cells need glucose?

While most of the cells in the body can adapt—at least temporarily—to using lipids (fats) and proteins as energy sources, the human brain cells require glucose in order to work well. In fact, the brain cells can get energy only from glucose. This means that when the body's blood glucose levels fall too low for that person, his or her brain cells shut down. This shutdown often results in fainting, which actually increases the flow of blood and glucose to the brain to compensate.

## Can diabetes contribute to short- and long-term memory loss?

Short-term memory loss and reduced brain function can occur during periods of low and high blood glucose (hypoglycemia and hyperglycemia, respectively). Over the long term, high blood glucose (hyperglycemia) can affect memory in people with type 1 and type 2 diabetes. This is because high glucose levels can damage nerves, including those of the brain, thereby increasing the risk of memory loss—and sometimes eventually contribute to dementia.

## What are the two forms of dementia most often mentioned in the media?

The term "dementia" describes a group of symptoms caused by changes in a person's brain function and is usually associated with advancing age. The two most common forms of dementia in older people—and the ones most often mentioned in our daily lives—are multi-infarct dementia (sometimes called vascular dementia) and Alzheimer's disease. These types of dementia are irreversible, which means they cannot be cured. Research on both types now center on mitigation or slowing down their progression.

In multi-infarct dementia, a series of small strokes or changes in the brain's blood supply may result in the death of brain tissue. The location in the brain where the small strokes occur determines the seriousness of the problem and the symptoms that arise. Symptoms that begin suddenly may be a sign of this kind of dementia. People with multi-infarct dementia are likely to show signs of improvement or remain stable for long periods of time, then quickly develop new symptoms if more strokes occur. In many people with multi-infarct dementia, high blood pressure is to blame. In Alzheimer's disease, nerve cell changes in certain parts of the brain result in the death of a large number of cells. The most common symptoms range from mild forgetfulness to serious impairments in thinking, judgment, and the ability to perform daily activities.

## What is the possible connection between diabetes, Alzheimer's disease, and something called "type 3 diabetes"?

In 2005, research suggested that there may be something called "type 3 diabetes," or a term proposed for Alzheimer's disease, which is thought to result (in part) from the brain's resistance to insulin. Other studies followed, including several in 2012, indicating that resistance to insulin—and resulting low levels of insulin in the brain—seemed to play a key role in the progression of Alzheimer's disease. Another study indicated that people with insulin resistance, especially those with type 2 diabetes, have an increased risk of eventually developing Alzheimer's disease—between 50 and 60 percent higher than people without type 2 diabetes.

Most researchers emphasize that not everyone with type 2 diabetes develops Alzheimer's disease, but type 2 could be a co-factor in the disease's progression. (In other words, having type 2 diabetes does not *cause* Alzheimer's disease but may contribute to an increase in impaired brain function and eventually Alzheimer's.) Other researchers suggest that diabetes and Alzheimer's disease may have the same source: An overconsumption of foods that cause problems with the many roles insulin plays in the body. And since such consumption often leads to obesity, several studies indicate that as the obesity rates have increased in the past several decades, so has the incidence of Alzheimer's disease. More studies need to be done. If there is a definite connection, some "cures" for type 2 diabetes and Alzheimer's may be as "simple" as eating the right foods, exercising, and keeping off excess weight.

# HOW DIABETES AFFECTS THE CIRCULATORY SYSTEM

## What are the main components of the circulatory system?

The main components of the circulatory system are the vessels, heart, and blood. The system also includes a person's blood pressure, as blood pressure involves the blood pumping through the body, and how it affects the heart and blood vessels.

## What is a pulse?

A person's pulse is the alternate expansion and recoil (contraction) of an artery, which can be felt in an artery close to the body's surface. The pulse occurs because of the rhythmic ejection of blood from the heart into a main artery called the aorta, which causes an increase and decrease of pressure in the artery. The pulse provides important information about the heart action, blood vessels, and circulation. For example, a fast pulse rate may indicate the presence of dehydration. And of course, in a medical emergency, a pulse will help determine whether a person's heart is pumping.

## DIABETES AND THE HEART

### In general, how does the human heart work?

The human heart (a muscle), located beneath the upper-left portion of a person's torso, is about the size of a clenched fist. On average, the heart beats about 70 to 75 times per minute (resting) and pumps about five quarts (just over five liters) of blood per minute. Within the heart, two atria receive blood, while two ventricles pump blood out of the heart. The heart also has a natural "pacemaker," called the sinoatrial node, or the part of the heart that times the contraction by generating and sending electrical signals to what is called the atrioventricular node. The impulses are sent to certain fibers, causing the ventricles to contract. These electrical impulses are also what are detected by an electrocardiogram (EKG) many people receive to check for irregularities in the heartbeat. Several factors can affect the heart's pacemaker, including two sets of nerves that speed up or slow down the heart, the release of hormones such as adrenaline, and the body's overall temperature.

### Does having diabetes increase the risk of heart disease?

Yes, for most people, diabetes increases the risk of heart disease. In fact, according to the National Institutes of Health, at least 65 percent of people with diabetes die of some form of heart or blood vessel disease. Other research indicates that type 2 diabetes is associated with a two- to fourfold excess risk of cardiovascular disease. This includes such conditions as elevated triglyceride levels and a decrease in HDL (the "good" cholesterol) levels. (For more about triglycerides and cholesterol, see this chapter.)

### What is atrial fibrillation?

Atrial fibrillation—often referred to as afib—is the most common abnormal heart rhythm reported. It is estimated that about 1 in 100 people, around 5 in 100 over age

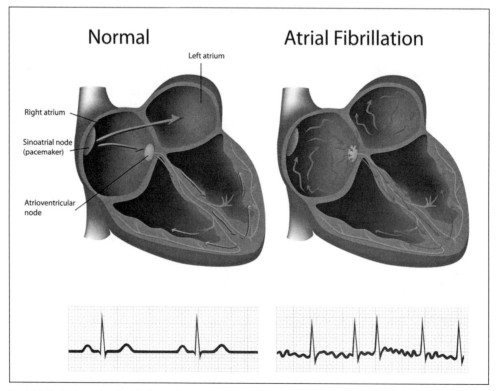

In atrial fibrilations, the electrical signals sent to the heart muscles are irregular, causing the atria (heart chambers) to not work well together. The resulting, fluttering heartbeat puts people at greater risk of heart attacks.

65, and around ten in 100 people over age 80 have this condition. It occurs when the heart beats irregularly in comparison to a normal heartbeat. The symptoms often include heart palpitations, fainting, fatigue, or congestive heart failure. It can also make the blood "pool" within certain heart chambers, causing the heart to "quiver" in a chaotic pattern, which slows the blood flow and creates irregular beats. If the pooled blood stagnates, it can sometimes cause clots to form, which can lead to embolic strokes. Atrial fibrillation is thought of as a problem with the heart's "electrical control," mainly a group of cells called the sinus node, also often referred to as the body's natural pacemaker. If for some reason—and many times, the reasons are difficult to diagnose—the electric signal has a problem, it can cause the heart to pump irregularly.

### Are people with diabetes at a higher risk for developing atrial fibrillation?

Some studies indicate that diabetes may be connected to atrial fibrillation (afib). In the past, there was disagreement as to whether diabetes and atrial fibrillation were linked. A study from the *Journal of General Internal Medicine* published in 2010 indicated that there is a connection, noting that people with diabetes seem to have an almost 40 percent greater risk of developing afib than people without diabetes. The study also found that the risk increases the longer a person has diabetes (with an estimate of afib increasing by 3 percent for each year the person has diabetes) and if the person has uncontrolled blood glucose levels (or if the HbA1c is more than 9 percent). But there is one thing no study has yet found: Which comes first, diabetes or afib?

# DIABETES, ARTERIES, AND VEINS

### What are the main types of vessels in the body that transport blood?

The following are the three types of vessels that transport blood throughout the body:

*Arteries and arterioles*—The arteries and arterioles always transport blood away from the heart (via rhythmic contractions known as the pulse) to the various organs in the body. These vessels are under enormous pressure. Thus, their walls are made of thick and elastic smooth muscles.

*Veins and venules*—Veins return blood to the heart after it circulates through the body. They are relatively thin-walled vessels that lack muscular tissues but are located within skeletal muscle—which means the blood is propelled upward and back to the heart as the body moves. They also contain one-way "valves" that prevent the backflow of blood within the vein.

*Capillaries*—The smallest vessels are the capillaries—mostly microscopic vessels that form an elaborate network conveying blood between arteries and veins (the walls are only one cell in thickness). They branch from the ends of small arteries and carry oxygen-rich blood to all tissues of the body—along with allowing for the diffusion of nutrients and wastes between cells and the blood.

## What is transcatheter aortic valve replacement?

Transcatheter aortic valve replacement (TAVR) is a surgical procedure for aortic valve stenosis. This is the narrowing of the heart's aortic valve (one of the main arteries at the top of the heart) that makes the heart muscle work harder, and that can eventually lead to heart failure. People with diabetes are at higher risk of aortic-valve stenosis and have an even higher risk of other cardiovascular complications than others without diabetes.

There are two procedures. One is the aortic valve replacement (AVR), which is usually performed during open-heart surgery (the aortic valve is physically replaced with a mechanical or tissue valve). The other method is the transcatheter aortic valve replacement (TAVR), in which a catheter is inserted with a balloon at the tip. As in a catherization, the catheter is inserted into an artery in the leg, or it can be inserted in a small incision in the chest. The instrument works its way to the damaged aortic valve, and the balloon—which carries a folded tissue or mechanical valve around it—is inflated, pushing the artificial valve into the body's own valve to fix the problem. TAVR is often used if the patient is at a high risk of complications with AVR as TAVR is a less-invasive procedure than AVR. In more recent studies, it has been shown that the TAVR procedure has a much higher survival rate than the AVR treatment.

## What is peripheral artery disease?

Peripheral artery disease, or PAD, is a condition in which the peripheral arteries narrow. The arteries that narrow can include those to the legs (the most common), stomach, arms, and head (brain). It is often caused by atherosclerosis, a disease in which fats, cholesterol, and other substances create plaque that builds up in the peripheral arteries, or the outer regions away from the heart. This buildup causes the arteries to become narrow, reducing or completely blocking the blood flow. The most common symptoms are cramping, pain, or tiredness in the leg or hip muscles during walking (called claudication) or climbing stairs. In many cases, the pain dissipates after resting and returns when the person walks or climbs stairs again. Those most at risk for developing PAD include smokers, people with high blood pressure or high cholesterol, older people, and those who have diabetes.

## Is there a connection between peripheral artery disease and diabetes?

Yes, there can be a connection between peripheral artery disease (PAD) and people with diabetes. In fact, if a person has diabetes (either type 1 and type 2), he or she is at a higher risk of developing atherosclerosis, the most common cause of PAD. In addition, PAD most commonly affects the legs and feet, places that may also be affected by diabetic peripheral neuropathy (for more about diabetic peripheral neuropathy, see the chapter "How Diabetes Affects the Nervous System"). PAD (along with diabetic peripheral neuropathy) may lead to pain in the legs (especially during walking), slow-to-heal foot wounds, one foot's being colder than the other, and, in severe cases, gangrene (in which there is a total loss of circulation), a condition that can increase the risk of foot or leg amputation.

## What is the risk that a person with diabetes will develop peripheral artery disease?

It is estimated that a person with type 2 diabetes has a three-times-higher risk of developing PAD than a person without blood glucose problems. If a person has a higher blood glucose level, it means an even higher risk. According to a 2010 study, it is estimated that every one-point increase in a diabetic's A1c level can increase the risk of having a PAD-related amputation by up to 44 percent for people with type 2 diabetes and 18 percent for people with type 1 diabetes.

## How can a person with diabetes lower the risk of peripheral artery disease?

There are several ways a person with diabetes can lower the risk of developing PAD, or peripheral artery disease. The most important, of course, is to monitor blood glucose levels and keep them as balanced as possible, as diabetes promotes the buildup of plaque in the arteries. In addition, exercise can help, as can medications such as statins (especially medicines that help keep the arteries free of plaque).

## What are varicose veins?

Varicose veins are enlarged or distended veins, usually occurring in the surface veins of the inside of the thighs and calves of legs. They are caused by the valves inside the veins becoming stretched so they no longer close completely. The affected veins then become filled with blood, often pushing on the skin and appearing as usually bluish or dark purple-colored veins that protrude or bulge through the skin.

## Are there any health concerns if a person who has diabetes also has varicose veins?

While varicose veins can be mildly uncomfortable for some, a proliferation of such veins can be accompanied by aching pain, swelling, itching, numbness, or a rash in the legs. In addition, if the veins gradually grow later, they may cause health problems that can require medical treatment. For example, if the pooling of the blood in the vein is significant, it can slow the return of the blood to the heart, possibly causing blood clots and severe infections. And if a varicose vein causes a rash or sore, it could eventually lead to an infection—which is why a person with diabetes and varicose veins should monitor his or her condition closely.

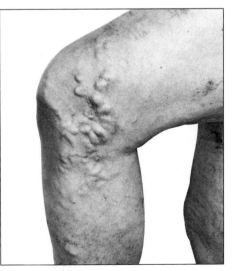

When valves in the veins no longer function properly, the veins get enlarged and distended. Diabetes can compound the problem because of the increased risk of infection it causes.

163

## Can varicose veins occur if a person frequently crosses his or her legs?

Contrary to popular belief, and according to Harvard Medical School, people are not at a higher risk of developing varicose veins if they frequently cross their legs. In fact, heredity is mostly to blame, and it is estimated that more than 80 percent of people are at risk for varicose veins if a parent has the same condition. There are other lesser factors, including high blood pressure, inactivity, smoking, hormonal changes that occur with puberty, pregnancy, and menopause, having a job that requires standing for prolonged periods, and obesity—the last of which often means a person who has type 2 diabetes (for more about obesity, see the chapter "Diabetes and Obesity").

### Are people with diabetes prone to varicose veins?

No, people with diabetes are not prone to varicose veins any more than the general population. But certain conditions may mean a higher risk for people with diabetes. For example, many overweight or obese people with type 2 diabetes have varicose veins, as both are associated with obesity. In addition, because it is estimated that roughly half of people age 50 and up have some degree of varicose veins, and type 2 diabetes is often considered age related, older people may suffer from both conditions.

# DIABETES AND BLOOD PRESSURE

### What is blood pressure?

Blood pressure, as the term implies, is the pressure of the blood in the bloodstream (circulatory system). This pressure rises with each heartbeat and falls when your heart rests between beats and can change from minute to minute, depending, for example, on whether a person is active, sleeping, resting, or under stress. Blood pressure is the lowest in veins and the highest in the arteries when the ventricles of the heart contract. This pumping of blood around the body gives it energy and the oxygen needed to survive. Blood pressure is most often used for diagnosis of certain heart- and blood-related problems in a patient. This is because it is closely related to the force and rate of a person's heartbeat and the elasticity and diameter of the arterial walls (depending, for example, on whether there is a buildup of plaque in a person's arteries that would narrow the vessels).

### What are the two numbers associated with blood pressure measurements?

Two numbers are associated with blood pressure: the systolic (top number) and diastolic (bottom number). For example, for a reading of 140/90, the top number is the systolic number (the measurement of the pressure when the heart's ventricles contract as blood pushes through the heart), or 140. The diastolic number (the measurement when the heart relaxes or the pressure maintained by the arteries between heartbeats) is 90. This is often stated as 140/90 mm Hg, or "140 over 90 millimeters mercury," or how blood pressure is measured by a blood pressure machine. Currently—a much debated topic—the blood pressure for normal resting adults (over age 20) is most often 140/90. These numbers have changed on the basis of new research. In fact, less than a half decade ago, most physicians suggested that a reading of 120/80 was considered healthy (see below about changing blood pressure reading guidelines).

## What new blood pressure guidelines were recently suggested?

According to the American Heart Association, a blood pressure reading below 120/80 for an adult over age 20 is recommended. But these numbers are currently being debated, and in 2014, the National Institutes of Health changed its blood pressure guidelines for the first time in 11 years. This was based on 2013 research presented in the *Journal of the American Medical Association* that suggested new guidelines for blood pressure readings depending on age and/or health conditions.

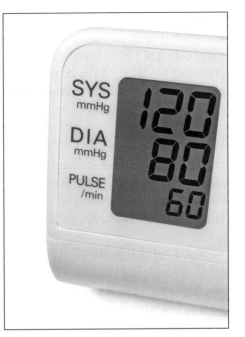

A blood pressure measurement of 120/80 is considered good for healthy adults in their twenties, but older adults may be fine with a reading of 15/90.

For example, the researchers recommended for the general population an increase from 140/90 to 150/90 mm Hg. It was suggested that among adults age 60 and older with high blood pressure, the goal should be a target blood pressure under 150/90; among adults ages 30 to 59 with high blood pressure, a target blood pressure under 140/90; and among adults with diabetes or chronic kidney disease, a target blood pressure under 140/90. Even though the systolic and diastolic numbers are "higher," doctors still recommend keeping blood pressure at a healthy low level and, if necessary, to make lifestyle changes to keep it low.

## What are hypertension and hypotension?

Hypertension is another way of saying high blood pressure. It is often referred to as a "silent killer." This is because it usually has no obvious symptoms, meaning not many people are aware they have it. In general, it occurs when a person's blood is pumping through the heart and blood vessels with too much force. It is usually found when a person has his or her blood pressure taken. If one or both of the numbers in the systolic and diastolic blood pressure measurements are high compared with what is considered normal in the overall human population, it can be an indication of hypertension. Although it is often a debated subject, it is thought that in healthy people, a blood pressure reading of 140/90 is considered normal (this often depends on whether the person's physician has adopted the new guidelines or not; see above). Hypotension means low blood pressure, in which a systolic pressure is below 100 mm Hg. Most commonly, it is caused by overly aggressive treatment for hypertension.

### Why is keeping a healthy blood pressure important to a person with diabetes?

High blood pressure is something a person with diabetes should try to prevent. This is mainly because high blood pressure can damage blood vessels, as does diabetes. Such damage from both conditions can greatly increase the risk of cardiovascular disease and other vascular problems.

### What are some risk factors for hypertension?

In the general population, several risk factors are connected to hypertension. For example, severe high blood pressure is three times higher for African Americans versus Caucasians. Older people are at a higher risk for hypertension (it is estimated that almost half of the people age 74 and older have hypertension, whether they have diabetes or not). If you are 35 or older, use oral contraceptives, or smoke, the risk of hypertension is increased. If you are obese or have a body mass index higher than 30 (which is often associated with type 2 diabetes), then the risk for hypertension is greater. And if you have diabetes or kidney disease, the risk of developing hypertension is greatly increased.

### Who is affected by hypertension?

High blood pressure can affect any human on the planet. Men, women, and children of all ages and all ethnic origins and races can have high blood pressure. But certain conditions increase a person's risk of developing hypertension. Some of the most common reasons are obesity, physical inactivity, and an unhealthful diet. High blood pressure has also often been tied to nicotine, salt, caffeine, and alcohol consumption in many studies. In addition, it can be genetic, as it is often common in various families and in certain ethnic groups. If a person's blood pressure is too high—often from the narrowing of the arteries because of the buildup of fatty deposits on the walls (plaque)—it can cause serious damage to the heart and blood ves-

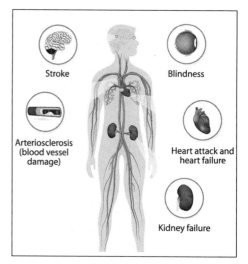

High blood pressure could lead to a number of serious ailments, from heart disease to even blindness and kidney failure.

sels. Such damage can cause the heart to lose its ability to pump well. It can also cause blood vessels to lose their elasticity and ability to carry blood efficiently. High blood pressure also increases the risk of stroke, heart attack, kidney failure, and congestive heart failure.

## Is there a "good" blood pressure reading for people who have diabetes?

The goal for patients with hypertension who do not have diabetes is usually 140/90 or below (not too low, but around that reading). For patients with hypertension and diabetes (or chronic kidney disease), the ideal goal has usually been a blood pressure of 130–135/80 (said as 130–135 [systolic] over 80 [diastolic]) or just below (readings depend on the study). But changes in blood pressure guidelines now propose a maximum target of 140/90.

## What percentage of people with diabetes have hypertension?

It is estimated that about 30 percent of people ages 50 and over have hypertension. Depending on the study, it is estimated that 20 to 60 percent of people with diabetes have high blood pressure. Overall, it is known that hypertension often affects people with diabetes. It is not known why there seems to be such a correlation between the two conditions. But it may be a "concurrent" or "simultaneous" effect in which factors associated with both diseases—such as obesity, a high-fat and high-sodium diet, and inactivity—lead to both hypertension and diabetes.

## Why are kidney disease, type 1 diabetes, and hypertension linked?

It is thought that hypertension in people with type 1 diabetes may be an indicator of kidney disease. In fact, it is known that hypertension is one of the principal causes of diabetic kidney disease and kidney failure. This occurs as blood vessels are damaged because of tension from high blood pressure. Along with the higher blood pressure, if a person has diabetes, then elevated levels of glucose can also damage blood vessels. And if the person also has high cholesterol, there is an even higher risk of blood-vessel damage. (For more about diabetes and kidney disease, see the chapter "How Diabetes Affects the Urinary System.")

## Does salt affect blood pressure, especially if a person has diabetes?

Most health care professionals agree that, for most people, ingesting too much salt can cause the body to develop high blood pressure over time. In fact, eating too much salt causes the body to hold extra water in order to eliminate the salt from the person's system. For some people, this causes extra pressure in the blood, causing a rise in blood pressure. The additional water also puts stress on the blood vessels and heart, and when the blood pressure increases, it puts even more pressure on the blood vessels and heart. Thus, the American Heart Association suggests that people with high blood pressure, or a tendency toward developing high blood pressure, should eat foods lower in salt, along with lower amounts of fats and calories. The AHA also recommends that a person ingest no more than 1,500 milligrams of sodium per day. To compare, a teaspoon of salt is about 2,400 milligrams of sodium. (This number has recently been highly debated; for more about the sodium controversy, see the chapter "Diabetes and Nutrition.")

For a person with diabetes, the effect of salt on blood pressure is also an issue. According to the Joslin Diabetes Center, having diabetes does not mean having to cut salt and sodium from the diet. However, people with diabetes should cut back on their sodium intake since they are more likely to have high blood pressure—a leading cause of heart disease—than people without diabetes.

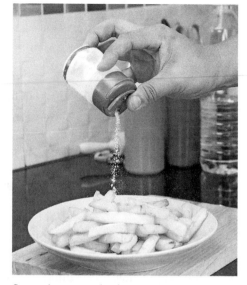

Consuming too much salt is never a good idea because it affects high blood pressure, which is also an issue with diabetics, of course.

### Do some high blood pressure drugs affect the body's insulin levels?

Yes. Drugs to lower high blood pressure can have different effects on insulin sensitivity in the body. The best way to find out which drugs have such effects is to ask a health care provider about the interactions of certain medications with the body's insulin. For a person who has prediabetes or diabetes, such questions are necessary, since insulin balance is so crucial to keeping the blood glucose in a healthy balance.

### What recent study showed a possible link between the time a person takes his or her high blood pressure medication and type 2 diabetes?

In a recent study, scientists uncovered a possible link between the time when a patient takes blood pressure medication and that person's risk of developing type 2 diabetes. Unlike people without high blood pressure (hypertension), people with high blood pressure do not experience a drop in blood pressure at night (called "non-dipping"). The researchers monitored people without diabetes, and a certain percentage of them had hypertension. After six years of monitoring the patients, the researchers found that the "non-dippers" were at higher risk of developing type 2 diabetes, while those whose blood pressure dropped at night were at a lower risk. The researchers also did a separate experiment, in which half the participants with high blood pressure took their blood pressure medication in the morning, while the other half took the medication before going to bed. They found that the participants who took their medications at bedtime not only lowered their nighttime blood pressure but also lowered their risk of developing type 2 diabetes by 57 percent compared with those who took the medication in the morning.

Overall, the scientists believe that the connections between type 2 diabetes and blood pressure may be hormonal. For instance, hormones such as adrenaline and angiotensin both contribute to high blood pressure and type 2 diabetes. Thus, for example, when angiotensin is targeted by blood pressure medications and therefore lowered, so is the risk of developing high blood pressure and diabetes. More studies have to be conducted before people change their medications, which is why it is best for a person with diabetes and/or high blood pressure to discuss such possible interactions with a health care professional.

## Can high blood pressure be "cured"?

According to most health care researchers, high blood pressure cannot be "cured," but it can be controlled in many ways. For example, most doctors treat high blood pressure patients with medication and/or through lifestyle modification, with both directed by the health care professional. Overall, a person with diabetes should discuss blood pressure goals with the health care professional.

# DIABETES AND BLOOD

## What are the main components of human blood?

Blood is considered a complex tissue—or group of similar cells—suspended in a fluid medium for easy transport through blood vessels. The following lists the four main components of human blood:

*Plasma*—Plasma is the liquid portion of the blood, and its principal component is water. Within the water are necessary elements that allow humans to live, especially dissolved salts, nutrients, and gases, along with molecular wastes being removed. It also contains clotting factors, hormones, enzymes, and antibodies.

*Red blood cells*—The red blood cells—scientific name, erythrocytes—are the most abundant cell type in the blood fluid. These dish-shaped cells measure about 8 micrometers in diameter. They lack a central nucleus like many other types of cells and cannot reproduce. But they have an extremely important job as they carry hemoglobin (a red, oxygen-carrying pigment that, when bound to oxygen, is called oxyhemoglobin) and

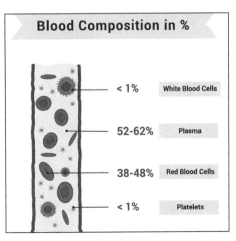

Human blood is composed of plasma, red blood cells, platelets, and white blood cells.

169

oxygen throughout the body. These cells only live about 120 days, forming in the bone marrow and being recycled in the liver.

*White blood cells*—White blood cells are also formed in the bone marrow. They die off fighting infections and are one of the major components of pus.

*Platelets*—Platelets—scientific name thrombocytes—are small, non-cellular components (actually cell fragments) that form in the bone marrow from megakaryocytes (large bone marrow cells) and are the main reason blood clots so well.

### How does human blood clot?

For most humans, the ability of blood to clot is vital. If it couldn't, then even a small cut could mean bleeding to death. Simply put, blood clotting (or thrombus) involves a mass of protein fibers that trap lymph and red blood cells, eventually hardening into a cap (generally called a scab) that protects the damaged area. The clotting reaction is thought to be platelets in the area of a cut releasing chemicals into the bloodstream, starting the formation of a clot through a series of enzyme-controlled reactions.

### What is the connection between blood clotting, arteries, and diabetes?

According to the American Heart Association, diabetes increases the risk of plaque buildup in the arteries, which can cause blood clots. In fact, some studies indicated that a very high percentage of people who have diabetes will eventually die of clot-related causes.

# DIABETES, BLOOD CHOLESTEROL, AND TRIGLYCERIDES

### What is blood cholesterol?

Blood cholesterol (or serum blood cholesterol) is a waxy, fatlike substance. Cholesterol is found in all the cells of the human body and helps to maintain the strength and flexibility of the cell membranes (thin layers of the cell). Cholesterol is obtained from food and is also naturally produced by the body. Humans need some cholesterol, but if found in excess levels in the body, cholesterol can often result in an increase in certain diseases, especially heart problems.

### Why is there a connection between cardiovascular disease and diabetes?

At this writing, researchers really do not know why there is such a strong relationship between diabetes and cardiovascular disease. This is because the majority of people with diabetes also have other heart disease risk factors, such as high blood pressure, high triglycerides, and obesity (some researchers would add higher levels of LDL, the "bad" cholesterol, and lower levels of HDL, the "good" cholesterol, to the list). But currently, many scientists are debating just how "bad" and "good" the two types of cholesterol are for people and just how much is detrimental.

## What are the so-called "good and bad cholesterols"?

There are, according to doctors, "good" and "bad" elements in the human body that can affect the body's healthy balance, especially in the circulatory system (or in other words, the heart and blood). In particular, if too much LDL, or low-density lipoprotein, often called the "bad" cholesterol, (although it is not a cholesterol; see sidebar) circulates in the blood, it can create a buildup of what is called plaque on

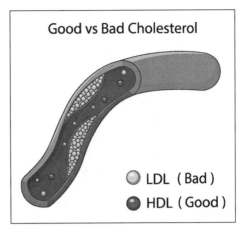

HDLs are the cholesterols in your blood that help prevent clotting, while LDLs can create blockage.

the inner walls of the arteries that feed the heart and brain. This in turn can cause the arteries to narrow and become less flexible (in excess, such plaque buildup is called atherosclerosis).

HDL, or what is often called the "good" cholesterol (although, again, it is not a cholesterol) or high-density lipoprotein, is thought to protect the body against heart attacks by carrying blood cholesterol away from the arteries and to the liver, where it is passed from the body. In addition, it may even slow plaque buildup. Yet another player in the body's cholesterol levels is Lp(a)—a genetic variation of LDL cholesterol. In particular, a high level of Lp(a) may be a high risk factor for the premature formation of fatty deposits in the arteries. Although not much is known about Lp(a) at this time, it may be connected to the buildup of fatty deposits.

## What are the suggested cholesterol levels for an adult?

Many factors affect our bodies—and one of them has to do with our cholesterol levels, especially in terms of the heart. The following, from the American Heart Association, lists what is currently thought to be the best cholesterol levels for an adult:

### Cholesterol Level Guidelines

| Total Cholesterol Level | Category |
| --- | --- |
| Less than 200 mg/dL | Desirable level that puts you at lower risk for coronary heart disease. A cholesterol level of 200 mg/dL or higher raises your risk. |
| 200 to 239 mg/dL | Borderline high |
| 240 mg/dL and above | High blood cholesterol. A person with this level has more than twice the risk of coronary heart disease as someone whose cholesterol is below 200 mg/dL. |

## Why are terms "HDL cholesterol" and "LDL cholesterol" often confusing?

The terms "HDL and LDL cholesterols" are often misnomers. This is because, although they are associated with cholesterol, they are truly not types of cholesterol. In reality, both are fat–protein compounds that transport cholesterol though the blood and thus throughout the body. HDL tends to carry blood cholesterol away from the arteries, and LDL tends to deposit cholesterol on the artery walls. One of the main problems with these terms is easy to see: When the blood cholesterol is *attached* to a lipoprotein—either HDL or LDL—the entire complex can be referred to as HDL and LDL cholesterol.

### What is the connection between atherosclerosis and diabetes?

Atherosclerosis occurs when lipids, particularly cholesterol, build up on the side arterial walls. Risk factors for atherosclerosis include cigarette smoking, a high-fat/high-cholesterol diet, and hypertension. For people who have either type 1 or type 2 diabetes—conditions that include inflammation and slow blood flow—the development of atherosclerosis can be dramatically accelerated.

### How do statin drugs work?

Statins are a group of drugs that work to lower cholesterol levels, particularly the "bad cholesterol," or the low-density lipoprotein known as LDL. The drugs work in two ways: They block an enzyme that is needed for cholesterol production, and they increase LDL receptors in the liver. (Cholesterol can only get into cells by binding to specific receptors that remove the LDL from blood. The extra receptors that statins create help decrease the cholesterol levels.) As Americans are more aware that high cholesterol is a major risk factor for heart disease, statins have become increasingly popular.

### What recent study indicated that certain statin drugs can lower the risk of amputation of the extremities, especially for people with diabetes?

Although giving cholesterol-lowering statins to people with type 2 diabetes has been around since 2010, the studies conducted have not been extensive. But a long-term study with close to 17,000 participants conducted in 2016 found that people with PAD (peripheral artery disease)—including many people with diabetes—seem to have a 22 to 33 percent lower risk of leg or other limb amputation when taking statins. The statins, many of them routinely supplied to people who have PAD, apparently lower cholesterol levels enough to cut back on the formation of arterial plaque. For many people with diabetes, the statin dosage has to be high, and if they can tolerate the medication—along with making other lifestyle changes (such as exercising and not smoking)—they can often lower their risk of amputation. (For more about PAD, see this chapter.)

## Can statins increase the risk of developing diabetes?

No one really knows, but a study presented in 2015 suggested that statins can increase the risk of developing type 2 diabetes. In particular, the drugs appear to increase a person's insulin resistance and also impair the ability of the pancreas to secrete insulin. But more research needs to be done, as this study pertained only to the risk of developing diabetes—and was limited to men.

## What are triglycerides?

Triglycerides are a type of fat (lipid) found in the blood. When a person consumes a meal or snack, the body converts any of the calories it does not need to use right away into triglycerides. This is stored in the fat cells. If a person needs energy, then certain hormones allow the triglycerides to be released into the bloodstream. Because, like cholesterol, triglycerides cannot dissolve in the blood, they circulate throughout the body with the help of proteins called lipoproteins.

## What is dyslipidemia (or dyslipidaemia)?

Dyslipidemia is a condition in which a person has an abnormal amount of lipids (mainly triglycerides), cholesterol, or both. It can also mean the person has high triglycerides, low HDL cholesterol, and often type 2 diabetes. (The most common type is called hyperlipidemia, or elevated lipid levels). Dyslipidemia is divided in two ways by researchers: by phenotype, or the way it is presented in the body (including the specific type of lipid that is increased in the body), and by etiology, or the reason for the condition (such as if it is genetic or secondary to another condition). Because of its connection to fats and to being overweight or obese, dyslipidemia is often associated with people who have type 2 diabetes—and vice versa.

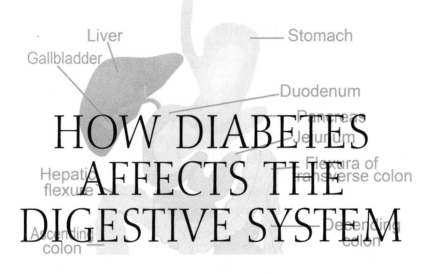

Liver

Gallbladder

Stomach

Duodenum

Pancreas

Jejunum

Hepatic flexure

Flexura of transverse colon

Ascending colon

Descending colon

# HOW DIABETES AFFECTS THE DIGESTIVE SYSTEM

## WHAT IS DIGESTION?

### How does human digestion work?

The purpose of digestion is to break down large food particles into smaller molecules that can be absorbed (as nutrients) and used by the cells of the body as a source of energy for growth and reproduction. For example, fats are broken down into glycerol and fatty acids and proteins into amino acids. The digestive tract, also called the alimentary canal, is approximately 30 feet (9 meters) long from the mouth to the anus. It is lined mostly with smooth muscles (involuntary) that push the food through the tract in a process called peristalsis.

### What are the major parts of the digestive system?

Humans have a special digestive system that allows them to break down large food particles into smaller molecules and absorb the nutrients within the food. The following lists the details of the major parts of the digestive system:

*Mouth*—The mouth, tongue, and teeth are responsible for breaking the food down with mechanical action. As omnivores, humans have teeth that include incisors for cutting, canines for tearing, and molars for grinding. As the food is in the mouth, salivary glands release saliva, which then chemically breaks down the starch in the food.

*Esophagus*—The esophagus is where the food goes after a person swallows. Food is directed into the esophagus by the epiglottis, or a flap of cartilage in the back of the pharynx (throat)—which essentially stops food from going into the windpipe (and which is why, in some circumstances, people choke on food).

*Stomach*—Food is churned mechanically in the stomach, an organ that secretes gastric juice, a mix of special enzymes and hydrochloric acid. A structure called a cardiac sphincter acts as a stop to prevent food in the stomach from backing up into the esophagus and thus burning it. A structure called the pyloric sphincter at the bottom of the stomach helps keep the food in the stomach long enough to be digested.

*Small intestine*—The upper part of the small intestine—about the first 12 inches (30 centimeters)—is called the duodenum. Bile from the liver (stored in the gallbladder) is released into the small intestine, breaking fats down and helping other digestive enzymes to work. The intestine is lined with millions of elongated projections called villi that absorb all the nutrients released from the digested foods.

*Large intestine*—The large intestine, also called the colon, has several functions. It removes undigested waste and excess water, and it harbors bacteria that create gas, digest some material, and help produce certain vitamins, such as biotin and vitamin K. All together, both intestines absorb 90 percent of the water that enters the mouth, with the small intestine absorbing most of that water. (But if too much water is removed, constipation results, or if not enough water is removed, diarrhea results.) The waste is finally released at the end of the digestive tract, or the anus.

### What are the general steps in the digestive process?

There are five major steps in the process of digestion—all of which can be affected if a person has diabetes. In general, the five steps are as follows:

*Ingestion*—The eating of any food.

*Peristalsis*—The involuntary muscle contractions that move the ingested food through the digestive tract.

*Digestion*—The conversion of the food molecules into nutrients that can then be used by the body.

*Absorption*—The passage of the nutrients into the bloodstream and/or lymphatic system to be used by the body's cells.

*Defecation*—The elimination of the undigested and unabsorbed ingested materials.

### How does digestion produce glucose?

During digestion, the fats, carbohydrates, and proteins that are consumed are broken down so they are easily used by the body's cells. One of the products from this process is glucose (sugar), one of the "fuels" that provide the energy needed to sustain all of the body's living cells.

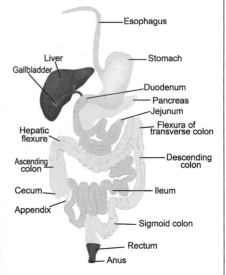

The human digestive system.

## What is the total average time from eating to excreting?

It takes an average of 53 hours, although this number is often debated, because food moves through the digestive system at different speeds. In addition, foods are not eliminated in stool in the same order in which people ingest them. For example, vegetables are easier to digest than meat, so fibrous plants typically move through the large intestines much faster.

## What is gastroparensis?

Gastroparensis is often a complication of diabetes in the digestive tract. It occurs when the nerves and muscles that help the stomach to empty do not work properly. Because there is no spontaneous movement of the muscles (motility) in the person's stomach, gastroparensis delays the emptying of the stomach contents into the small intestine after a meal. Not only does the condition interfere with a person's normal digestion, but it can also cause nausea and vomiting, along with poor nutrition and blood glucose-level problems, especially in people with diabetes.

## How does the body normally metabolize glucose?

A person without diabetes metabolizes glucose in certain ways. First, the energy for the body's cells is provided by food. When that person consumes food with carbohydrates— bread, pasta, cakes, fruits, vegetables, and legumes—the carbohydrates are converted to simple sugars (for example, glucose) in the small intestine. As the level of glucose in the blood (often referred to as blood sugar) begins to rise, the pancreas produces insulin. This insulin helps muscles and the liver absorb the glucose, preparing it to be used for energy. When a person has diabetes, the normal process of breaking down sugar goes awry, stopping the body's cells from receiving the energy they need to function properly.

## What is meant by the body's metabolism?

Metabolism (from the Greek *metabole,* meaning "change") refers to all the physical and chemical processes involved in the activities of the body. It includes changing nutrients into usable energy for the body, the synthesis of proteins, helping with the physical construction of the body's many cells and cell parts, eliminating cellular wastes, and helping with the production of body heat (in other words, it regulates the body's temperature).

## In general, how does the body respond after eating carbohydrates in terms of blood glucose levels?

The body does several things when a person eats a food containing carbohydrates. In general, the process is as follows:

1. As the blood glucose level rises, the pancreas produces insulin. This hormone prompts the cells to absorb blood sugar for energy or storage.
2. As the cells absorb blood glucose, levels of sugar in the bloodstream begin to fall.

3. As the blood glucose levels fall, the pancreas starts making glucagon. This hormone signals the liver to start releasing stored sugar.

4. The glucose and glucagon travel throughout the body, ensuring that cells—especially brain cells—have a steady supply of blood sugar.

# DIABETES AND FATS

## What happens when a person ingests foods containing fats?

When a person ingests fats, many processes take place. In particular, if a person eats food that contains fat (mostly triglycerides), the fats go through the stomach and intestines. When the fat reaches the small intestine, it goes through a series of changes to make the fats easier to be used by the body, mainly for energy. An excess of fat in the system, especially if a person becomes overweight or obese, can lead to many health problems, including cardiovascular disease and diabetes. (For more about fats, diabetes, and obesity, see the chapter "Diabetes and Obesity.")

## How does insulin help many of the body's cells?

Insulin produced by the pancreas helps many of the body's cells, especially those in the liver, muscles, and fat tissue. The main activities insulin "tells" the cells to do are: 1) to absorb glucose, fatty acids, and amino acids and stop breaking down glucose, fatty acids, and amino acids; 2) to turn glycogen into glucose, fats into fatty acids and glycerol, and proteins into amino acids; 3) to start building glycogen from glucose, fats (triglycerides) from glycerol and fatty acids, and proteins from amino acids.

## How does the body store fat?

The body stores fat through the activity of many components. In particular, after insulin is secreted (see above), fatty acids are absorbed from the bloodstream into fat, liver, and muscle cells. The insulin acts on the cells, turning the fatty acids into fat molecules, which are stored as fat droplets. The fat cells can also take up glucose and amino acids, converting them to fat molecules. (For more about insulin and the pancreas, see below.)

## What is the link between lipoprotein lipases and insulin in the body?

There is a definite link between lipoprotein lipases—the enzymes that break fats into fatty acids—and insulin in the body. In fact, the activity of the lipoprotein lipases greatly depends on the level of insulin in a person's body. If insulin is high, then the lipoprotein lipases enzyme activity is also high; if the insulin is low, then so is the lipoprotein lipases enzyme activity.

## Why does the body "prefer" to store fat rather than carbohydrates for energy?

The body's fat cells grab fat from the system (after a person eats certain fats) more readily than carbohydrates. This is because of how much energy is expended to store fats versus carbohydrates. For example, if a person has around 100 calories in extra fat in the bloodstream, the fat cells only use up about 2.5 calories of energy to store that fat. If the person has 100 calories in extra glucose in his or her bloodstream, then it takes about 23 calories of energy to convert the glucose for the body's fat stores.

# DIABETES AND THE PANCREAS, LIVER, AND GALLBLADDER

## What are accessory organs in the digestive system?

The pancreas, liver, and gallbladder are considered to be accessory organs in digestion. They are "accessory" in that none of these organs is a part of the digestive tract (beginning at the mouth and ending at the anus). But overall, they contribute important chemicals, enzymes, and lubricants necessary for the functioning of the digestive system.

## What cells in the pancreas are important to digestion?

The pancreas has both endocrine and exocrine cells, supplying hormones and enzymes for digestion, respectively. The acinar cells (also called *acini,* from the Latin, meaning "grapes," as their structure resembles clusters of grapes) are responsible for secreting digestive enzymes. (For more about how the pancreas acts as an endocrine gland, see the chapter "How Diabetes Affects the Endocrine System.")

## How are the enzymes in the pancreas involved in the small intestine?

The enzymes in the pancreas are responsible for a major part of chemical digestion in the small intestine. They reach the small intestine through a long tube that links the bile duct with the pancreatic duct. The secretions of digestive juices from the pancreas are highly alkaline (generally the opposite of acidic; a pH of 8) and are composed of many enzymes. These enzymes break down all types of food and neutralize what is called the chyme, or the acidic, soupy mixture of partially digested food that forms in the stomach (it's the ingested food that sits in the stomach for one to three hours after eating). In most adults, nearly 1.6 quarts (1.5 liters)—sometimes more—of these digestive juices are secreted by the cells of the pancreas daily.

## What is the function of the liver?

The liver is the second-largest organ in the body (the skin is the largest). It weighs 3 pounds (1.4 kilograms) in adults and represents about 2.5 percent of the total body weight. This large organ has more than 500 vital functions, too many to examine in this

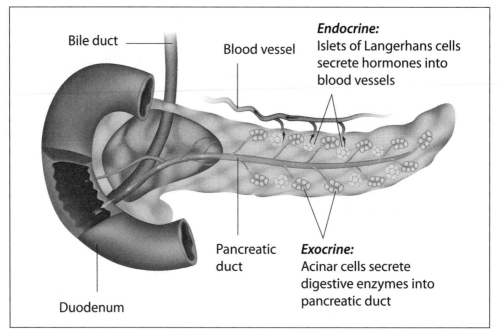

Bile duct

Blood vessel

**Endocrine:**
Islets of Langerhans cells secrete hormones into blood vessels

Pancreatic duct

**Exocrine:**
Acinar cells secrete digestive enzymes into pancreatic duct

Duodenum

The pancreas not only provides vital hormones to the blood, it also excretes digestive enzymes.

text. It is often called the "wastebasket" of the human body because it collects and processes so many substances essential for the body to function properly. For example, the liver is responsible for filtering the blood, making special proteins that protect the body from infection, removing alcohol and poisons from the blood, and producing proteins that help the blood to clot. In terms of the body and diabetes, the liver plays a crucial role in managing blood sugar levels.

### What is a unique feature of the liver?

The liver is unique in the human body, as it is the only organ that can regenerate itself. As much as 75 percent of the liver may be removed, and in most people (usually not people with hepatitis C; see sidebar), it will grow back to the same shape and form within a few weeks.

### What are the digestive functions of the liver?

The liver's major function in the digestive tract is to produce and secrete bile. Other liver functions that help digestion include separating and filtering waste products from food nutrients, storing glucose until it's needed, and producing many chemical substances—such as cholesterol—that the body and cells need to survive.

### What is hepatitis, and can a person with diabetes contract it?

The most common forms of hepatitis are A, B, and C (there are also hepatitis D and E)—
and all have to do with the liver. According to many studies, there is often a connection

between diabetes and hepatitis. The connection varies depending on the type of hepatitis. The following gives a general description and how it may be linked to diabetes:

*Hepatitis A*—This type of hepatitis is a virus that is transmitted from person to person mainly through feces, causing an inflammation of the liver. The most common transmission occurs when a person ingests food or water contaminated with the feces of an infected person. It can also spread from contaminated shellfish and from foods or drinks prepared by someone with the virus. It is divided by type into acute (with short-lived symptoms that usually begin suddenly) and chronic (in which the liver is inflamed for at least six months, producing mild symptoms). Acute symptoms can include stomach pain, jaundice, light-colored stools, and dark yellow urine. Hepatitis A can be transmitted to a person with diabetes, but there is thought to be no solid connection between the two conditions. Studies are being conducted to see whether a person with acute viral hepatitis also has underlying diabetes—and whether that can cause the hepatitis to become chronic.

*Hepatitis B*—This type of hepatitis is a virus usually spread when blood or other body fluids from an infected person enters another person's body. For example, decades ago, when the blood supply was not as diligently screened, people could contract hepatitis B through routine blood transfusions. It is also spread through sexual contact and from an infected mother to her baby during childbirth. For people with diabetes, hepatitis B has been spread through the sharing of glucose meters, lancets, and other supplies such as syringes and insulin pens, which is why it is best for a person with diabetes not to share diabetic supplies.

*Hepatitis C*—This type of hepatitis is a virus and is the leading cause of liver damage in the United States. It often takes decades to manifest itself. Once it develops, the disease can lead to scarring of tissues that can eventually destroy the liver. At this stage, a liver transplant is often necessary, but even so, it will not eradicate the virus from the body. There is also a hepatitis C–diabetes connection: People with hepatitis C have a higher prevalence of type 2 diabetes, and people with diabetes are more likely than most people to have hepatitis C. In fact, some researchers suggest that type 2 diabetes is often a symptom of hepatitis C.

## What does the liver produce if a person's body runs low on glucose for energy?

If a person needs energy and is low on glucose, then the liver produces ketones. The ketones are made from fatty acids in the body in a process called ketogenesis. Ketones circulate in the body at any given time but their levels seem to be higher when a person is exercising for sustained periods or is fasting.

## What is the connection between ketones and diabetes?

For a person with diabetes, the level of ketones increases when the body fails to produce enough insulin. Ketones are also produced when there is not enough insulin available to increase the glucose in the body. If glucose levels are not brought into balance, a condition called diabetic ketoacidosis can occur.

## What is fatty liver disease?

Fatty liver disease is caused by an increase of fat buildup in the liver. It is usually broken down into two types: alcoholic and nonalcoholic fatty liver disease (NAFLD). As the name implies, alcoholic fatty liver disease is prevalent in alcoholics. Nonalcoholic fatty liver disease is most often found in overweight people, including those who have type 2 diabetes. In fact, it is estimated that of all overweight people, around 54 percent to as high as 74 percent have NAFLD. This disease can harm the liver and may add to a person's risk for heart disease. In the United States alone, this disease affects around one in five American adults—some research suggests one in three—especially those who are overweight, obese, and/or who suffer from diabetes.

## What conditions can cause a fatty liver?

At one time, it was associated with people who drank excessively, but now, between lack of exercise and poor diet, more people are experiencing the disease. In addition, research has shown that certain people may carry a special genetic variation called single nucleotide polymorphism (or SNP) that make them more susceptible to developing a fatty liver. Even the types of fat a person eats can play a part in developing a fatty liver. For example, some fats can cause inflammation that can increase the risk of liver disease, such as some polyunsaturated fats in red meat that contain omega-6 fatty acids. The best way to stave off nonalcoholic fatty liver disease is obvious: lose weight and eat more healthful foods.

## Do only overweight or obese people with diabetes have fatty livers?

No, even people who have diabetes and are at a normal body weight can have a fatty liver, although overweight people are more likely to have the disease. Research has

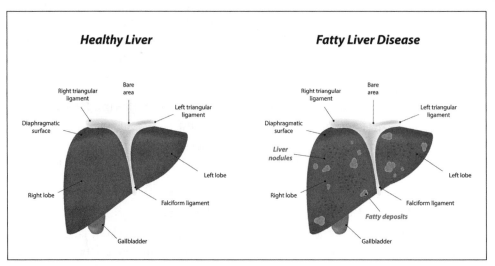

When fat builds up in the liver, it can cause fatigue and abdominal pain. If left untreated, the next stage can be cirrhosis, liver failure, and cancer.

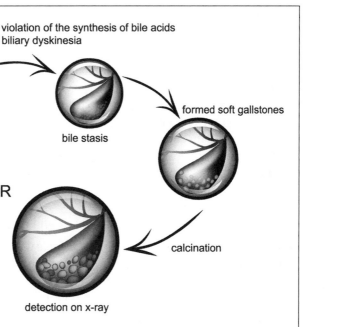

Too much cholesterol or bilirubin in the blood can lead to the formation of gallstones. The material builds up in the gallbladder, then calcifies to form the stones.

shown that the type of diabetes a person has can affect the health of the liver. For example, people who have type 1 diabetes with controlled hyperglycemia (high blood glucose levels) are much less likely to have a fatty liver. But there is a 70 percent correlation between liver disease and type 2 diabetes. In fact, some studies estimate that around 98 percent of people with any type of diabetes have some form of fatty liver disease.

## What is bile?

Bile is an alkaline liquid composed mostly of water, bile salts, bile pigments (bilirubin), fats, and cholesterol. It is essential for digestion of fats because it breaks down fats into fatty acids, which can then be absorbed by the digestive tract. Bile gets its color from bilirubin, a waste product from the breakdown of worn-out red blood cells.

## What is the major purpose of the gallbladder?

The gallbladder (from the Latin *galbinus,* meaning "greenish yellow"), a pear-shaped, small sac, is mainly a storage vessel. It is connected by ducts to both the liver and small intestine. It stores bile until it is needed in the duodenum. Its name is derived from its usual color of green from the accumulation of bile. The gallbladder is a nonessential organ. It may be removed surgically—in a procedure called a cholecystectomy—if it is diseased or injured. Once the gallbladder is removed, bile flows from the liver directly to the small intestine, where it continues to aid digestion. The excess bile is then stored 183 in the bile duct. This is why individuals who have had their gallbladder removed usually lead normal lives and enjoy a regular diet.

## What are the two types of gallstones?

Gallstones are hardened masses (stones) of bile. Gallstones form when bile contains too much cholesterol, bile salts, or bilirubin. The two types of gallstones are cholesterol stones and pigment stones. Cholesterol stones are more common, accounting for nearly 80 percent of all instances of gallstones. They are usually yellow-green in color and are made primarily of hardened cholesterol. An insufficient amount of water may also contribute to the development of cholesterol gallstones. Pigment stones are small, dark stones made of bilirubin.

## Is there a connection between gallstones and diabetes?

No one understands why, but in general, people with diabetes have more gallstone problems than the general population. One possible reason may be that people with diabetes—in particular, type 2—are often overweight or obese, both conditions being linked to the formation of gallstones. In addition, triglycerides are linked to type 2 diabetes and are thought to encourage gallstone formation.

## How serious are gallstones?

Many individuals who have gallstones are asymptomatic, and treatment is not necessary. However, if the stones block a duct, bile may be prevented from entering the small intestine. Surgery is then often recommended to remove the gallbladder. Women between ages 20 and 60 are twice as likely to develop gallstones as men.

Kidney

Infection

Ureter

Bladder

Prostate

Urethra

Wh
blo
cell

# HOW DIABETES AFFECTS THE URINARY SYSTEM

## THE URINARY SYSTEM

### What are the major parts and functions of the urinary system?

The functions of the urinary system include regulation of body fluids, removal of meta-bolic waste products, regulation of the volume and chemical makeup of blood plasma, and excretion of toxins from the body. The major parts of the urinary system are the kid-neys, the urinary bladder, two ureters, and the urethra, and in men the prostate. Each component of the urinary system has a unique function. Urine is manufactured in the kidneys. The urinary bladder serves as a temporary storage reservoir for urine. The ureters transport urine from the kidney to the bladder, while the urethra transports urine from the bladder to the outside of the body (it also carries semen; for more about the urethra and male reproduction, see the chapter "How Diabetes Affects the Repro-ductive System").

### Why is it important for a person with diabetes to drink enough water each day?

One reason that a person with diabetes—or even without diabetes—needs to drink enough water each day is dehydration. If a person with diabetes becomes dehydrated, then major problems can occur with blood glucose levels (and vice versa). The kidneys need water to eliminate the body's excess glucose and some wastes, so if a person does not drink enough water, the kidneys will look elsewhere in the body for fluid in order to function—which means a person will become drier, usually first in the eyes and mouth. In addition, the higher the glucose level, the more fluids a person drinks (and why thirst is one of the symptoms of diabetes). The symptoms of mild dehydration in-clude thirst, headache, dry mouth and eyes, dizziness, fatigue, and dark-colored urine. Severe dehydration causes all those symptoms plus low blood pressure, sunken eyes, weak pulse and/or rapid heartbeat, confusion, and lethargy. It is interesting to note, too, that older people with or without diabetes do not get dehydration symptoms as readily as younger people. Thus, if an older person has diabetes or uncontrolled glucose levels, he or she may not be diagnosed with dehydration as readily.

### Does drinking water lower a person's blood glucose level?

No, this idea is a myth. Drinking an adequate amount of water helps eliminate toxins and supports a person's kidney function. What lower a person's blood glucose level are insulin, exercise, and the body's kidney function.

# DIABETES AND THE KIDNEYS

### What are the kidneys?

The kidneys are located on each side of the spinal column in the lumbar region, just underneath the ribcage. The kidney has two layers: the outer layer, called the cortex, which is reddish brown and granular, and the inner zone, the medulla, which is a darker, reddish brown in color. The medulla is subdivided into six to 18 cone-shaped sections called the pyramids. The pyramids are inverted so that each base faces the cortex and the tops project toward the center of the kidney. Separating the pyramids are bands of tissue called renal columns. A renal lobe consists of a renal pyramid and its surrounding tissue.

### What are the major roles of the kidneys?

The kidneys have several important roles in the human body. The two kidneys most people have (people have been born with one kidney or may have a kidney in the "wrong" place, such as low in the pelvic area) are responsible for filtering the blood. They help control blood pressure by producing rennin, an enzyme that regulates the volume of fluid in the body. They are important to maintain healthy levels of minerals, such as potassium, chloride, and sodium. They also are responsible for regulating concentrations of phosphate, which is necessary in maintaining the body's pH by making sure the body does not become too acidic. They also process two major hormones, erythropoietin and vitamin D (yes, bioactive vitamin D is considered a hormone). These hormones help produce red blood cells and help the body convert vitamin D through the skin by the action of sunlight on the skin, respectively.

## How much blood is filtered daily by the kidneys, and how much is filtered in an average lifespan?

The kidneys filter about 120 to 150 quarts (113 to 142 liters) of blood daily and produce about 4 ounces of filtrate per minute. Each day, about 1.5 to 2 quarts (1.4 to 1.9 liters) of urine are eliminated by the kidneys and eventually excreted. The entire blood supply is filtered through the kidneys 60 times per day, with the kidneys receiving 20 to 25 percent of the total heart output, or approximately 2.5 pints (1,200 milliliters) of blood per minute. This means kidneys in a person living 73 years have filtered almost 1.3 million gallons of blood.

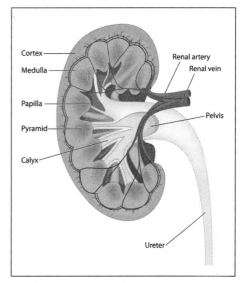

Anatomy of the human kidney.

## What are kidney stones?

Most people who have had a kidney stone attack (called renal lithiasis) will tell you it is a very painful experience. The stones are usually small, hard deposits that form inside the kidneys and are made of minerals and acid salts. They often affect many places along the urinary tract from the kidneys to the bladder—and can be in one or both kidneys. They seem to form when the urine becomes concentrated and/or when the urine contains more crystal-forming substances, such as calcium or uric acid, than can be diluted by the fluid in the urine. The stones are most commonly classified as calcium, struvite, uric acid, and cystine stones—all of which form for various reasons.

## Are kidney stones connected to diabetes?

For some people, yes, there may be a connection between the development of kidney stones and having diabetes. The common risk factors include diet (especially a high intake of animal protein, sodium, and sugar—along with not drinking enough fluids); some medications (for example, in some people who take calcium supplements); a family history of kidney stones (although no one agrees upon this factor versus the influence of diet and environment); and certain health conditions, including gout, obesity—and diabetes.

## Is there a rise in the number of people with kidney stones?

According to a recent study published in the *Clinical Journal of the American Society of Nephrology,* there appears to be a rise in the number of people with kidney stones.

The researchers analyzed data from more than 150,000 people in South Carolina who experienced kidney stones from 1997 to 2012. They found that the frequency of kidney stones increased 16 percent over the study period, with the biggest increases in children, women, and African Americans. They also noted that, as past studies have shown, more men have kidney stones than women, but women in this study outnumbered the men with kidney stones among those under age 25.

According to Harvard Medical School, there seems to be no direct reason for the rise in kidney stones. There are some speculations, including the rise in obesity in recent years (and also connected to type 2 diabetes). Some scientists even mention climate change, citing that warmer temperatures may increase dehydration, one of the factors often mentioned as a contributor to kidney stones.

## In the United States, what percentage of people who have diabetes develop chronic kidney disease (CKD)?

Even when it is controlled, diabetes can lead to chronic kidney disease (CKD) and eventual kidney failure. In the United States alone, it is often said that diabetes is the most common cause of kidney failure. And even though most people with diabetes do not develop CKD that is severe enough to lead to kidney failure, it is estimated that of the nearly 25.8 million people in the United States with diabetes, around 180,000 are living with CKD as the result of their diabetes.

## What are the major causes of kidney failure in the United States?

According the National Institutes of Health's National Institute of Diabetes and Digestive and Kidney Diseases, to date, diabetes affects 25.8 million people of all ages in the United States, and around 40 percent of people who have diabetes may eventually develop kidney disease (CKD). This accounts for 44 percent of all the new cases of kidney failure each year. The main reasons for kidney disease are as follows:

- 1.4 percent urologic diseases
- 2.3 percent cystic kidney

### What is eGFR?

The term eGFR stands for estimated glomerular filtration rate, or flow rate in the kidneys. Doctors will often use the eGFR when assessing kidney damage, including in people who have diabetes and may have symptoms of kidney disease. For example, an eGFR of less than 60 milliliters per minute is often indicative of kidney disease. Doctors may also use other tests, such as looking for protein in the person's urine, as even a small amount may indicate trouble with the kidneys (although everyone is different in terms of protein in the system, which is why other tests are used).

- 6.6 percent glomerulonephritis (or glomerular disease, an acute inflammation of the kidney's tiny filters called glomeruli, which remove excess fluid, electrolytes, and waste from the blood and pass them into the urine)
- 17.6 percent other reasons
- 28.4 percent high blood pressure (the second major cause of kidney failure; it is important since many people with diabetes also find controlling blood pressure to be a major problem. For more about high blood pressure, see the chapter "How Diabetes Affects the Circulatory System.")
- 43.7 percent diabetes

## How is it determined that a person with diabetes has kidney disease?

There are five stages of kidney disease, with kidney failure the final and most severe stage. Certain numbers are associated with kidney disease, called the glomerular filtration rate, or GFR. This is a reflection of how the kidneys are filtering fluid per minute. The lower the number, the less efficiently the kidneys are working. It is estimated that if a person has a GFR of around 60 milliliters per minute, it could be indicative of kidney disease. And if a person has a GFR of 15 milliliters per minute or less, he or she is a candidate for renal-replacement therapy, or, in other words, either a kidney transplant or some type of kidney dialysis.

## What is kidney failure?

Kidney failure is a condition in which the kidneys fail to rid the body of waste products. It is also considered to be end-stage kidney disease (ESRD, or end-stage renal disease). It is most often treated with a kidney transplant (if a kidney can be found and/or the patient is strong enough for a transplant) or dialysis, a blood-filtering treatment (see below). Each year in the United States, more than 100,000 people are diagnosed with kidney failure.

## What are the symptoms of kidney failure?

There are several symptoms of kidney failure, including excess fluid buildup (most often seen in the legs) and a buildup of salt in the body. This is because the kidneys cannot excrete enough water and salt (in urine) from the body. This causes an increase in blood pressure, which often leads to hypertension. An indirect symptom of kidney failure is anemia owing to the decreased production of erythropoietin, a hormone secreted by the kidney that increases the rate of red blood cell production in response to falling levels of oxygen in the body's tissues. Without adequate red blood cells, a person will have fatigue and shortness of breath, two major symptoms of anemia.

## What is kidney dialysis?

Kidney dialysis is a procedure that uses a special machine to eliminate wastes, salt, and excess fluids from the blood. Dialysis is usually done because the kidneys are not functioning properly, either because of disease or injury. One of the major causes of kidney

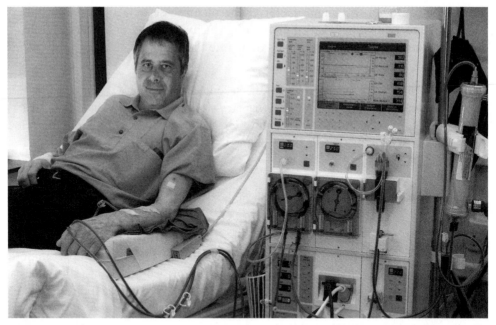
When a patient's kidneys fail and they have not been able to get a transplant, dialysis is really the only option left. Typically, patients require three treatments a week.

failure that leads to dialysis is diabetes, owing to high blood glucose levels. This excess amount of glucose damages the millions of nephrons, the small filtering units in the kidneys. A person usually needs dialysis when he or she develops end-stage kidney failure, or has lost about 85 to 90 percent of their kidney function.

### Is there any way doctors can potentially identify kidney disease in a person with diabetes?

Yes, there are ways in which doctors can potentially identify kidney disease in a person with diabetes. They use what are called markers, or chemicals produced by the body that help determine possible problems with the kidneys. In particular, doctors look at A1c values to see whether a person who has diabetes has been controlling his or her blood glucose levels in the long term. They also can assess damage to blood vessels of the kidneys (and the heart) by checking on advanced glycation end products (AGEs). Doctors also check on the kidney levels themselves, including the glomerular filtration rate (GFR) and serum albumin.

Doctors are also using several new markers to determine possible kidney disease in people with type 1 and type 2 diabetes. For example, neutrophil gelatinase-associated lipocalin (NGAL) is a protein that is produced in response to a decrease in blood flow to the kidneys or a trauma to the kidneys. Another is the enzyme N-acetyl-beta-D-glucosaminidase (NAG). An increase in activity of this enzyme may be connected to uncontrolled diabetes.

# DIABETES AND URINE

## What is a ureter?

There are two ureters, which are tubes extending from the kidney into the urinary bladder. Each ureter is 10 to 12 inches (25 to 30 centimeters) long. They begin in the kidneys as thin, hollow, narrow tubes and widen to 0.5 inches (1.7 centimeters) as they enter the bladder. Urine is transported to the bladder via the two ureters.

## Where is the urinary bladder located?

The urinary bladder is located in the abdominal cavity. In males, it is behind the rectum and above the prostate gland. In females, it is located much lower, behind the uterus and upper vagina.

## How much urine can the urinary bladder hold?

The urinary bladder is highly distensible and can vary in its capacity. As urine fills the bladder, at moderate capacity, it expands to about 5 inches (12 centimeters) long and hold 1 pint (473 milliliters) of urine. The bladder can expand to twice that capacity if necessary. It usually accumulates 0.63 to 0.85 pints (300 to 400 milliliters) of urine before emptying, but it can expand to hold 1.27 to 1.69 pints (600 to 800 milliliters).

## How does the urethra differ in males and females?

Urine is transported to the outside through the urethra, which is a thin, muscular tube that extends from the urinary bladder to the exterior of the body. The length and structure of the urethra differ between males and females. In males, the urethra is about 8 inches (20 centimeters) long and extends from the urinary bladder to the exterior. It has the dual function of transporting semen as well as urine out of the body. The female urethra is only about 1.5 inches (3 to 4 centimeters) long and extends from the bladder to the exterior opening.

## What is urea, and where is it produced?

During the process of metabolizing proteins, the body produces ammonia. Ammonia combines with carbon dioxide to form urea. Urea is the major organic component in the urine; it is eliminated by the kidneys. Humans generate about 0.75 ounces (21 grams) of urea each day.

## What is the composition of human urine?

Human urine is composed mostly of water containing organic wastes as well as some salts. The composition of urine can vary according to diet, time of day, and diseases, but overall, it is mostly water (95 percent) and organic waste products (5 percent), such as urea, uric acid, and creatinine, along with some other organic chemicals.

## How are urine tests used in diabetes diagnoses?

Urine tests were once used to detect glucose in a person's body. In addition, many doctors would taste a person's urine for sweetness—an indication of diabetes (the excess glucose, or sugar, eliminated in the urine)—or pour the urine into sand to see whether it was sweet enough to attract insects. Now most health care professionals rely on blood tests, which are much more accurate to determine diabetes. That being said, urine tests do have a place in diabetes diagnoses. For example, tests for protein in the urine may be conducted if a person with diabetes is suspected to have kidney damage. Tests for ketones in the urine may indicate hyperglycemia, too.

### Is urine always yellow in color?

Normally, dilute urine is nearly colorless. Concentrated urine is a deep yellow; colors other than yellow are not normal. Food pigments can make the urine red, and drugs can produce colors such as brown, black, blue, green, or red. Urine may also be brown, black, or red owing to disorders or diseases such as severe muscle injury or melanoma. Cloudy urine suggests the presence of pus, due to a urinary tract infection, or salt crystals from uric acid or phosphoric acid.

### Is frequent urination one of the signs of diabetes?

Yes, among other symptoms, frequent urination is often one of the signs of type 1 and type 2 diabetes. It is a symptom of high blood sugar, or hyperglycemia, or an overall rise in blood (or plasma) glucose. (For more information about the fasting plasma glucose test to measure glucose levels, see the chapter "Coping With Diabetes.")

### Is there a connection between high uric acid levels and diabetes?

Uric acid is a chemical that is created when the body breaks down substances known as purines. These are found in some foods and drinks, including liver, seafood, dried beans and peas, and beer. In people without high uric acid problems, the uric acid dissolves in the blood and travels to the kidneys, and most of it is excreted in the urine. But often, the body produces too much uric acid or the kidneys don't excrete enough, causing uric acid to build up in the blood. This buildup can create sharp crystals that eventually form in joints, causing pain and inflammation. (If a person has an excess of uric acid in the body, it is called hyperuricemia, with a blood uric acid level greater than 7 considered to be uncontrolled.) One of the more common results of such a buildup is gout.

Recent studies have shown that people who have problems with uric acid in the blood also have a nearly 20 percent increased risk of developing diabetes, along with a more than 40 percent increased risk of developing kidney disease (also often associated

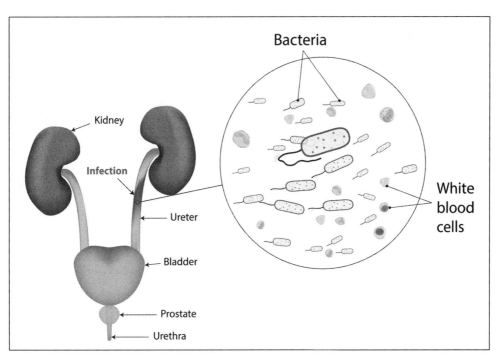

Bacteria

White blood cells

Kidney

Infection

Ureter

Bladder

Prostate

Urethra

Diabetics are more prone to urinary tract infections, which occur when bacteria contaminate the bladder, ureters, or kidneys.

with diabetes). The studies do not prove that uncontrolled uric acid levels cause these health problems, but there seems to be an association between high uric acid levels and the risk of developing these two diseases.

## What is a urinary tract infection?

A urinary tract infection, or UTI, is caused by different types of bacteria (usually *E. coli*), most often from the bowels. The bacteria often travel up the urethra to the bladder, the most commonly affected organ. If the infection is in the bladder, it is called cystitis (a lower urinary tract infection), and if it is in the kidneys and ureters, it is called pyelonephritis (an upper urinary tract infection). Symptoms include a burning sensation when urinating, strong-smelling urine, fever or chills, a pain in the back or abdomen, and cloudy, dark, or bloody urine.

## Why are women more prone to urinary tract infections?

Women are ten times more likely to suffer from urinary tract infections (UTI) than men. More than 50 percent of women will have a UTI at some point in their life. The main reason is that the urethra in women is much shorter, making it easier for bacteria to reach the bladder and cause an infection. It also becomes more of a health problem if the woman has diabetes.

193

## Do people with diabetes have more urinary tract infections?

Yes, people with diabetes seem to be more prone to developing urinary tract infections (UTI) than people who do not have diabetes. Some statistics indicate that people with type 1 and type 2 diabetes are about twice as likely to experience urinary tract infections as people without diabetes. This increased risk of UTI for diabetics may be due to several reasons. The person may have poor circulation because of diabetes, which lowers the ability of white blood cells to travel in the bloodstream and fight off infection. And if he or she has high blood glucose, it can damage the nerves of the bladder, so the person cannot sense when the organ is full. The person also may have trouble controlling the muscles that help release urine, causing bacteria to grow within the bladder.

# HOW DIABETES AFFECTS THE REPRODUCTIVE SYSTEM

## DIABETES, MENSTRUAL CYCLE, AND FEMALES

### What are the female reproductive organs?

The organs of the female reproductive system include the ovaries, the uterine tubes, the uterus, the vagina, the external organs called the vulva, and the mammary glands. The paired ovaries are the female gonads. Each ovary is approximately 1 to 2 inches (2.5 to 5 centimeters) long, 0.6 to 1.2 inches (1.5 to 3.0 centimeters) wide, and 0.24 to 0.6 inches (0.6 to 1.5 centimeters) thick, similar in size and shape to an unshelled almond. They produce the female gametes, called ova, and secrete the female sex hormones.

### What is the female reproductive cycle?

The female reproductive cycle is a general term to describe the ovarian cycle and the uterine cycle as well as the hormonal cycles that regulate them. The ovarian cycle is the monthly series of events that occur in the ovaries related to the maturation of an oocyte. The menstrual cycle is the monthly series of changes that occur in the uterus as it awaits a fertilized ovum. The reproductive cycle averages 28 days, but it may last from 24 to 35 days. A cycle of 20 to 45 days is still considered within normal range. The menstrual phase lasts five to seven days.

### In what way does diabetes affect a woman's menstrual cycle?

Diabetes' effect on a woman's menstrual cycle mainly involves the hormones that regulate the cycle—estrogen and progesterone. These hormones interact with the insulin hormone and may make a woman's body more resistant to its own insulin or injected insulin (if the woman has type 1 diabetes). This causes a rise in blood glucose either before, after, or during menstruation and lasts for about three to five days. The actual number of days and times varies from month to month and person to person. The number of days can also change because of certain conditions, such as eating a food that makes the person's blood glucose levels become unbalanced.

## How are menstruation and diabetes linked?

Unusually long, extremely irregular, or infrequent menstrual cycles may be linked to insulin resistance and the development of type 2 (or adult-onset) diabetes. In addition, there are changes in a woman's menstruation if she has type 1 diabetes, including starting menstruation a year later (on average) than women without diabetes and being more likely to have menstrual problems before age 30. Diabetes also increases a woman's chances of having longer menstrual cycles and periods, heavier periods, and an earlier onset of menopause.

## What is polycystic ovary syndrome?

Polycystic ovary syndrome (PCOS) is a disease of hormones. It affects between 5 and 20 percent of American and European women, depending on the study, and is the most common reproductive hormone disorder for women of childbearing age. It is also the number one cause of female infertility. Symptoms include ovaries with a large number of "cysts," skin discoloration, depression, fatness around the waist, and painful periods.

PCOS is often thought of as a form of prediabetes, as some of the symptoms—especially the early ones—are similar. For example, PCOS, like prediabetes, often starts with insulin resistance, which causes the body to produce high levels of insulin. (In some women, the insulin stimulates the production of male sex hormones, such as testosterone.) There are also crossovers to both diseases, such as irregular or absent periods and a link to heart disease. As with diabetes, PCOS is thought to be caused by several factors, including genetics, exposure to certain environmental conditions, and/or eating refined carbohydrates.

# DIABETES AND SEX

## How does diabetes affect female and male sexual activity?

Diabetes can cause autonomic neuropathy, or damage to nerves that take care of everyday functions. Such nerve damage can also gradually decrease sexual response in men and women, although the sex drive may be the same. Such damage may also mean a man may be unable to have erections or may reach sexual climax without ejaculating normally. Women with such nerve damage may have difficulty with arousal, lubrication, or having an orgasm.

## Do birth control pills affect a woman who has diabetes?

If a woman takes a birth control (contraceptive) pill, she may experience a difference in blood glucose levels from before she started taking the pill. But taking birth control pills is a highly debated subject, as many health care professionals believe they have a potentially harmful effect on women with diabetes. This is because many studies indicate that diabetic women who take contraceptives—or use other methods that contain estrogen—have higher blood glucose and cholesterol levels than women who are on the pill and do not have diabetes.

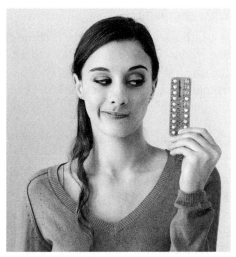

Contraceptive pills can affect blood glucose levels in women with diabetes.

## Why do some pregnant women experience gestational diabetes?

This type of diabetes occurs in about 4 percent of pregnant women and usually disappears after the baby is born. But some studies show that if a mother has gestational diabetes, both she and her child may have a higher risk of type 2 diabetes later in life. (For more details about gestational diabetes, see the chapter "Other Types of Diabetes.")

## What is the main function of the male penis?

The penis is an external organ of the male reproductive system. It consists of three parts: the root, which is where the penis is attached to the wall of the abdomen; the shaft or body; and the glans, also known as the tip of the penis. The main body of the penis has a tubular, cylindrical shape and surrounds the urethra, which transports urine to the outside of the body. Spongy tissue that can expand and contract fills the body of the penis. There is also a slit opening at the tip of the glans through which urine is excreted and semen is ejaculated.

## What is retrograde ejaculation and its connection to diabetes?

Although it is frequently, but not always, caused by diabetes, some men experience retrograde ejaculation. This is when the man's semen is not ejected through the penis but goes backward into the bladder. It is not harmful, but it can cause male infertility (in other words, the man may need help in order to father a child).

## What is erectile tissue?

The penis contains three main cylindrical bodies of erectile tissues, called the corpus cavernosa (which are two lateral bodies) and corpus spongiosum (which also contains the urethra). The three bodies are bound by a stocking of the more vascular, dense, and sensitive tissue called deep perineal fascia (tissue). Upon stimulation, blood flow to the erectile tissue is increased, resulting in an erection.

## What are sperm?

It is estimated that during the lifetime of a normal male, he will produce $10^{12}$ sperm, or one trillion sperm, equivalent to about 300 million sperm per day. Sperm are some of the smallest cells in the human body and are about 0.002 inches (0.05 millimeters) long from the head to the tip of the tail. Each sperm cell has three distinct regions: the head, the middle piece, and the tail.

## Can diabetes affect a man's sperm?

Yes, in some cases, if a male has diabetes, he will have a lower sperm count. One study found that 25 percent of men with type 2 diabetes were infertile mainly because high blood glucose had damaged the sperm. Another study indicated that men with diabetes had less sperm mobility, or the ability of the sperm to move.

## Is erectile dysfunction connected to diabetes?

Yes, it is estimated that as many as half of men with diabetes may develop erectile dysfunction (impotence), especially if they have had diabetes for many years. This is thought to be mainly because of a type of nerve damage called autonomic neuropathy (for more about autonomic neuropathy, see the chapter "How Diabetes Affects the Nervous System"). For men with diabetes who experience this problem, such drugs as sildenafil (Viagra), tadalafil (Cialis), vardenafil (Levitra), and avanafil (Stendra) are often prescribed. Other solutions include injecting medications directly into the penis, the use of certain devices to help with an erection, and surgical implants.

## Is there a connection between testosterone and diabetes?

Low testosterone is known to trigger erectile dysfunction, reduce physical strength, cause mood changes, and lower a man's sex drive. There are several connections be-

---

### What are some causes of erectile dysfunction?

Erectile dysfunction (ED, or impotence) is the inability to achieve or sustain an erection. It is often the result of disease, injury, or a side effect of certain drugs, including blood pressure drugs, antihistamines, antidepressants, tranquilizers, appetite suppressants, and cimetidine (an ulcer drug). Damage to nerves, arteries, smooth muscles, and fibrous tissues of the penis are the most common physical causes of erectile dysfunction. In addition, it is estimated that about 70 percent of ED cases are caused by some of the major diseases, including diabetes, kidney disease, chronic alcoholism, multiple sclerosis, atherosclerosis, and vascular and neurological diseases. Treatment may include lifestyle changes, adjusting medications to alleviate side effects, medications to induce erection, surgery, and testosterone-replacement therapy (see below).

tween low testosterone and diabetes. For example, one recent study showed that obesity (based on body mass index, or BMI) was strongly associated with low testosterone levels in men, a problem that often accompanies type 2 diabetes. It also showed that erectile dysfunction in men with type 2 diabetes could be caused by impaired circulation from blood vessel damage and neuropathy, or nerve damage. According to another study conducted at the University of Buffalo, men with type 2 diabetes and low levels of testosterone may benefit from TRT, or testosterone-replacement therapy. The study showed that TRT helped by improving insulin sensitivity in men, alleviating many problems associated with low testosterone.

# DIABETES AND OBESITY

## OBESITY, FAT, AND DIABETES

### In general, what is obesity?

According to the Centers for Disease Control and Prevention, in general, obesity results when a person's body fat accumulates over time, mainly as a result of what is called a chronic energy imbalance. In other words, the calories consumed exceed the calories expended in such activities as exercise. Obesity is a major health hazard worldwide. It is also extremely costly, as it is associated with workplace absenteeism, mainly because of obesity's association with other diseases, such as diabetes, hypertension, heart disease, and some cancers. Of course, eating is only part of the story when it comes to obesity. Other conditions may exist, such as thyroid disease, genetic predisposition, and/or taking certain medications.

### What is the health care definition of obesity?

According to the National Heart, Lung, and Blood Institute (in cooperation with the National Institute of Diabetes and Digestive and Kidney Disease), obesity is most often defined in terms of body mass index, or BMI. These numbers are based on a person's weight and height, with most health care professionals agreeing that there is a strong correlation between BMI and total body fat content. A person who is overweight is usually considered to have a BMI of 25 to 29, while a person who is obese has a BMI of 30 or higher. (For more about BMI, see this chapter.)

### What are some reasons for so many people being overweight or obese in the United States?

Although the subject is highly debated, a great deal of research has indicated that there are several major reasons for the overweight and obesity problems in the United States.

And the list of reasons is very long and often convoluted as not everyone has the same chemistry, eats the same, or lives under the same conditions. But there are some suggestions for why people have gained so much weight over the past several decades. For example, serving sizes have changed over that time both in homes and in restaurants (in other words, people often eat more now, mainly because food is often plentiful and available). In addition, the average American diet tends to include many foods that are high in fats and sugars. The standard portion size for many foods has increased over the past several years, including "supersized" portions at fast-food restaurants that offer

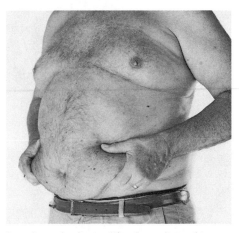

Poor diet and sedentary lifestyle are the two biggest reasons for being obese. America is facing an obesity epidemic, with nearly 36% of Americans falling into this category.

more calories, sugars, and fats. This type of diet, coupled with a lack of physical activity, often leads to people's becoming overweight and obese. In addition, life has become more stressful for many people. Stress often leads to a change in eating habits (mainly eating more) in response to negative emotions such as sadness, anger, and boredom.

## What is fat in the human body?

Fat in the human body is medically called adipose tissue and is found in several places in the body. Fat is made up of unique cells, simply referred to as fat cells. In general, fat cells are found beneath the skin and on top of both kidneys, along with some that is stored in the liver and a small amount in the muscles. In most people, the number of fat cells remains the same after they reach puberty (exceptions are if an adult has liposuction or if the person gains a significant amount of weight). And while the number of fat cells remains the same, each cell can get larger, which is why people "gain weight" without increasing the number of fat cells. (For more about how fats are metabolized—after ingestion—by the digestive tract, see the chapter "How Diabetes Affects the Digestive System.")

## What are white and brown fats?

In general, fat cells are divided into white and brown fats. Overall, a person carries white fat, or fat that cushions the body near the surface and makes up around 90 percent of body fat. These fat cells are large and have little cytoplasm and a small nucleus, with a fat droplet making up around 85 percent of the cell's volume. They are most important to energy metabolism and heat insulation in the body. Brown fat is mostly found in newborn babies between the shoulders and is important to making heat (called thermogenesis) as newborns do not have much white fat to insulate their bodies and retain heat. The cells have a small amount of fat droplets and many mitochondria, or cell organelles (structures within the cell) that can generate heat. Adults usually have little or no brown fat, but if they do, it is most often found around the upper back, the nape of the neck, the armpits, between the shoulder blades, and deep in the chest cavity.

## Is there a connection between white and brown fat, obesity, and diabetes?

According to some studies—and even though most adults carry few or no brown fat cells—some researchers believe that the proportions of white and brown fat cells may be connected to being overweight or obese. They suggest that because brown fat primarily burns calories and white fat stores calories, some overweight and obese people may have less brown fat than adults who are not obese, or the brown fat in a person who is overweight or obese is not as efficient in burning calories. Either way, the fat is more readily stored in these people than burned off.

Exercise may also change a person's white fat. In a 2016 study, researchers found that exercise may help to control weight and to fend off diabetes by changing white fat into brown. This may be due to a boost in a hormone, irisin, that is produced during exercise. This previously unknown hormone apparently migrates mostly to fat and, through several biochemical processes, causes some of the normally white fat cells to turn to brown fat cells—fat that is known to burn calories and improve control of insulin and blood glucose.

## Where does fat collect in the abdomen, especially fat that can lead to obesity?

Two types of fat associated with obesity collect in the upper body (abdomen). The intra-abdominal fat—also called visceral or organ fat—collects around organs and represents about 10 percent of the upper-body fat. Around 90 percent is called regular, organ, or abdominal subcutaneous fat and is found under the surface of the skin. It is the type of fat that can be grasped with a hand and is located between the skin and the outer abdominal wall. While fat found under the surface of the skin may be in some ways connected to abdominal obesity and metabolic risk factors, the intra-abdominal fat is thought to be a much stronger indicator—even predictor—of metabolic abnormalities, diseases, and a person's mortality.

### Who discovered the connection between upper-body obesity and the risk of such diseases as diabetes?

In 1947, French physician Jean Vague (1911–2003) was the first person to mention that upper-body obesity was somehow linked to such diseases as gout, atherosclerosis, and diabetes. Later, this finding was further attached to the metabolic syndrome, the clustering of at least three of five conditions, with upper-body obesity being one of the five conditions.

## Why is intra-abdominal (visceral or organ) fat thought to affect a person's health?

Research indicates that fat cells (in particular, intra-abdominal [visceral] fat cells) are considered to be biologically active, with some scientists thinking of the fats as similar to an endocrine organ or gland. This is because the fats can produce hormones and other substances in a person's body—along with affecting other hormones in the body—that can affect the person's overall health. The following are some of the connections researchers have made between visceral fat and health:

*Cardiovascular disease*—Visceral fat pumps out immune-system chemicals called cytokines that can contribute to the increased risk of cardiovascular disease. The cytokines, along with other chemicals in the body, are believed to have a bad effect on cells' sensitivities to insulin, blood pressure, and blood clotting.

*Diabetes*—Visceral fat is connected to many of the conditions included in diabetes. For example, it is associated with glucose intolerance and insulin resistance (see next on the list)—which are in turn connected to type 2 diabetes.

*Insulin resistance*—Research indicates that visceral fat secretes more of retinol-binding protein 4 (referred to as RBP4), a molecule that increases insulin resistance (when the body's muscle and liver cells don't respond to the normal levels of insulin and blood glucose levels rise). Thus, if the visceral fat increases, the RBP4 level also increases.

*Portal vein connection*—Intra-abdominal fats can also be harmful depending on their location in the body. For example, if the excess visceral fat is located near the vein that carries the blood from the intestinal area to the liver, it can cause a problem. (The vein is called the portal vein and has other functions, too.) In particular, intra-abdominal fat can release substances such as free fatty acids that can travel to the liver, where they influence the production of blood lipids. This condition is often associated with higher LDL (the "bad" cholesterol), lower HDL (the "good" cholesterol), and insulin resistance. (For more about cholesterol, see the chapter "How Diabetes Affects the Circulatory System.")

*Women's health*—Other research suggests that for some women, intra-abdominal fat may also be associated with breast cancer and the need for gallbladder surgery.

*Dyslipidemia*—Dyslipidemia is a condition in which the body has an abnormally high amount of lipids, mainly triglycerides, cholesterol, or both. It is thus connected to intra-abdominal fat.

*Inflammation*—Research indicates visceral fat is often associated with inflammation in various parts of the body. Thus, because this fat can trigger low-level inflammation, it is usually considered a risk factor for certain chronic conditions associated with inflammation, such as asthma.

*Other disease connections*—Some research has recently tied several other diseases with visceral fat. One is dementia—one study found people in their early 40s with high levels of visceral fat (compared with those without such fat at that age) were nearly three times more likely to develop dementia, including Alzheimer's, by their mid-70s to early 80s. Another is colorectal cancer. Some studies indicate that a person with a great deal of visceral fat may have three times the risk of developing colorectal adenomas (or what are usually referred to as polyps) than people with much less intra-abdominal fat; it was also found that these types of polyps in a person's colon are connected to insulin resistance.

## Can intra-abdominal fat be measured?

Yes, there are several ways to measure intra-abdominal (visceral) fat, although some are more accurate than others. The most accurate ways to date are CT scans and full-body MRIs, but not everyone can afford to pay for these methods. Another procedure uses a bioelectrical impedance machine that uses an electric current to differentiate between fat tissues in the abdomen. Still another approach can be done at home, although it is not as accurate as a CT scan or bioelectrical impedance machine. It entails measuring the person's waist and hip circumference with a tape measure, then dividing the waist by the hip measurement. In most cases, a number greater than 1.0 for men and 0.85 for women is considered excessive amount of visceral fat, whereas a lower number (for example, for a man a result of 36/40, or 0.9) means there is not as much in terms of intra-abdominal fat. But this is only an estimate because some of the fat will be subcutaneous fat. To make the number more accurate, measure the waist when you are lying down, then divide by the hip measurement. Since the subcutaneous fat usually will fall to the side of the body when it is lying down, the visceral fat will remain.

Overall, the main reason for understanding a person's visceral fat measurement is not to "stay within the numbers." It is merely to let a person know if he or she has a problem with intra-abdominal fat—and then decide what to do if the fat needs to be reduced. This knowledge, in turn, will usually help the person lower his or her risk of such conditions as cardiovascular disease—and diabetes.

## What do the terms "apple-shaped" and "pear-shaped" indicate in terms of health?

In terms of health—and abdominal fat—the terms apple-shaped and pear-shaped have certain meanings. Both terms are associated with how a person's waistline often seems to grow as the person gets older, which also means a possible increase in a variety of health problems. (These terms usually refer to intra-abdominal fat, not the subcutaneous fat.) The big difference is that people who have subcutaneous fat that accumulates in the abdominal area are considered apple-shaped; people who have fat that accumulates in the lower body are considered to be pear-shaped. Thus, apple-shaped people seem to have more health

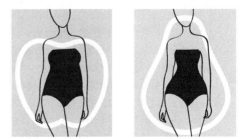

Apple- (left) or pear-shaped bodies are the result of too much fat being stored in the abdomen or hips, respectively.

problems associated with their intra-abdominal fat than pear-shaped people, including a higher risk of developing type 2 diabetes.

### Do some races seem to have more intra-abdominal fat than others?

Yes, there appear to be certain connections between a person's race and intra-abdominal fat. Many studies have shown that Asians have more intra-abdominal fat than Caucasians. And Caucasians have more of the fat than African Americans. But because most of the studies of intra-abdominal fats stress Caucasian populations, it is difficult to determine any more possible racial differences.

### What are two of the best and most healthful ways to lose intra-abdominal fat to reduce the risk of developing such diseases as diabetes?

Most research suggests there are two major ways that a person can lose intra-abdominal fat and reduce the risk of developing diseases such as diabetes (especially type 2). These are exercise (individuals who are more physically active have lower amounts of intra-abdominal fat) and reducing calories. Both are considered equally effective in producing moderate weight loss. In addition, although weight loss is the desired outcome of exercise in overweight people, research suggests that even when the person's body mass does not change, regular exercise can still reduce intra-abdominal fat and shrink the waist size. (For more about exercise and weight loss, see the chapter "Exercise and Diabetes.")

For example, some studies showed that, if an overweight or obese person exercises around 20 minutes a day for three months, intra-abdominal fat can be reduced by 10 percent. If an overweight or obese person exercises around 60 minutes a day for around that same amount of time, it can translate to a 30 percent reduction in intra-abdominal fat. In addition, the amount of intra-abdominal fat that is lost is, in general, greater than abdominal subcutaneous fat lost.

---

### Can performing sit-ups help get rid of intra-abdominal fat?

For most people, doing sit-ups is good for tightening abdominal muscles. But such spot exercise will not get rid of intra-abdominal (visceral or organ) fat, or what is often referred to in the media as a "beer belly" or "spare tire." This is because this type of fat lies under the abdominal muscles and within the organs, not just below the surface of the skin as with subcutaneous fat. Thus, doing sit-ups will strengthen abdominal muscles, but unless visceral fat is reduced, the "six-pack abs" won't be noticed. In fact, it is difficult to do any spot exercise to target fat loss in the body. This is because the body stores fat in a random way, and those locations are usually dictated by the person's genetics. And, according to some studies, as a person loses weight, the body will most often lose fat in the reverse order in which it was put on.

When it comes to calories, if a person (subject to an individual's overall health and doctor's advice) reduces his or her caloric intake by 400 to 700 calories a day, it can mean a 15 to 30 percent reduction in intra-abdominal fat. By focusing on energy intake (calories in), an overweight or obese person can often lower intra-abdominal fat.

Although it is possible to drastically restrict calorie intake, it is often not practical or healthful to do so. Thus, most researchers suggest a more moderate approach to reducing calories. In most overweight or obese people, reducing calories often leads to a reduction in body weight and intra-abdominal fat. The total percentage of loss depends on many factors, but on the average, there is often not only a weight loss but also a reduction in intra-abdominal fat that ranges from 15 to 30 percent.

## Do overweight or obese males and females differ in their ability to lose weight and intra-abdominal fat?

Although both males and females can be overweight and obese, there are thought to be some gender differences when it comes to intra-abdominal fat reduction and weight loss. For example, some studies suggest that exercise and/or diet reductions to get rid of intra-abdominal fat may not work as well for women as for men. Yet other research indicates that women can significantly reduce intra-abdominal fats though exercise and diet. Thus, many researchers believe that the studies may be confounded by gender differences involving exercise and expended energy, differences in exercise intensity, and duration of the activity. They also cite the fact that women generally have less intra-abdominal fat than men. All of this means that no one truly knows whether males or females have more trouble reducing intra-abdominal fat—and more studies, of course, are needed.

## Why doesn't liposuction work in terms of visceral fat?

Liposuction is the surgical procedure that uses a suction technique to remove fat from various places on the body. Most people who choose to have the procedure wish to enhance and change the contours of their body, including the abdomen, arms, buttocks, calves and ankles, chest and back, hips and thighs, and neck. It is purely cosmetic and is in no way a weight-loss method or treatment for obesity. This is because the fat that is removed is subcutaneous, and the procedure does not reach the inside of the abdominal wall. In other words, liposuction will not get rid of intra-abdominal (visceral) fat.

It is interesting to note that people who have the procedure are permanently getting rid of fat cells—or those cells that they have had all their lives. They cannot be replaced, and if the person does not lead a healthful lifestyle after the operation, there is a risk that the remaining fat cells will grow bigger and he or she will gain weight. This is because when a person gains weight, it's actually the fat cells increasing in size and volume. Conversely, if the person exercises and eats a healthful diet, the fat cells will decrease in size and volume, and the person will lose weight.

All this may be a moot point if the person has diabetes, too. In most cases, and because of possible complications from the surgery, liposuction is usually not recommended for people who have coronary artery disease, a weak immune system—or diabetes.

## What is bariatric surgery?

Bariatric surgery is a somewhat generic term that means most surgeries conducted on people who wish to lose weight. It is not for everyone who wants to lose weight, and in most cases, it is suggested only for extremely obese patients, or obese people who have other severe weight-related health problems, such as type 2 diabetes, heart disease, very high blood pressure, and extreme sleep apnea. It is only used as a "last resort" for most obese cases and only after attempts to lose weight, by eating more healthfully and nutritionally, along with exercise, fail.

In most bariatric surgeries, the person has his or her digestive system altered in such a way as to limit the ability to eat, slow down the absorption of nutrients, or a combination of both. The following lists the most common forms of bariatric surgery performed in the United States at this writing:

*Adjustable gastric band (AGB)*—In this operation, a small band is placed around the top of the stomach to shrink the opening between the esophagus and stomach and reduce a person's food intake.

*Bilopancreatic diversion with duodenal switch (BPD-DS)*—This operation (which is usually only conducted on severely obese patients) involves three procedures: removing much of the stomach, making the person feel fuller after eating; changing the effects of bile and other digestive juices to reduce a person's digestion and absorption of nutrients; and rerouting food around part of the small intestine in order to lessen the absorption of nutrients.

*Roux-en-Y gastric bypass (RYGB)*—In this operation, a small part of the stomach is stapled, creating a small pouch. This causes the food to go directly from the pouch to the small intestine, bypassing part of the gastrointestinal tract to limit the amount of food it absorbs.

*Vertical sleeve gastrectomy (VSG)*—Here, most of the stomach is removed, lessening the amount of food eaten and absorbed by the gastrointestinal tract.

## What study linked weight-loss surgery and diabetes remission?

A 2013 study reported in the *Annals of Surgery* noted possible benefits for some people with type 2 diabetes and weight-loss surgery. The researchers looked at 217 severely obese people with type 2 diabetes, with an average body mass index (BMI; for more about BMI, see this chapter) of 49, an indication of extreme obesity. The participants had weight-loss surgery between 2004 and 2007, and six years later, the researchers found that 24 percent of them were in complete diabetes remission, meaning they had an A1c of less than 6 percent and were not taking any diabetes medication. In addition, 26 percent of the participants were in partial remission, or an A1c of 6 to 6.4 percent and not taking diabetes medication. The researchers also noted that people who had diabetes

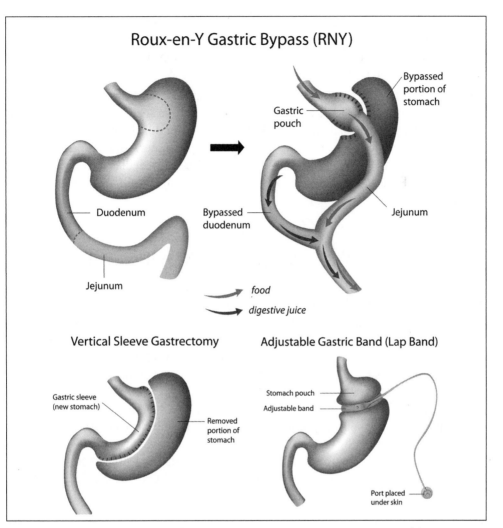

## Roux-en-Y Gastric Bypass (RNY)

Gastric pouch

Bypassed portion of stomach

Duodenum

Bypassed duodenum

Jejunum

Jejunum

*food*

*digestive juice*

### Vertical Sleeve Gastrectomy

Gastric sleeve (new stomach)

Removed portion of stomach

### Adjustable Gastric Band (Lap Band)

Stomach pouch

Adjustable band

Port placed under skin

Three types of bariatric surgery are shown above. (Not pictured is BPD-DS surgery.) Such surgeries should only be considered when all other options for weight loss have proven to be ineffective.

for less than five years had the most health improvements. Although this is not an endorsement for weight-loss surgery, it may be a possibility for people who have other severe health problems and diabetes. The best way to find out is for the patient to ask his or her health care professional if such surgery is an option.

### How has recent research explained why bariatric surgery is associated with type 2 diabetes remission?

Researchers have known for many years that patients who have bariatric surgery—or stomach surgeries that concentrate on weight loss—often experience type 2 diabetes remission. In 2016, a Cornell University-led study on mice written up in, appropriately, the journal *Gut,* suggested why the diabetes goes into remission, even days after the surgery and before the weight is lost. The researchers discovered that TGR5, a bile-acid receptor, along with an increase in bile-acid concentrations known to occur after these surgeries, both help to balance glucose levels in the blood.

This does not mean the researchers advocate bariatric surgery to combat type 2 diabetes, as such surgery is not without risks. Most of these surgeries are conducted on people who have a body mass index (BMI) from 35 to over 40, along with other obesity-related health problems (for more about BMI, see this chapter). But the researchers do want to concentrate on methods other than weight loss to treat diabetes. Thus, they are looking at TGR5 as a possible clue to treatment, especially the link between the TGR5 and bile acid.

# OBESITY AND BODY MASS INDEX

### What is body mass index, or BMI?

Body mass index is a way of measuring your body's mass—a statistical measurement that gives an estimate of a healthy body weight based on the height of a person. Overall, it gives you and your doctor a good idea of how you stand weight-wise. In general, for an adult female (males have slightly higher BMI numbers), if you have a BMI of less than 18.5, you are considered underweight; 18.5 to 24.9 means normal weight; 25 to 29.9 means overweight; and over 30 is considered obese. To determine your BMI, take your weight in pounds and your height in total inches. Then multiply your weight times 703, and divide that number by your height squared. For example, if you are 5 feet, 4 inches tall (or 64 inches tall) and weigh 133 pounds, the calculation would be as follows: 133 x 703 = 93,449; 64 inches squared = 4,096; divide 93,449/4,096 = 22.83—your BMI is in the normal range.

### What are some of the health risks of having a high BMI?

There are numerous health risks if a person has a high BMI, or body mass index, meaning over 30. Risks include hypertension, dyslipidemia (for more about dyslipidemia and diabetes, see the chapter "How Diabetes Affects the Circulatory System"), type 2 diabetes, cardiovascular disease, stroke, gallbladder disease, osteoarthritis, sleep apnea and respiratory problems, gout, and even certain types of cancer, such as endometrial, breast, and colon cancers.

### Is a high BMI the only factor in obesity?

No. Health care professionals also cite genetic, environmental, psychological, and underlying medical problems—all of which may be factors that lead to obesity. Underlying medical conditions may include hypothyroidism, Cushing's syndrome, depression, and certain neurological problems that can lead to overeating. Drugs, such as steroids, used to treat certain medical conditions may cause weight gain, too. Scientific study has also indicated that obesity may be linked to heredity, but many researchers note that in terms of a "family unit" that shares the same basic diet, it is often difficult to separate genetics from environmental factors.

## Why are many doctors concerned about BMI in terms of diabetes?

Health care professionals are usually concerned if a person's BMI is too high, which often indicates that the individual is very overweight or obese. In addition, many studies have found that a person's BMI is strongly and independently associated with the risk of being diagnosed with type 2 diabetes.

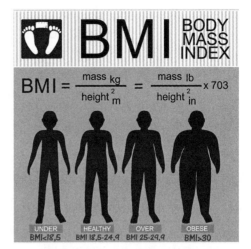

$$BMI = \frac{mass\ kg}{height^2\ m} = \frac{mass\ lb}{height^2\ in} \times 703$$

A simple calculation based on your weight and height will give you your BMI and tell you whether you are at a healthy weight or not.

## What is an example of a good BMI for a certain height?

Depending on your height, which is usually considered to be a constant, you can also determine what weight range will send you into another BMI category. For example, here are the weight ranges, the corresponding BMI ranges, and the weight-status categories for a sample height of a man who is 5 feet, 9 inches:

### BMI for 5'9" Tall Male

| Weight Range | BMI | Weight Status |
|---|---|---|
| 124 lbs. or less | Below 18.5 | Underweight |
| 125 lbs. to 168 lbs. | 18.5 to 24.9 | Normal |
| 169 lbs. to 202 lbs. | 25.0 to 29.9 | Overweight |
| 203 lbs. or more | 30 or higher | Obese |

# STUDIES IN OBESITY

## Do researchers believe that obesity is inherited?

To date, researchers studying obesity genetics have identified more than 30 candidate genes on 12 chromosomes associated with body mass index—or how much weight we carry around (for more about body mass index, see this chapter). For example, in 2007, the first "fat mass and obesity-associated" gene (or FTO) was found on chromosome 16;

## How reliable is BMI as a health indicator?

For several reasons, not everyone thinks that the BMI is a person's best indicator of health. For example, although the connection between the BMI number and the fatness of a person is fairly strong, the numbers all vary by gender, race, and age; for instance, at the same BMI, older people (on average) tend to have more body fat than younger adults, and highly trained athletes may also have a high BMI, but it is more because of muscles than body fat. Another objection is that the BMI is only one factor related to risk for certain diseases. Thus, some organizations look at other factors to understand a person's likelihood of developing overweight- or obesity-related diseases. For example, the National Heart, Lung, and Blood Institute guidelines recommend looking at two other factors: A person's waist circumference (because abdominal fat is often a predictor of risk for obesity-related diseases) and other possible risk factors a person has for diseases associated with obesity (for example, high blood pressure or physical inactivity).

it's estimated that people who have this gene variant carry a 20 to 30 percent higher risk of obesity. Another obesity-associated gene is located on chromosome 18. But as many researchers mention, even when the genes are found, they only account for a small part of the gene-related susceptibility to obesity. According to Harvard University's School of Public Health, recent research shows that genetic factors identified so far in obesity make only a small contribution to a person's obesity risk—and that our genes are "not our destiny." In other words, many people who do have the so-called "obesity genes" do not necessarily become obese or even overweight—and often can counteract potential overweight problems owing to genes with exercise and healthful eating habits.

## Why are carbohydrates the center of a debate about type 2 diabetes?

Some researchers believe that it is actually carbohydrates in our diets that have made many people overweight and eventually obese, both of which conditions can lead to type 2 diabetes. They believe that insulin resistance in many people is caused by the pancreas's "wearing out," as it sends out more and more insulin, so more sugar is stored as fat, which leads to obesity.

The researchers' solutions seem drastic to some, as they often contradict some commonly "accepted" dietary guidelines. The researchers believe that several foods should be replaced in the diet, as they cause such rapid sugar spikes after eating. These foods include whole grains (which raise the blood sugar drastically after ingestion and can be replaced with such flours as coconut or almond), potatoes, and sugar. This way, the body will not be flooded with sugar followed by insulin and, thus, will lower fat stores in the body. The researchers also believe that a person with type 2 diabetes, or even prediabetes, should eat more protein and fats instead of most carbohydrates. This is because proteins—especially fats—do not cause a spike in blood glucose levels after eating.

Overall, the researchers' message is that most (especially Western) diets have not cut back on carbohydrates; they also stress that obesity may be linked not to which carbohydrates a person eats but to how much the person eats for his or her particular body. They also note that much of the information about treating diabetes tends to mention the medications as opposed to such alternatives as maintaining a health lifestyle. They do admit, too, that some people do have a genetic predisposition to type 2 diabetes—but their main concern is that along with the increase in type 2 diabetes has come an increase in obesity.

### Is type 2 diabetes a problem for low-income people?

Yes, in many cases, type 2 diabetes is a major problem for low-income people, and it can sometimes afflict entire families. A recent study found that at the end of a month, low-income people are admitted to hospitals with low blood sugar more than people with higher incomes. It is thought that this is because without money, the low-income people cannot buy enough to feed their families. This lack of stable access to food can cause a person to have unstable blood glucose levels.

# OBESITY RESEARCH AND STATISTICS

### What is the "obesity paradox"?

In the past decade or so, researchers have noticed that there are people who are not obese or overweight but still develop diseases most often associated with excess weight. The phrase "obesity paradox" refers to these normal-weight people who are not obese but still develop diseases such as type 2 diabetes—and those diseases seem to affect them more than they do obese people *with* diabetes. In one 2016 study from the *Journal of the American Medical Association,* it was found that normal-weight people who develop type 2 diabetes often have double the risk of dying from heart disease and other causes over people who have type 2 diabetes and are overweight. The paradox comes from the idea that excess weight can "protect" certain people—though the opposite is more often true.

The researchers do not suggest that people become overweight to stave off certain diseases like type 2 diabetes. This is because statistics show that around 85 percent of people who do develop type 2 diabetes are overweight or obese. What they believe is that something other than weight gain is causing the onset and severity of type 2 diabetes in these "normal-weight" people. Some suggest it may be certain conditions not yet researched as much, such as the amount of fat a person carries around his or her waist. Another suggestion is that such conditions for these people may not be the amount of fat itself but how the person stores it in the body. Still another study points to hormones that tell the brain when to eat or when the person has had enough to eat.

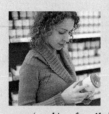
### What study found a possible connection between certain chemicals in the body and obesity?

In a study presented in 2007, researchers found that many obese people in the study actually had higher amounts in their systems of leptin, a hunger-suppressing hormone, but in most cases, the participants' systems were also resistant to leptin. This hormone is released by fat cells and travels through the bloodstream to the brain. In general, the more fat a person has on his or her body, the more leptin is released. But when a person's fat level is low—which means the leptin levels are low—it causes the brain to increase the person's appetite, so he or she eats more and gains weight.

The researchers also discovered that obese people had suppressed ghrelin levels, a chemical the stomach secretes when it is empty to tell the brain that it's time to eat. Both leptin and ghrelin may contribute to a person's propensity to eat too much at meals—and they are thus associated with hunger and craving, along with the possibility of contributing to obesity. They may also contribute to the reasons behind the "obesity paradox" (see above), in which the fat, brain, and leptin do not respond correctly—and many times lead to type 2 diabetes without the person's being obese.

### How many Americans are thought to be obese?

Currently, it is thought that overweight (meaning a body mass index, or BMI, of 25 to 30) and obese (meaning a BMI of over 30) Americans represent about 65.2 percent of the population. Although it is a worldwide problem, in the United States alone, it is estimated that one in four people are obese. Still another statistic states that more than half of the adults in the United States are overweight.

## What does air pollution have to do with obesity—and perhaps diabetes?

**A**lthough more research needs to be done, in yet another study on obesity, researchers working jointly from Duke and Peking Universities suggested that air pollution may play a part in diet-associated weight gain, inflammation in the body (thought to be a contributing factor to obesity), and insulin resistance. They base their suggestions on studies conducted on rats, in which the animals were exposed to the polluted city air of Beijing or air cleaned by an air filter that removed most of the pollutants. The scientists found that after 19 days, the animals in the polluted air showed signs of inflammation and had a 50 percent higher level of LDL (low-density lipoprotein, considered "bad") cholesterol, 46 percent higher triglycerides, and 97 percent higher total cholesterol, all thought to be contributors to obesity. In terms of diabetes, the rats also had an increase in insulin resistance. The animals' offspring did no better and were heavier than the offspring in the filtered air, even with eating the same diets. If this study can be translated to humans, it may show how major air pollution can contribute to the growing numbers of people who are not only obese but who also develop diabetes.

## How many people who develop type 2 diabetes are obese or overweight?

According to Harvard Medical School, it is estimated that around 85 percent of people who develop type 2 diabetes are overweight or obese. Although this estimate applies to the U.S. population, it is no doubt close to the percentage of people worldwide who develop type 2 diabetes.

## What are the three major conditions associated with obesity?

According to some statistics, one in three Americans and one in four adults worldwide have at least three conditions that often accompany obesity. These three major conditions include type 2 diabetes, high cholesterol, and high blood pressure. These disorders, usually found in combination, double a person's risk of heart attack and strokes. Another condition called fatty liver—when a large amount of fat accumulates in the liver—is also caused by obesity and can lead to liver failure.

# COPING WITH DIABETES

## DIABETES AND EMOTIONAL HEALTH

### Can stress cause diabetes?

No, contrary to some reports, there is no evidence that stress can cause diabetes. But it can affect a person with diabetes, as stress does raise blood glucose levels.

### How does diabetes cause stress?

Experts often say that stress can affect diabetes (mainly by raising blood glucose levels), and diabetes can cause stress. Most people with diabetes do not realize this double connection, especially when they are first diagnosed with the disease. In particular, having diabetes puts a burden on the person because it requires many lifestyle changes, not only for that person, but also for those around him or her (and especially when a child is diagnosed with diabetes). There is the stress of making sure the person's blood glucose stabilizes to a level that is good for that person. And there is the stress of making sure that he or she eats, exercises, and works comfortably while maintaining a healthy blood glucose level. Many people without the disease do not understand the challenges of the disease—and such a lack of understanding can also cause stress in the person with diabetes.

### How do the many stresses in life affect a person's blood glucose levels?

The double whammy, as it is often called, is that stressful events are tough on the body (mentally and physically) and, in turn, affect blood glucose levels, whether a person has diabetes or not. With or without diabetes, the stress hormones (usually cortisol and catecholamines) can counteract the effects of the body's insulin (stress can even affect injected insulin for a person with type 1 diabetes). This stress effect makes blood glucose levels rise, sometimes to dangerous levels.

### What problems may people with diabetes face in relation to others who do not have the disease?

If you talk with people who have diabetes, they'll often say that communication or "people problems" can lead to stress or bad feelings. For example, many people will tell a person with diabetes what he or she should eat (even though they themselves do not have the disease) or treat the person differently when a diagnosis is made. Most people with diabetes want practical and emotional help, but they also want others to understand the many difficult challenges they face with diabetes.

### What study indicated that people with diabetes may be more prone to depression and vice versa?

It is well established that diabetes and depression often occur together. It is unknown why this link exists, but according to a study of 55,000 women conducted by researchers at Harvard School of Public Health, the link appears to be bidirectional, meaning either condition can cause the onset of the other. The study showed that over a ten-year period, there was a 29 percent higher risk of developing depression for women who had diabetes than for those who did not. Contrarily, women who had depression were 17 percent more likely to develop diabetes than those who were not depressed. Both results took into account risk factors for both conditions, such as excess body fat and inactivity.

The researchers speculated that depression may result from biochemical changes that occur if a person develops diabetes. It could also be that diabetes occurs as a result of the treatment for the depression, as antidepressant drugs may affect a person's glucose levels or cause weight gain that puts the person at risk for diabetes. They also suggest that depression may develop after someone develops diabetes because the person has to live with the stresses of the chronic disease. These suggestions are all speculation so far, and more studies need to be done.

# DIABETES AND VACCINATIONS

### What is the purpose of a vaccination?

The purpose of vaccination, or immunization, is to artificially induce active immunity, so there will be resistance to the pathogen upon natural exposure in the future. Vaccinations are prepared under laboratory conditions from either dead or severely weakened antigens.

### Should people with diabetes obtain a flu and/or pneumonia shot each year?

Most health care professionals suggest that a person with diabetes obtain a flu shot each year, usually in the fall. According to the CDC, people with diabetes (types 1 or 2), even when the disease is well managed, are at higher risk of developing serious flu complications than most other people. These can include such conditions as pneumonia, bronchitis, and sinus and ear infections, which may lead to hospitalization. Such susceptibility occurs because the immune system of a person with diabetes is less able to fight off infections, and an illness makes it more difficult to control blood glucose levels. For example, when people are sick, they may not feel like eating, and if they have diabetes, lack of food can cause blood glucose levels to become unbalanced.

In addition, people with type 1 or type 2 diabetes should ask their health care professional if they need a pneumonia shot—also called pneumococcal vaccination—as they are at increased risk of developing pneumonia if they do contract the flu. Overall, a person with diabetes should contact his or her health care provider to understand what shots are needed and the best way to obtain them.

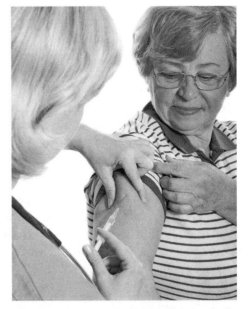

Because diabetics are at higher risk of getting the flu or pneumonia, it is recommended they get a flu shot every year without fail.

### Why does a new flu vaccine have to be prepared each year?

A new flu vaccine is prepared every year because the strains of flu viruses change from year to year. Nine to ten months before the flu season begins, scientists prepare a new vaccine made from inactivated (killed) flu viruses. The vaccine preparation is based on the strains of the flu viruses that are in circulation at the time. It includes those A and B viruses expected to circulate the following winter. Another reason to get vaccinated for the flu every year is that immunity after a flu shot declines and may be too low to provide protection after one year.

## ENJOYING THE OUTDOORS

### Can sunburn affect a person with diabetes?

Yes, sunburn can affect a person with diabetes, whether the individual gets burned while hiking, walking in the sunshine, or skiing at a ski resort. Sunburn can stress the body, and for a person with diabetes, such stress can raise blood glucose levels. Sunshine can also put stress on the eyes, causing eye strain. The best way to counteract these problems is not to quit going outside but to use a broad-spectrum sunscreen and to wear protective eye gear.

## What SPF (sun protection factor) is best?

For people with or without diabetes, it is best to use sunscreen lotion to protect against the sun's ultraviolet rays. When it comes to sunscreen, the SPF number located on a lotion's container is the most important. Most experts generally recommend that a sunscreen with an SPF of at least 30 is usually sufficient, since it blocks out around 97 percent of the sun's ultraviolet rays. For those with fairer skin or who have a history of skin cancer, dermatologists often recommend an SPF closer to 60. In addition, those who are outside for more than two to three hours—especially from 10 A.M. to 2 P.M., the peak sun-exposure hours—can often benefit from a higher SPF number.

Of course, the use of sunscreen is often debated, especially in association with vitamin D. Although the seasonal change in sunlight is one of the major reasons for fluctuations in a person's vitamin D levels, another culprit is clothing that covers the arms and legs, limiting the sunlight that helps the body produce vitamin D. In addition, using sunscreen may affect vitamin D levels to a certain extent, although in reality, few people use enough sunscreen to block all of the UV rays.

## Is there a connection between skin cancer and diabetes?

Although more studies are needed, a study from 2013 indicated there may be an association between skin cancer and diabetes, especially if a person has had diabetes for 15

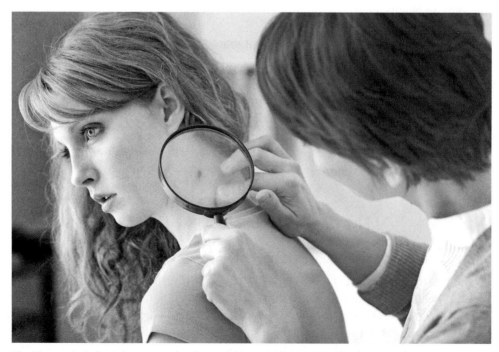

Checking regularly for melanoma or other forms of skin cancer is important for everyone, so take precautions and schedule an appointment with a dermatologist to be safe.

years or longer. But the study raised many questions, and no one truly knows whether there is a higher risk of skin cancer for people with diabetes or whether it is just that the older a person becomes, the more he or she is exposed to environmental conditions that cause skin cancer. Overall, health care professionals suggest that people with diabetes follow the same guidelines as those without diabetes, such as using sunscreen, wearing light clothing to cover the arms and legs, and being aware of how much time they are exposed to sunlight.

## What is Lyme disease?

Lyme disease is caused by a bacterium transmitted to humans through the bite of various types of infected ticks. The smaller, immature tick nymphs usually spread the disease because they are so small and difficult to see. In most cases, the tick must be attached for 36 to 48 hours or more before the Lyme disease bacterium can be transmitted. If infected, a person can experience flulike symptoms, such as fever, headache, and fatigue, and in about 80 percent of the cases, a "bull's-eye" skin rash can be seen around the bite area. The typical treatment is a few weeks of antibiotics. If the infection is not treated, it can eventually affect joints, the heart, and the nervous system. According to the Centers for Disease Control and Prevention, it is estimated that children ages five to nine face the greatest risk of contracting Lyme disease, with about 75,000 children diagnosed annually. It is also considered the most common tick-borne disease in the country, with about 300,000 new cases (all ages) per year. But the numbers may be higher as many cases mimic other illnesses and are not diagnosed.

## What happens if a person with diabetes contracts Lyme disease?

Few studies have been conducted on how a person with diabetes can cope with Lyme disease. In addition, if there is no telltale rash, the symptoms often mimic other diseases. Some of the symptoms, if the infection is not treated, seem as if they would exacerbate diabetic conditions, as the infection often involves inflammation (from the infection) and neuropathy-type symptoms—both of which are not only symptoms of diabetes but also conditions that worsen if a person has diabetes.

## What is the West Nile virus?

According to the Centers for Disease Control and Prevention, the West Nile virus is a seasonal problem that is commonly transmitted by infected mosquitoes. It is found widely on other continents, including Africa, Europe, and Asia, and was first detected in the United States in 1999. The insects become infected with the virus when they feed on other contaminated animals, especially birds. From there, the insects spread the virus to humans and other animals. The virus has an incubation period of about three to 14 days (which means that the symptoms will not start until three to 14 days after a bite). But most people—around 70 to 80 percent—do not develop any symptoms. Others who are infected can develop a fever, along with a headache, body aches, joint pains, vomiting, diarrhea, or rash. Most people recover completely. It is estimated that less than 1 percent of people infected develop serious neurological illness, such as encephalitis (inflammation of the brain) or meningitis (inflammation of the lining of the brain and spinal cord). As of this writing, there is no treatment or vaccine for the virus.

## What happens if a person with diabetes contracts West Nile virus?

For people with diabetes, there is a known risk factor for contracting a severe case of West Nile virus. In addition, it appears that people who also had high blood pressure were more likely to develop a serious case of West Nile virus in comparison with healthier individuals who contracted the virus. It is estimated that people with diabetes were four times more likely to have serious complications from the virus, while people with high blood pressure were twice as likely to have serious complications. This is why health care professionals suggest that people with diabetes use insect repellent while outdoors in the summer, especially in areas in which West Nile virus has been reported (or when traveling to mosquito-infested areas, including some overseas spots). Because mosquitoes are most active at dusk and dawn, people should wear long sleeves and pants if they go outdoors during these times. Finally, anyone with diabetes who experiences any hyperglycemia or symptoms noted above should seek medical attention.

## Are people with diabetes sensitive to temperature?

Yes, a person with diabetes can be temperature-sensitive, especially when it is hot. In fact, people with diabetes have to be extra cautious when the temperatures go up as extreme heat can affect their blood glucose levels, depending on what they have eaten, whether they are well-hydrated, and their level of physical activity. For example, studies have shown that older people with type 2 diabetes have a more difficult time cooling down in hot temperatures. One study also found that exercise and a subsequent rise in body temperature could be a difficult challenge to those with diabetes—indicating that people without diabetes were able to cool down twice as well as people with diabetes. The researchers believe this is because diabetes damages blood vessels, including those involved in regulating body temperature. (For more about diabetes and exercise in hot and cold conditions, see the chapter "Diabetes and Exercise.")

## How can extremely high temperatures affect diabetes medications and equipment?

Not only do extreme temperatures affect a person with diabetes, but they can also cause a problem with a person's medications and testing equipment. Heat—especially combined with high humidity—can affect certain medications, especially long-term exposure to high temperatures. For example, many types of insulin are fine in temperatures ranging from 93–95° Fahrenheit (34–35° Celsius), but any higher, and the medication rapidly degrades. When temperatures are about 80° Fahrenheit (27° Celsius), with humidity higher than about 40 percent, not only are diabetes medications affected, but so also is diabetes-testing equipment, causing the equipment (including insulin pumps) to malfunction or batteries to stop functioning. In addition, a disconnected pump or supplies should not be left in a hot car, by a pool, in direct sunlight, or on the beach. According to the American Diabetes Association, it is best, in these conditions—or in any climate and temperature—to protect and take precautions to maintain medications, supplies, and equipment.

## Can cold weather affect a person with diabetes?

Yes. In particular, people with diabetes often have problems with slower blood flow (vascular problems), especially to the extremities. For a person with diabetes who already has "sluggish" blood flow, cold weather can cause major problems, especially with staying warm. Because the blood flow in their extremities is less, the cold may further cause problems with feet and hands. Thus, people with diabetes who attend outdoor events or enjoy cold-weather activities should be aware of frostbite.

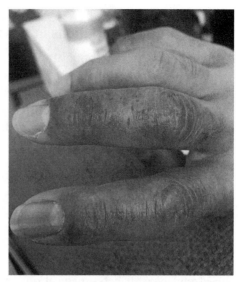

Because of the circulation problems diabetics suffer, frostbite is of special concern.

The cold can also affect the monitoring of a person's blood glucose levels. For instance, if diabetes test strips are used to monitor glucose, the strips need a certain level of oxygen and blood flow to calculate the level accurately. Thus, a person who is too cold may obtain an incorrect blood glucose reading. And if the person attempts to get blood from his or her fingertip to test blood glucose levels, cold fingers make it more difficult to obtain a good blood sample. In such cases, warming the hands—many suggest holding the hands under their armpits—becomes necessary for a good reading.

## What is Raynaud's phenomenon or syndrome?

Raynaud's phenomenon or syndrome is an autoimmune condition that causes a person's hands and feet to become extremely cold. It is usually brought on by cold weather and/or stress, with symptoms ranging from extreme cold in the feet, toes, and/or hands to numbness. It is mostly due to the constriction of blood vessels in the extremities. If a person also has diabetes, the blood flow to the extremities is slower, thus creating an even colder (or numb) feeling in the hands and feet. This can also cause problems with blood glucose readings. Raynaud's can cause a false reading if blood is taken from the hands or feet and will not represent the person's blood glucose levels throughout the body. Thus, efforts to "correct" a blood-sugar level may be in error.

## How can extremely cold temperatures affect diabetes medications and equipment?

Like extremely hot temperatures, cold temperatures can affect the medications and testing equipment (such as glucose monitors and test strips) of a person with diabetes. As

## How are variations in temperature detected by the body?

Temperature sensations are detected by specialized free nerve endings called cold receptors and warm receptors. Cold receptors respond to decreasing temperatures, and warm receptors respond to increasing temperatures. Cold receptors are most sensitive to temperatures between 50°F (10°C) and 68°F (20°C). Temperatures below 50°F (10°C) stimulate pain receptors, producing a freezing sensation. Warm receptors are most sensitive to temperatures above 77°F (25°C) and become unresponsive at temperatures above 113°F (45°C). Temperatures near and above 113°F (45°C) stimulate pain receptors, producing a burning sensation. Both warm and cold receptors rapidly adapt. Within about a minute of continuous stimulation, the sensation of warmth or cold begins to fade.

in extreme heat, diabetes medications are affected by cold, especially liquids such as insulin. Diabetes-testing equipment can also be damaged by extreme cold, causing it to malfunction (especially insulin pumps and glucose monitors) or batteries to stop functioning. As with extreme heat, it is best to protect all diabetes medications and equipment from the cold if at all possible. If possible, take the medicines and equipment inside, as even leaving them in a car could cause problems in freezing temperatures.

### Is there any seasonal variation in diabetes?

It is truly unknown whether there is any seasonal variation in diabetes. But there are some interesting observations. For example, according to several studies, it appears that type 1 diabetes develops more often in the winter than in the summer. In addition, it is thought that type 1 diabetes is more common in cold climates. This fact is often thought to be why Northern Europeans have more type 1 diabetes than Southern Europeans. But more research needs to be done. After all, one of the warmest islands in the Mediterranean is Sardinia, where people have a high risk of developing diabetes.

# DIABETES AND TRAVELING

### What should a person with diabetes think about before driving a vehicle?

One of the major things a person with diabetes can do when driving is to make sure his or her blood glucose level is stable. This means the driver's glucose levels are in a safe target range—not too low, causing a possible hypoglycemic episode, or too high, possibly causing a hyperglycemic episode. In addition, most people with diabetes carry certain items in their car, including snacks and supplies in case they are delayed in traffic. Some also carry a blood glucose meter and/or a glucagon kit in case of an emergency. (For details about glucagon kits, see the chapter "Taking Charge of Diabetes.")

## How can a person let local law officials know he or she has diabetes?

People with diabetes often experience episodes of hypoglycemia or low blood glucose. When that happens, the person seems to slur his or her words, may be irritable and pale, and may stagger and sweat—much like someone intoxicated or on drugs. If the person with diabetes is stopped by police during such an episode, officers may not know the difference. And although many communities have trained or are training first responders (police, firefighters, and emergency medical technicians) to spot and care for people with diabetes, there are things a person with diabetes can do to help.

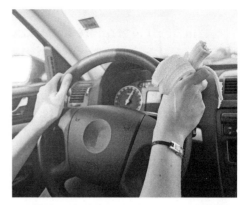

It might be a good idea to have a snack available in the car in case you get stuck in traffic and need something edible to control your sugar levels.

Although wearing a medic-alert bracelet, necklace, or tattoo is good for identifying a diabetic in an emergency, many police officers suggest also carrying a card that identifies a person as diabetic (one in a wallet with the driver's license and one with the car registration in case the other gets misplaced). There are several medic-alert cards that a diabetic— types 1 and 2, and gestational—can use, including those offered by the American Diabetes Association. Not only should the identification include information about the signs of low and high blood glucose (hypo- and hyperglycemia, respectively), but it also should carry a list of suggestions as to how the first responder can help treat both conditions.

## Is it better for a person with diabetes to bring his or her own food when traveling?

This is a matter of personal preference. Some conditions do not warrant bringing foods, and there are even certain airlines—especially those from overseas—that do not allow certain foods to be carried on board owing to contamination risks.

## What items should a person with diabetes carry on a trip?

Most people don't leave behind their medicine when they embark on a trip, and a person with diabetes will need to remember not only medicine but also several items that may be vital to keep his or her blood glucose at a safe level. Bringing the proper supplies takes some planning, especially for people on insulin. On an extended trip, most people with diabetes carry snacks and supplies. They also have their blood glucose meter available and often a glucagon kit in case of a hypoglycemic episode.

## How can a person with diabetes handle eating on a long trip?

For most diabetics, eating is often a trial when traveling long or short distances, and longer distances are the most challenging. Thus, most health care professionals suggest that a person with diabetes should stop frequently for meals if possible in order to keep his or her blood sugar levels balanced or should carry enough food to keep levels even. For insulin-dependent diabetics, knowing how their glucose levels respond to insulin and meals is necessary. And for those on oral medication, how much and what can be consumed in terms of food is necessary to know. This does not mean people with diabetes cannot celebrate on a trip, but it is important that they know how certain foods affect them. (For more about eating out, see the chapter "Shopping for Food and Eating Out.")

## What are some conversion tables for blood glucose monitoring during travel outside the United States?

Not all glucose monitors are created equal. Therefore, it is necessary when traveling outside the United States (or for people coming into the United States) for diabetics to understand the differences in glucose monitoring. In the United States, monitors use milligrams per deciliter; in other countries, it is thousandths of a mole (mmol; a mole is the amount of any chemical substance that equals the number of atoms in 12 grams of carbon–2) per liter. The following chart gives some of those conversions:

### Converting Moles per Liter to Milligrams per Deciliter

| Mmol/l | mg/dl |
| --- | --- |
| 0.06 | 1 |
| 0.07 | |
| 0.28 | 5 |
| 0.29 | |
| 0.55 | 10 |
| 0.56 | |
| 2.2 | 40 |
| 2.3 | |
| 2.8 | 50 |
| 2.9 | |
| 3.3 | 60 |

| Mmol/l | mg/dl |
|--------|-------|
| 3.4 | |
| 3.9 | 70 |
| 3.10 | |
| 1.4 | 80 |
| 1.5 | |
| 5.5 | 100 |
| 5.6 | |
| 6.1 | 110 |
| 6.2 | |
| 7.2 | 130 |
| 7.3 | |
| 8.3 | 150 |
| 8.4 | |
| 9.4 | 170 |
| 9.5 | |
| 11.1 | 200 |
| 11.2 | |
| 13.9 | 250 |
| 13.10 | |
| 16.6 | 300 |
| 16.7 | |
| 20.0 | 360 |
| 21.0 | |
| 22.2 | 400 |
| 22.3 | |
| 27.7 | 500 |
| 27.8 | |
| 40.0 | 720 |
| 41.0 | |
| 50.0 | 900 |

## Is there a cruise line that caters to people who need dialysis?

Yes, as of this writing, there is a cruise line that offers dialysis (link to http://www.dialy sisatsea.com). But it does take planning. In addition, the services are usually not covered by insurance, and the times of travel vary widely. Another option for people who need dialysis may be to arrange for dialysis ahead of time at the cruise ship's ports of call—something that a person's home dialysis center may be able to help set up.

## Do cruise lines cater to people with diabetes?

For many people, going on a cruise is a lifetime dream. But for a person with diabetes, it's vital to understand what the cruise line of choice has to offer in terms of accommodations, foods and beverages, and medical facilities. For example, some cruise lines provide nutritional information, especially carbohydrate counts, that is important to a

227

person with diabetes to maintain blood glucose levels. Thus, according to many diabetes organizations, the best way for a person with diabetes to approach a cruise is to ask questions and be prepared.

# PREPARING FOR DISASTERS AND EMERGENCIES

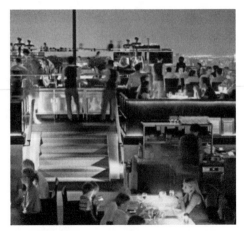

Cruise ships will make arrangements for the dietary needs of vacationers.

### Why should a person with diabetes prepare for possible disasters?

Disasters force people to leave their homes or offices quickly. Such emergencies can include train derailments or gas explosions or natural disasters, such as hurricanes, earthquakes, or tornadoes. Because a person with diabetes needs certain foods and medicine, diabetes organizations recommend that a diabetic have an emergency package to grab in times of emergency or disasters. Also, in temporary shelters, people with diabetes should identify themselves as such so they can get proper care if it's available.

### What are some tips to help people with diabetes plan for emergencies?

According to the Centers for Disease Control and Prevention, there are ways for a person with diabetes to prepare for a possible emergency or disaster. This is particularly important if the person lives in an area with the potential for natural emergencies (such as floods, snowstorms, tornadoes, hurricanes, or earthquakes). The following lists some of these suggestions, which can apply not only to an adult with diabetes but also to a family who has a child with diabetes (for more about websites that help a person with diabetes plan for an emergency, see the chapter "Resources, Websites, and Apps"):

• Prepare an emergency supply of food and water, along with an adequate supply of medicine and medical supplies in an emergency kit. This should be a three-day supply for most areas, but amounts depend on the needs of the person. For more disaster-prone areas, it is probably best to have at least a week's supply or more. (The person with diabetes should ask a pharmacist or health care provider—if the medications come from them—how to properly store the prescription medicines during an emergency.)

• Keep a list of all the medicines (and any other medical information that may be important) handy. Most people keep such information on the refrigerator or on a kitchen or bathroom cabinet door. In case the person with diabetes cannot communicate during an emergency, a list is especially helpful to emergency personnel or others assisting the person with diabetes.

- Keep a copy of all prescriptions and other important medical information in the emergency kit, along with the name and phone number of the health care provider(s) of the person with diabetes.

- Keep a list of the types, model numbers, and number of medical devices used by the person who has diabetes.

- Before an emergency happens, the person with diabetes, especially if he or she needs insulin, should plan how to handle medicine that normally requires refrigeration.

- Periodically check the expiration dates on the medicines and supplies in the emergency kit, so there is not a problem if there is an emergency.

- The person with diabetes—or a person who is providing him or her health care— should keep the emergency kit in easy reach in case of an emergency. The last thing a person wants in an emergency is to be unable to find necessary medications and equipment.

- If a person with diabetes needs certain medical treatments—for example, kidney dialysis—it is best to ask the health care provider (or the person who administers the treatment) about emergency plans to care for the patient.

- A person with diabetes should always wear identification that says he or she has diabetes. In addition, a person with diabetes should carry an emergency identification card at all times, especially when traveling—whether close to or far away from home.

- A person with diabetes who takes insulin should find out from the health care provider what to do if the insulin (or any other necessary medication) runs out during an emergency.

## How can parents protect their child with diabetes at school before an emergency happens?

If a parent has a child with diabetes at school, there are additional preparations that can be made in case of an emergency. According to the Centers for Disease Control and Prevention, parents can add several items to the adult emergency preparedness list (above) in order to help their child:

- If a child has diabetes, and is in school or day care, understand the school's emergency plans, so there will be no added confusion in an already-confusing emergency situation.

- Make sure the school or day care has the supplies needed for the child with diabetes before an emergency happens.

- Ask the school or day care whether anyone there could help the child with diabetes in case medications or injections are needed during an emergency.

## What is geoenvironmental diabetology?

Geoenvironmental diabetology is the name for studies of how environmental stressors have negative effects on people with diabetes. It also includes studies of the interaction between the environment and people with diabetes. An even more specific definition of the research in this field is the study of how geophysical phenomena affect people with diabetes, including effects on metabolism; equipment, medications, supplies, access to care, and how people with diabetes cope with extreme natural circumstances. Researchers in this field examine such events as natural disasters (for example, earthquakes) and extreme weather (hurricanes, extreme cold, and heat waves). The study does not include how events in the physical world might trigger the disease but how environmental factors affect people with the disease.

For example, geoenvironmental diabetology studies of the Kobe and Mid-Niigata earthquakes in Japan (January 17, 1995, and October 2004, respectively) indicated a significant worsening of HbA1c levels in people with diabetes for up to six months following the disasters. In these cases, people with diabetes could not get to their medications and supplies, and medical care was disrupted. Most people lost insulin vials, needles, and other diabetes equipment because of the destruction. Such studies help officials and nongovernmental organizations determine and anticipate the best way to provide people with diabetes relief after natural disasters. These studies do not apply only to one area of the world but to many places that experience natural disasters. This field is in its infancy; many researchers believe it has a place in the modern world, especially with an expanding population exposed to extreme geologic and weather events. In addition, in many places, there is the threat of global climate change that many people—and many with diabetes—face.

## How can a person with diabetes help prevent falls in the home?

According to many diabetes organizations and studies, falls, especially in the home, are the number-one cause of injury for people age 60 and older, as well as the second-likeliest cause of injury for people ages 40 to 59. According to a recent study, older adults with diabetes—especially those using insulin—are more likely to fall, causing injury and possible hospitalization. The researchers stressed that those people with diabetes were more likely to experience falls because of poor standing balance, a history of falling, and often an A1c of 8 percent or higher (for more about the A1c test, see the chapter "Taking Charge of Diabetes").

Because of this risk of falling, health care professionals offer several suggestions to people with diabetes. These include controlling blood glucose levels; practicing balance and strength exercises (ask your doctor for suggestions as to the type of exercises needed); and keeping hallways,

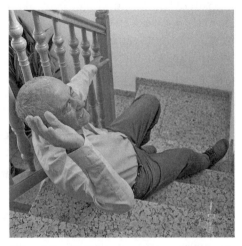

Older adults with diabetes are even more likely to suffer injury from falls than those without the disease.

stairs, and major pathways in the home clear of boxes, cords, and sundry other items that are easy to trip over. If possible, have grab bars, railings, and nonslip rugs throughout the house (especially in the bathroom) to make navigation easier. Finally, see an eye care professional at least once a year. (Diabetics have more problems with vision loss than people without diabetes.)

### How can a person with diabetes help family and friends understand what to do in a diabetic emergency?

The best thing people with diabetes can do for themselves and their friends, families, and neighbors who check on them periodically is to leave a note of instructions on their refrigerator in case of a diabetic emergency. (Be sure to tell others where the list is located!) On the note, the person with diabetes should legibly list the emergency number (911 in most places), the hospital he or she would like to be taken to in an emergency, the location of the glucagon kit (with quick, visual instructions inside the kit), the primary-care physician's name and telephone number, the insurance company (perhaps even a copy of the insurance card), and emergency contact numbers (family, friends, caregivers, etc.).

# DIABETES AND BLOOD AND ORGAN DONATIONS

### Can a person with diabetes give blood?

Yes, a person with diabetes can donate blood, platelets, and plasma. According to the American Red Cross (an organization that controls about 45 percent of the blood supply in the United States), people with type 1 or type 2 diabetes that is well controlled by insulin or oral medications are eligible to donate. Of course, other qualifications have to be met, such as being in good health, weighing over 110 pounds, and being over age 17. Some states also have their own specific restrictions, such as different age requirements, or, for example in California, refusing blood donation from a person who has diabetes and uses bovine-derived insulin.

### Why are some people with bronze diabetes often not allowed to donate blood?

According to the American Red Cross, people with bronze diabetes, a form of diabetes caused by hemochromatosis (excess iron in the blood), are currently prohibited from giving blood donations. It is not necessarily the bronze diabetes that stops a person from donating but the overall hemochromatosis disease, which usually begins before bronze diabetes develops. (For more information about hemochromatosis and bronze diabetes, see the chapter "Other Types of Diabetes.")

Not everyone agrees. Although there is no risk of passing on this genetic disease to other people through blood transfusions, the Red Cross still does not allow such donations. Yet the Food and Drug Administration does permit people with hemochromatosis to donate blood, as long as the blood is specially marked and there are certain restrictions and rules about how blood banks can use this blood. Because of such regulations, most blood banks in the United States currently do not accept donations by people with hemochromatosis. Most other countries do not have such rules and have no restrictions on people with hemochromatosis that keep them from donating blood.

## Can a person with diabetes donate an organ—such as a kidney—to a relative?

No, in most cases, a person with diabetes cannot donate an organ to a relative. This is because the disease—whether type 1, type 2, or other type of diabetes—affects the kidneys, pancreas, and other organs to a certain extent depending on the person's condition. In addition, the surgery for such operations often puts the person with diabetes at risk, mainly owing to a weakened immune system.

## Can a person with diabetes donate an organ (or organs) upon death?

Yes, according to the National Kidney Foundation, if a person who had diabetes had normally functioning organs, then he or she can donate those organ(s) after death. But there is an exception: An insulin-dependent diabetic cannot donate the pancreas after death.

# TAKING CHARGE
# OF DIABETES

## WHO HELPS A PERSON WITH DIABETES?

### Who are "trained diabetes personnel"?

Trained diabetes personnel are nonmedical people who have received in-depth training about diabetes and diabetes management. They are often hired by school systems to help students with diabetes take care of certain tasks, such as blood glucose monitoring, administering insulin, and helping to recognize possible emergencies, such as hypoglycemia and hyperglycemia. They can also help the school nurse or diabetes-trained health care professional test urine or blood for ketones, if necessary. They are also often referred to as unlicensed assistive personnel, assistive personnel, paraprofessionals, or trained nonmedical personnel.

### What is the Diabetes Complications Severity Index?

The Diabetes Complications Severity Index is a tool used to predict deaths and hospitalizations among people with diabetes. It was developed to model the severity of diabetes complications at any one point in time and is used by researchers (used to predict mortality, hospitalizations, and severity of these complications), by hospitals, and even to understand health care costs. The severity index includes seven categories of complications: cardiovascular disease, nephropathy, retinopathy, peripheral vascular disease, stroke, neuropathy, and metabolic problems.

## HEALTH–CARE TESTS AND DIABETES

### What is the fasting plasma glucose (or fasting blood glucose) test?

The fasting plasma glucose test is a test that measures blood glucose levels after a person has not eaten for at least eight hours (some suggest 12 to 14, depending on the test-

233

ing lab). Thus, no foods interfere with the results. According to the American Diabetes Association and Harvard Medical School, for the majority of people, a fasting plasma glucose level of less than 100 mg/dL (milligrams per deciliter) is considered normal.

If the blood glucose level is at or above 126 mg/dL, it is an indication of diabetes. If a person's reading suggests diabetes, most health care professionals suggest a second test to confirm the results, as various conditions (such as excessive stress) can cause blood glucose levels to fluctuate. A person with a blood glucose level between 100 and 126 mg/dL is thought to be prediabetic (for more about prediabetes, see the chapter "Prediabetes and Type 1 Diabetes").

### What is a random plasma glucose (or random blood glucose) test?

A random plasma glucose (also called random blood glucose) test measures the glucose in a person's blood. For this test, the person does not have to fast. But overall, the amount of carbohydrates, and the amount of time since the person had a snack or meal, can affect the outcome of the test. Although it is usually not as reliable as other tests (see below), it is most often used for emergencies (for example, in a hospital emergency room) or if a doctor needs a faster result of a person's glucose level. In this case, if the glucose reading is over 200 mg/dl, the person probably has diabetes, although there may be other circumstances that result in a high measurement. If the number is high, then a fasting glucose test (see above) is usually ordered by the person's health care professional.

### How is an oral glucose-tolerance test used to determine blood glucose levels?

An oral glucose-tolerance test is used to determine blood glucose levels after a person has fasted overnight (the usual length of the fast is around 12 hours). The person then drinks a sugar solution, and another reading is taken two hours later. If the levels rise and fall quickly, then the person usually does not have indications of diabetes; if the levels rise above normal and decrease slowly, then it may indicate that the person has diabetes.

While this test is thought to be accurate, it is mostly used for determining gestational diabetes in pregnant women. This is because the fasting plasma glucose test is less time consuming than the oral glucose-tolerance test (the fasting test is done after fasting for around 12 hours only). If an oral glucose-tolerance test is taken, a blood glucose measurement less than 140 mg/dL when the two-hour blood sample is taken is normal; if the reading is 200 mg/dL or higher, then the person is thought to have diabetes. If the number is between 140 and 200 mg/dL, then the person is thought to have prediabetes.

### What is a glycated hemoglobin (HbA1c, or more often seen as A1c) test?

A glycated hemoglobin (also called glycosylated hemoglobin or glycohemoglobin) test, or HbA1c, often abbreviated as A1c, measures a person's blood glucose levels over the preceding two to three months. Glucose in the blood attaches itself to hemoglobin (an oxygen-carrying protein in red blood cells). Thus, the higher a person's blood glucose level, the more hemoglobin is bound to glucose. Because red blood cells have a lifespan of about three months, the HbA1c measurement—as a percentage—reflects the blood glucose control over that period.

The A1c percentages are often used by health care professionals to diagnose diabetes, and no fasting is required. The percentages are as follows: Normal (no diabetes), when the reading is less than 5.7 percent; prediabetes, when the reading is 5.7 to 6.4 percent; and diabetes, when the reading is 6.5 percent or higher. (The test result may be in error if a person has anemia, kidney disease, or certain blood disorders.) If the level is 7 percent and the person has diabetes, then it often indicates that his or her blood glucose levels are not well controlled.

## How can a person with diabetes convert HbA1c (A1c) data into average blood glucose level?

There is a general way for a person with diabetes to convert HbA1c data into average blood glucose level. The following lists this conversion:

### HbA1c to Blood Glucose Level Conversion

| HbA1c | Blood Glucose Level |
|---|---|
| 6.0 % | 135 mg/dl |
| 6.5 % | 153 mg/dl |
| 7.0 % | 170 mg/dl |
| 7.5 % | 188 mg/dl |
| 8.0 % | 205 mg/dl |
| 8.5 % | 223 mg/dl |
| 9.0 % | 240 mg/dl |
| 9.5 % | 258 mg/dl |
| 10.0 % | 275 mg/dl |
| 10.5 % | 293 mg/dl |
| 11.0 % | 310 mg/dl |
| 11.5 % | 328 mg/dl |
| 12.0 % | 345 mg/dl |

# SELF–MONITORING DIABETES
# WITH METERS

## How does a person with either type 1 or 2 diabetes monitor blood sugar levels?

Most people with diabetes—types 1 and 2 and even some with prediabetes—monitor their blood glucose levels using a blood glucose meter. In general, the glucose meter measures a person's blood glucose in milligrams per deciliter (seen as mg/dl or mg/dL).

## What are test strips?

Most glucometers require what are called test strips in order to obtain a reading of a person's blood glucose level. The strip contains special enzymes designed to react with the person's blood.

## What is a glucometer?

A glucometer is a meter that measures blood glucose levels. Today's meters come in all kinds of forms, from talking and large-display meters to those that light up (for testing in the middle of the night, if necessary). Some also have built-in food databases and record-keeping systems. Almost all glucometers measure plasma glu-

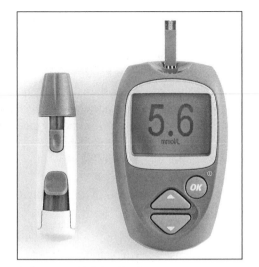

A glucometer (right) and syringe.

cose results by taking the value derived from a drop of whole blood and adding 12 percent to the measured value. For most meters, this is equivalent to a reading that a laboratory obtains.

## Where does one purchase glucometers?

Most glucometers are found at pharmacies and clinics, and many of them are free through special offers from the manufacturer. (It is the test strips used in the glucometers that often are the more costly items, since many people with diabetes have to test their blood glucose levels several times a day.) Some meters also have mail-in rebates after the meter is purchased, and some even offer trade-in rebates if a person has an older machine. For the coverage of diabetes supplies, such as test strips, patients should contact their insurance company to see what is covered (if anything). At this writing, for people on Medicare, the program will cover the costs of blood testing supplies for people with diabetes.

## What is a continuous glucose monitor (CGM)?

A continuous glucose monitor tracks a person's glucose levels every few minutes. It is also often used in conjunction with a regular blood glucose meter (that does not continuously monitor glucose levels). Once used mainly for young children (especially for nighttime monitoring) and less mobile people, the technology has improved enough for many others to use the device, such as diabetics who travel extensively, who have an active lifestyle, or who can't stop and monitor their blood glucose levels as much. The monitors have a small filament with a sensor that is inserted just below the skin, usually in an unobtrusive spot, such as just above or below the waist. Using a small radio transmitter, the sensor sends information to a handheld receiver; an iPhone, tablet, or computer can receive the data. The receiver displays the person's glucose level every few minutes. Depending on the model, special alarms can alert the person to fluctuations in blood glucose levels, especially drops in levels that can lead to hypoglycemia.

## What should a person look for when choosing a glucometer?

Choosing a glucose meter is mostly a personal choice (but not always, especially when certain health insurance companies cover only specific types of glucometers). There are some features to think about before picking a meter, including the speed (meters can take anywhere from five to 20 seconds to show results); a beeping or silent monitor for prompts; type of test strips (wrapped or not); or a meter with a memory. Other things to consider include how much the meter has to be cleaned; how portable it is (especially for travel); whether the meter checks for glucose and ketones; the size of blood sample the meter needs; and the types of (and ease of finding) batteries the meter uses. There are more considerations, but these are the most common.

## In general, how much fluctuation is there in glucometer readings?

No machine is perfect, and glucometers are no exception. Even if a glucometer is cleaned and calibrated regularly, it may vary in accuracy from other meters, perhaps by as much as 20 percent. If a person with diabetes has any question about the accuracy of a glucometer, it is best to have the device checked out by a health care professional, pharmacy, or diabetes educator.

## Can test strips give erroneous readings?

Yes, test strips can give a person with diabetes erroneous readings for a number of reasons. For example, the test strips may be too old. The enzymes that are embedded in the test strip can lose their activity and cause bare spots on the strips, giving an erroneous reading.

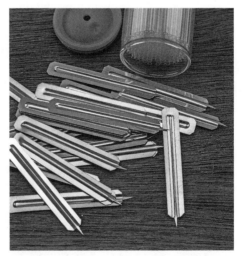

A person may use the wrong test strips for the glucometer, giving a false or inaccurate reading, or no result. (This is usually because every machine has its own special test strips.) Abnormal readings may also occur if the temperature is too low. Low temperatures often affect the ability to draw blood for testing (blood does not circulate as close to the skin's surface in lower temperatures as it does in higher temperatures).

## What is a lancet?

In order for patients to get a clean prick of the finger to obtain a blood sample for a glucometer, many companies provide a lancing device, commonly called a lancet. This tool for pricking a finger is usually ad-

Lancets allow you to make a clean, safe prick on the finger to draw a blood sample for testing.

justable to varying depths into the skin, depending on the individual's need. The lancet needle has a release button, pricking the finger quickly. For most people, this way of obtaining a drop of blood is easy, fast, and clean.

## What are some general steps when a person with diabetes takes his or her blood glucose level?

There are some very general steps a person with diabetes can take when using a blood glucose meter. Some people may have to take other steps, so it is best to check the procedure with a health care professional).

- The first step is having everything out that the person will need to take his or her levels, such as the meter, unused test strips, unused lancets, and alcohol swabs. (Make sure the meter's batteries are charged.)

- Next, the person should make sure his or her hands are clean and free of anything that could influence the meter's reading. (It is best to wash the hands in warm water.)

- After drying the hands, the person may shake the hands below the waist, then squeeze (some people refer to it as "milking") the fingers a few times before using the lancet. This helps to bring the blood flow to the fingertip. (Blood samples are most often taken at the fingertips, where there are fewer nerve endings.)

- The lancet device is then put on the side of the fingertip, and the release button on the lancet is pushed. As a small drop of blood appears, it can be helped along if the person gently squeezes from the base of the finger toward the tip until a good drop of blood appears.

- From there, the test strip essentially sucks up the drop of blood, and the meter is set to read the blood glucose level.

- At this point, some meters will digitally record the person's blood glucose data for each day. Other meters just give the blood glucose number, meaning it is up to the person to record and keep track of the blood glucose numbers each day (many glucometers come with a free log book).

## What events and actions can often throw off blood glucose levels?

Several events and actions can throw off a person's blood glucose levels, no matter how well the person monitors his or her blood glucose. Ordinary or non-ordinary events such as stress, certain illnesses, unanticipated activity, menstruation, eating, alcohol, or medications can throw the blood glucose levels off balance and cause (sometimes dangerous) fluctuations.

## What medical conditions can lead to erroneous readings on a glucometer?

Several medical conditions a person with diabetes can have affect the readings on a glucometer. For example, blood disorders can cause inaccurate readings, such as in people who are anemic whose readings are often falsely high. A person with high levels of he-

## Do blood glucose meters measure ketones?

**Y**es, some blood glucose meters measure ketones. This is important to people with diabetes, especially for people with type 1 diabetes. The meters use special blood ketone strips, with the level of ketones shown as a number on the meter display. In most cases, if the ketone reading is moderate or high, and a person's blood sugar is also high, the person should receive medical attention immediately as high ketones indicate possible diabetic ketoacidosis (for more about diabetic ketoacidosis, see the chapter "Type 1 Diabetes").

moglobin in the blood (polycythemia) can experience false low readings. If a person is dehydrated or in shock, he or she may also have false or abnormal glucometer readings.

### What other things can interfere with blood glucose readings on a glucometer?

Many things can interfere with blood glucose readings on a glucometer. For example, acetaminophen (commonly referred to as Tylenol) and acetaminophen-containing drugs (some over-the-counter cough and cold medications contain the drug, as do some prescription pain medications such as Zutripro) can interact with certain chemicals used in various medical devices. This interaction can cause the person's blood glucose levels to rise, interfering with the correct readings. In addition, if a person does not clean his or her hands before collecting a blood sample, incorrect readings can result (the more recent meters only need a small sample, and if it is contaminated with other chemicals or dirt, it can throw off the reading). Other more technical conditions may lead to false blood-sugar readings. For example, glucose meters vary in the way they work and are calibrated. Failure to calibrate the meter regularly can lead to false blood glucose readings.

### Why do many doctors suggest that blood samples for a glucometer be taken from a person's fingertips?

For some blood glucose meters, there is a reason for taking most of the blood samples from the person's fingertips—obtaining it in almost any other part of the body (unless it is necessary) can result in a false reading. That being said, many of the more modern glucose monitors require a tiny blood sample, some as small as a third of a microliter. For many of these machines, the small sample can be taken from other sites on the body, such as the forearm or thigh.

### How many times a day should a person with diabetes test his or her blood glucose levels?

There is no set number of times a day that blood glucose levels should be tested. This is because everyone's needs and blood glucose levels are different. Some health care professionals suggest monitoring after a meal; others advocate testing as many times as possible throughout the day. Most believe it is a good idea to check glucose levels before a person drives, exercises, uses heavy equipment, or performs any high-risk task. But overall, the number of times a person monitors glucose levels depends on the individual, the extent of the diabetes, and the recommendations of health care professionals and diabetes-care team.

## Who should test their blood glucose levels on a regular basis?

Although not all people with diabetes need to diligently self-monitor their blood sugar levels, whether they should or not seems

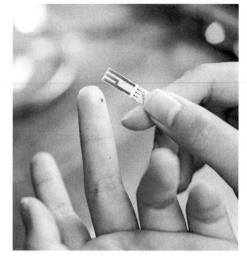

Taking blood from the tip of one's finger provides the most accurate readings of glucose levels.

to depend on what type of diabetes a person develops. Most health care professionals suggest that people who take insulin should test their blood sugar regularly. Those who take oral diabetes medication for type 2 diabetes should test their levels frequently, especially if they are taking sulfonylureas or glinides, both of which can occasionally cause low blood sugar.

In addition, Harvard Medical School suggests that certain situations warrant more frequent testing of blood sugar levels, including very high levels at the time diabetes is diagnosed, recent weight gain or loss (not explained by dieting or stress), exercising more than usual (or even less than usual), a change in a person's diabetic medications (especially sulfonylureas and glinides), and during an illness, such as a gastrointestinal virus (because even a flu or cold can cause blood sugar levels to fluctuate).

## Are there any Internet tools a person can use to manage diabetes?

Yes, thanks to current technology and the Internet, there are many tools that a person with diabetes can use to manage diabetes. For example, there are websites that help keep track of blood glucose readings, which is important for the patient and the health care professionals who are helping their patient to stay healthy. There are also websites that offer diabetes-management assistance, and some clinics and health care providers can send your lab results directly to a patient's account. The Internet also offers many personal health-management or electronic health record websites, some for free (but such sites may have online advertising) and some for a price. It is up to the individual to decide how much information he or she is willing to provide when signing up for an account. For security purposes, a person with diabetes interested in such a service should do some research on the company before choosing. (For more about the websites, see the "Resources, Websites, and Apps" section of this book.)

# DIABETES AND MEDICATION

## What types of medicines are used to treat diabetes?

Two main types of medications are used. The first are oral medications, or those that are taken by mouth; these are most often associated with type 2 diabetes. The second type is insulin that is injected or administered using an insulin pump or pen and is most associated with type 1 diabetes. (Insulin cannot be taken as a pill because the acid and digestive enzymes in a person's stomach destroy the hormone.) According to the Centers for Disease Control and Prevention, the medicines used by adults with diabetes (both type 1 and 2) can be broken down by how they are taken. Among adults, 57 percent take oral medications only, 14 percent take only insulin, 14 percent take a combination of insulin and oral medication, and 15 percent take no medication (mostly people with prediabetes).

## How long will it take before someone with diabetes can see an improvement in blood glucose levels—after taking medications and/or making lifestyle changes?

Everyone differs when it comes to how long it takes to see an improvement (or a worsening) in blood glucose levels. And, of course, everyone is different when it comes to taking medications and making lifestyle changes after being diagnosed with diabetes. But, on the average, most people with diabetes will see an improvement in three to four months. Therefore, a follow-up blood glucose test is usually administered three to four months after a diagnosis. There is one caveat: according to the American Diabetes Association, if a person has had uncontrolled diabetes for a long time and has just been diagnosed, most doctors will test the person's blood glucose levels after two to three weeks to make sure there is an improvement.

## Does a person with diabetes always have to take some type of medication?

Unfortunately, if a person has type 1 or type 2 diabetes, then he or she will probably have to take some medication for the rest of his or her life. Diabetes is a progressive disease, and the longer a person has it, the more likely the person will need pharmaceutical help to manage it. Most people with prediabetes—people who have blood glucose levels above the normal range but not high enough to be called diabetes—will not need to take diabetes medication or will take medication only for a short time (until their blood glucose levels are lower and/or stable). And if a per-

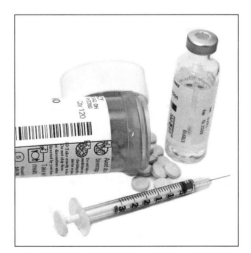

Insulin is only one medication diabetics can take to control blood sugar. For example, metformin works for those with less pronounced cases.

241

son who has prediabetes can maintain normal blood glucose levels and not develop diabetes, then he or she will never need any diabetic medication.

## What diabetes medications have recently been approved by the U.S. Food and Drug Administration?

For the past few decades, the U.S. Food and Drug Administration (FDA) has approved many different types of diabetes medications. These include medicines that are taken orally, injected, or inhaled. The following chart lists the diabetes medications that were approved between 2013 and 2016:

### Recently Approved Diabetes Medications

| Brand Name | Generic Name | Approval Date |
| --- | --- | --- |
| Basaglar | insulin glargine injection | December 16, 2015 |
| Tresiba | insulin degludec injection | September 25, 2015 |
| Ryzodeg | insulin aspart: insulin degludec | September 25, 2015 |
| Toujeo | insulin glargine injection | February 25, 2015 |
| Lucentis | ranibizumab | February 6, 2015 |
| Glyxambi | empagliflozin and linagliptin | January 2015 |
| Trulicity | duglaglutide | September 18, 2014 |
| Invokamet | canagliflozin and metformin hydrochloride | August 8, 2014 |
| Jardiance | empagliflozin | August 1, 2014 |
| Afrezza Inhalation Powder | insulin human | June 27, 2014 |
| Tanzeum | abliglutide | May 2014 |
| Farxiga | dapaglifozin | January 2014 |
| Invokana | canagliflozin | March 29, 2016 |
| Nesina | alogliptin benzoate | January 25, 2016 |
| Duetact | pioglitazone hydrochloride and glimepiride | January 2013 |

Source: FDA website. All FDA-approved medicines used in the treatment of diabetes are either taken orally, injected, or inhaled and can be found listed at what is called Drugs@FDA (http://www.access-data.fda.gov/cder/drug-satfda/). For drug-labeling information, go to the National Library of Medicine database of current drug information called DailyMed (http://dailymed.nim.nih.gov/dailymed/about.cfm).

## What is the common procedure if a person is diagnosed with type 2 diabetes?

According to Harvard Medical School, people who have been newly diagnosed with type 2 diabetes should start by concentrating on lowering their blood glucose levels. The two most frequent steps are making lifestyle choices—mainly eating better and exercising more—and to start taking a medication called metformin. Initially, traditional treatment started with lifestyle changes, and if that did not work, then the person was treated with medications. In the meantime, the disease would progress. Now, most doctors recommend that both lifestyle changes and medication be started when a person is first diagnosed. This is because research has shown that many times, in the early stages of the disease, the insulin-secreting cells in the pancreas that are "wearing out" may be saved. This results in either slowing down the disease's progression or even, for some people, mitigating the disease before it can take over.

## What is metformin?

The type of drug most often used to treat a person who has just been diagnosed with diabetes is called by the generic name metformin (one brand name is Glucophage). It is known to lower a person's HbA1c by about 1.5 percent and, in most cases, does not

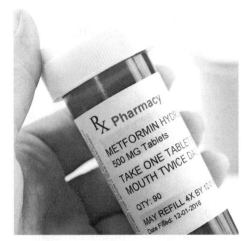

Metformin lowers your HbA1c without causing weight gain or hypoglycemia.

cause weight gain or hypoglycemia. It acts by reducing glucose secretion by the liver, lowering the organ's resistance to insulin, and it decreases blood glucose levels without stimulating the secretion of insulin. It is considered a biguanide (see above for other types of medications), a type of oral diabetes medication, and is most often taken twice a day (usually with breakfast and dinner) or one to two times a day if an extended-release formula is taken. There are some side effects, such as nausea and diarrhea, and in rare cases, it may cause lactic acidosis. In addition, there are often some restrictions to metformin that a person should discuss with his or her health care provider, especially if the person has kidney, heart, or liver disease.

## Does metformin have a peculiar smell?

Yes, there is one aspect of the diabetes drug metformin that no one expected. According to most people who take metformin, it has a distinctive smell that some describe as a "fishy" odor. Some doctors are concerned that this characteristic may cause a person to stop taking the drug. And since the drug works so well for most people with type 2 diabetes, stopping metformin would be detrimental to the person's health! There are potential solutions. One study indicated that switching to certain extended-release versions of the drug may help (these drugs are said to have less smell, if any at all). But the best solution if the smell is a concern—without holding one's nose as they take the drug—is to contact a health care professional about possible alternative formulations.

## Do any non-diabetic medicines affect a person with diabetes?

According to the Centers for Disease Control and Prevention, some non-diabetic medications can affect a person's blood glucose level. This is a concern if a person already has type 1 or type 2 diabetes. This is also why health care professionals must know the various medications a person with diabetes is taking, including those taken without a prescription (for example, vitamins and herbal supplements). The following are only some types of medications that can cause a problem with blood glucose levels:

- barbiturates
- thiazide diuretics (given mainly for high blood pressure)
- corticosteroids
- birth control pills and progesterone
- decongestants containing beta-adrenergic agents, such as pseudoephedrin
- vitamin $B_3$, also called niacin (but the risk of high blood sugar from niacin decreases after it has been taken for a few months)

## Is type 2 diabetes always treated with oral medications?

Most people with type 2 diabetes are commonly treated with oral medications. But if the drugs no longer work, then the person may have to turn to insulin injections. This means either insulin only or oral medications augmented with insulin injections.

## What are some possible ways to get off or lower diabetic medication if a person has type 2 diabetes?

Some health care professionals suggest that there are certain specific conditions in which a person with type 2 diabetes may be able to take less diabetes medication or even stop taking medication. One of the major problems in coping with diabetes is that the

### What combination drug was recently approved by the U.S. Food and Drug Administration for type 2 diabetes?

In 2016, the U.S. Food and Drug Administration approved a combination drug that includes metformin (a common treatment for type 2 diabetes) and empagliflozin (an SGLT2 inhibitor). The medicine, called Synjardy, is a joint effort by Boehringer Ingelheim Pharmaceuticals and Eli Lilly and Company. When the kidneys filter blood, they usually reabsorb all the filtered glucose and return it to the bloodstream. One of the primary proteins responsible for reabsorption is called SGLT2. What empagliflozin does is block this reabsorption, causing glucose to be lost in the urine and lowering a person's blood glucose levels. At the same time, with this combination pill, the metformin decreases the amount of glucose made by the liver. It also improves insulin sensitivity in the liver and in muscle and fat cells. Through trials, researchers found that this combination significantly lowered the HbA1c levels compared with the same dose of either medicine alone. But there are some restrictions. It cannot be used by people with type 1 diabetes or who have diabetic ketoacidosis or severe kidney disease.

person usually has to make conscious lifestyle changes. In fact, certain lifestyle changes may help immensely. These include more healthful eating habits, starting or maintaining better exercise routines, and keeping excellent track of blood glucose levels. The following lists some target glucose levels to reach in order to reduce, possibly, or even stop a person's type 2 diabetes medication (of course, getting off medication also depends on other health conditions and what the health care provider says):

*126 to 140 or 150 mg/dl*—This is still above the normal level, but if these readings are consistently low enough, the person may be able to eventually stop taking medication.

*150 to 200 mg/dl*—This is above the normal level, but with lifestyle changes, eventually the medication dosage may be lowered. But most people who have levels between these numbers will still need medication, and some may eventually need occasional doses of insulin.

*Above 200 mg/dl*—At and above this level means that the person with diabetes may need medication or full-time insulin coverage—and maybe even both. If the person with diabetes makes some or all of the above lifestyle changes, it may mean a reduction in medication dose or other adjustments. But it is likely that he or she will need medication for the rest of his or her life.

## What are some popular oral medications for people with type 2 diabetes?

A huge range of oral medications has been developed for people with type 2 diabetes—too many to mention in this text. There is a good reason for so many choices as every person who has diabetes has a different body composition and diabetic condition. (For more about listings of the most current medications from government sites, see the chapter "Resources, Websites, and Apps.") In general, there are several general types of medications. They include the following:

*Biguanides*—The most commonly prescribed biguanide medication for type 2 diabetes, especially for a person who has just been diagnosed with the disease, is metformin. (For more about metformin, see above.)

*Sulfonylurea*—The sulfonylureas are the oldest class of oral diabetes medications (often seen as antidiabetic) and often a second choice after metformin. They work by stimulating the pancreas to make more insulin. There are some side effects that must be considered. For example, there is the risk of hypoglycemia, especially for the elderly or those who take a long-acting sulfonylurea (such as glyburide), and even if a person drinks a certain amount of alcohol or skips a meal. It also should not be taken by a person who is allergic to sulfa drugs.

*Alpha-glucosidase inhibitors*—These diabetic medications slow down the digestive enzyme that breaks down carbohydrates into smaller sugars, so they are more easily absorbed by the intestines. This action causes sugar levels to rise more slowly, and the insulin the body produces has more time to work efficiently, which helps slow down the surge in blood glucose after a meal. Side effects include flatulence and diarrhea, but if the dosage can be built up slowly, then such effects often slowly diminish over time.

*Thiazolidinediones*—These diabetes medications, also called glitazones, reduce a person's insulin resistance and are frequently used in conjunction with other diabetes medicines. They help a person with diabetes by making the body's muscles, fat, and liver more sensitive to insulin and thus more able to absorb nutrients from the blood. There are several side effects, such as weight gain and fluid retention, meaning this drug is not for everyone. Because of these side effects, thiazolidinediones (especially rosiglitazone and pioglitazone) have been linked to increased risk of heart failure and possible increase in bone fractures and loss. Thus, it is best to discuss this type of drug with the health care provider to understand these side effects.

*Meglitinides*—These drugs work by increasing the amount of insulin produced by the pancreas, thereby lowering blood sugar. They act quickly and do not stay in the body long. Therefore, they are usually ingested at or just before each meal. They are often used for people with type 2 diabetes who eat healthfully and exercise but still cannot sufficiently lower their blood glucose levels. There are several side effects in some people, including weight gain and low blood sugar.

## What is lactic acidosis and its connection to some diabetes medications?

Lactic acidosis occurs when the body cannot get rid of lactic acid from the blood. During strenuous exercise, lactic acid (lactate) is created in the muscles and blood as a natural byproduct of the body's metabolism, primarily because the cells are not getting enough oxygen. Normally, this acid is cleared from the blood by the liver, kidneys, and muscles. Although it rarely happens, if lactic acid builds up to very high levels in the body, then it can cause a life-threatening condition called lactic acidosis.

In some people, lactic acidosis can occur—again, rarely—if they take metformin (Glucophage) to control diabetes, especially if they are experiencing heart or kidney failure and if there is a severe infection present. (Because of this, the FDA states that the drug must carry a warning about its possible lactic acidosis side effect.) It is thought that since the liver filters acid from the body when it produces sugar, and metformin decreases the organ's ability to produce sugar, lactic acid buildup results. Metformin is not the only drug to have this effect. Two other diabetes medications, phenformin and buformin, also have lactate side effects and have been banned from use in the United States.

## What are some of the more recent oral medications for people with type 2 diabetes?

There are several more recent oral medications prescribed for people with type 2 diabetes. The following lists some of them:

*DPP-4 inhibitors*—These drugs work by blocking an enzyme called DPP-4. DPP-4 normally deactivates a protein (GLP-1, or glucagon-like peptide) that keeps insulin circulating in the blood, and by blocking the enzyme, it helps reduce sugar production, lowering blood glucose levels. The first DPP-4 that was approved by the Food and Drug Administration was Januvia (sitagliptin phosphate), an oral medication taken once a day, either alone or with diet and exercise or in combination with other oral diabetes medications.

*Incretin mimetics*—These drugs work by mimicking the action of incretin hormones (which help the body make more insulin). They also slow the rate of digestion so that glucose enters a person's bloodstream more slowly. This medicine makes the person feel full longer, thus reducing food intake, which can help people lose weight while on the medication.

*Byetta (exenatide)*—This drug is an injectable medication used in combination with other oral diabetes medications. It is not an insulin, and it does not take the place of insulin. It is used for type 2 diabetes only and cannot be given with insulin. It comes in a pre-filled injector pen, with dosages taken twice a day within an hour before morning and evening meals.

*Antihyperglycemic synthetic analogs*—These drugs are synthetic versions of human substances. For example, there is a human hormone drug called amylin, which is used by the pancreas to lower blood glucose levels.

*Symlin (pramlintide acetate)*—Symlin is an injectable medication used with insulin for tighter blood glucose control. It can also increase the risk of severe hypoglycemia; therefore, patients who are put on Symlin are selected carefully and monitored closely by their health care providers.

# INSULIN

## What are the main types of insulin?

There are several types of insulin you can take. Each type serves a different purpose, and you might need to take a combination of the following (note: some references show different times to take effect; thus, the following is only a general guide):

### What two ingredients in some type 2 diabetes medication now have FDA warnings?

Not all diabetic medications can be used by people with type 2 diabetes, and some even carry warnings on their labels. For instance, diabetic medications containing saxagliptin (for example, Onglyza) and alogliptin (for example, Nesina) are known to increase the incretin hormones, which increase insulin production after a person eats. But as with any medication, nothing is perfect. In 2014, the Food and Drug Administration added warnings and precautions to diabetes medications containing saxagliptin and alogliptin, as clinical trials linked the substances to an increased risk of heart failure, especially in patients who already had heart or kidney disease.

*Rapid-acting insulin*—This type of insulin takes effect in 15 minutes or less and is taken before a meal. In someone without diabetes, the body releases the right amount of insulin when the person eats. This insulin helps someone with diabetes process and use the carbohydrates in the food. (The release of insulin at mealtime is called the bolus secretion; thus, rapid-acting insulin imitates the bolus secretion; see below.)

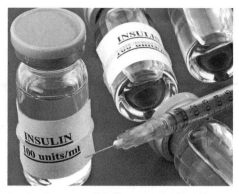

People who are not diabetic may not realize that there are actually several types of insulin. Some take effect more quickly than others.

*Regular or short-acting insulin*—Regular insulin takes effect within 30 minutes of injection. It is also taken before a meal, but its effect lasts longer than rapid-acting insulin. (Regular or short-acting insulin imitates the bolus secretion; see below.)

*Intermediate-acting insulin*—This type of insulin lasts for 10 to 16 hours, and is generally taken twice a day. (It imitates basal secretion; see below.)

*Long-acting insulin*—Long-acting insulin is similar to intermediate-acting insulin, as it imitates the basal secretion. Long-acting insulin lasts for 20 to 24 hours, so the person with diabetes needs to take it only once a day (whereas intermediate-acting insulin is injected twice a day).

*Pre-mixed insulin*—A pre-mixed insulin combines two other types of insulin. For example, it may include rapid-acting and intermediate-acting insulin. This combination ensures that the person with diabetes has enough insulin to cover bolus and basal secretions.

## What is basal insulin?

Another name for slow-acting insulin is basal insulin. It is also called background or long-acting insulin and is used to keep blood glucose levels stable during times when the person with diabetes is not eating, meaning during "fasting" times (the basal secretion is the small amount of insulin that should always be in your blood). Between meals in someone without diabetes, the body steadily releases glucose into the bloodstream, where it provides the body's cells with energy. In a person with diabetes, the injected basal insulin keeps blood glucose levels under control, as long as it is injected once or twice a day (depending on the insulin).

## What is the timing of insulin's action in the body?

In general, the various types of insulin react in different ways in the body. The following chart shows the type of insulin, how long it takes to begin working, how long it takes to peak, and the estimated duration of the medication. These various medications can be used alone or in combination (see below). In addition, there is no guarantee that each insulin type will work the same for everyone and under every condition. (*Note*: Some medications, such as the long-acting insulins Lantus and Levemir, differ as to when they start working and their peak and duration. Thus, there are two listings in the chart below):

### Types of Insulin

| Type | Starts Working | Peaks | Estimated Duration |
|---|---|---|---|
| Very rapid-acting | 15 minutes | 1–2 hours | 3–5 hours |
| Rapid-acting | 30–60 minutes | 1–2 hours | 5–6 hours |
| Intermediate-acting | 1–2 hours | 4–8 hours | 8–12 hours |
| Long-acting | 1 hour | none | 24 hours |
| (brand dependent) | 3–4 hours | 6–8 hours | 6–23 hours |

## What is bolus insulin?

A bolus insulin dose is one that is taken specifically at mealtimes (either before, during, or just after meals) in order to keep a person's blood glucose level under control following a meal. This type of insulin needs to act quickly to prevent hypoglycemia, and thus, short-acting or rapid-acting insulin is used.

## What is a basal-bolus injection regimen?

People with type 1 diabetes and some with type 2 diabetes will often maintain a basal-bolus injection regimen. This schedule combines both the basal insulin and bolus insulin methods. In particular, a basal-bolus injection regime includes an injection at each meal (bolus) and a longer-acting form of insulin (basal) once or twice a day. In this way, the regimen emulates somewhat how a person who does not have diabetes naturally delivers insulin throughout the day. For many people with type 1 diabetes, taking rapid-acting insulin at mealtime and a long-acting insulin once or twice a day is a good way to control their blood glucose levels.

### What is the difference between long-acting peaking and long-acting peakless?

Although these terms seem similar, long-acting peaking is a form of insulin that does not begin to lower blood glucose levels until four to six hours after it is injected. It works mostly from eight to 30 hours after injection and continues to work for up to 24 to 36 hours. One example is ultralente insulin. The long-acting peakless is a basal type of insulin. It lowers blood glucose within one to two hours after injection and continues for 24 hours. One example is glargine insulin.

There are several advantages to this regimen, including that it simulates the natural release of insulin in the body. It can often give a person flexibility as to when he or she can eat a meal—and even, if the insulin is adjusted correctly, how many carbohydrates a person with diabetes can consume. (Depending on the person's condition, he or she may be able to eat more carbohydrates.) There are also some disadvantages to the regimen. For example, it involves taking several daily insulin injections. Hypoglycemia is often a common occurrence on a basal-bolus regimen (which is why it is recommended to keep a blood glucose testing kit and a fast-acting carbohydrate available in case of a low blood glucose level). And depending on a person's diabetic condition, not everyone will be able to use this regimen. In addition, children who are on this regimen would have to be comfortable getting injections at mealtimes, either at school or other functions—and would have to understand that they need several injections each day.

## What is inhalable insulin?

Inhalable insulin is a powdered form of insulin (or dry insulin) that is delivered via inhalation, sending small particles of insulin into the lungs. From there, it is absorbed by the cells in the lungs and then into the bloodstream. It can be used by people with type 1 or type 2 diabetes. The delivery system may be a nebulizer, meaning a device using compressed air that allows the particles to be inhaled (a process called aerosolization), or inhalers that can be activated with the breath (the insulin is inhaled directly through the mouth and into the lungs). The suggested advantage of inhaled insulin is that, because it enters the lungs, the dose can enter the bloodstream more quickly than injected insulin. One form of inhaled insulin called Afrezza has been said to have "peak activity" 12 to 15 minutes after taking the dose, while insulin injections average between 30 and 90 minutes after injecting.

Insulin inhalers are not to be used all the time. They are meant to be used mainly at the start of a meal to help with blood-sugar control. Most research shows inhalers to be safe to use with basal insulin (for more about basal insulin, see above). Of course, there are some warnings. In particular, inhalers are not recommended if the person with diabetes has chronic lung problems or if the person smokes. In addition, the most common adverse reaction with inhalable insulin (or any insulin) is hypoglycemia.

## What new manmade version of insulin has recently been approved in the United States?

Research has developed a long-acting, manmade version of natural human insulin, referred to as insulin glargine. Insulin glargine not only replaces the body's natural insulin but also moves glucose into the tissues and prevents the liver from making extra sugar. This type of insulin was developed by the pharmaceutical company Sanofi US (also known as Sanofi-aventis) and called by the brand name Lantus®. It was already on the market in 2000, but the patent expired in 2015. This meant that other drug companies could start making their own types of insulin glargine, also referred to as "biosimilar insulin."

## Which inhalable insulin was eventually taken off the market?

In January 2006, an inhalable insulin called Exubera, developed by Inhale Therapeutics (later Nektar Therapeutics), was commercially introduced to the public by the pharmaceutical company Pfizer. But because of poor sales, by October 2007, it had been taken off the market.

Thus, in 2016 the U.S. Food and Drug Administration (FDA) approved the first "copycat" version of insulin glargine called Basaglar from Eli Lilly. (It was also the first company to come out with commercially available insulin in the 1920s; for more about the company and the first commercial insulin, see the chapter "Introduction to Diabetes.") Similar to Lantus®, the newest biosimilar insulin is administered by daily injection. It is used mainly for children and adults with type 1 diabetes and under certain conditions in adults with type 2 diabetes. Other biosimilar insulins will no doubt follow, as long as the pharmaceutical companies who want to develop the insulin go through a rigorous FDA approval process. It is too early to tell whether more insulin glargines on the market will mean lower prices for many of the 10 million Americans with diabetes who use insulin.

## Do people with type 2 diabetes need injectable medication that is NOT insulin?

Although some people with type 2 diabetes take oral medication and insulin, there are some who need injectable medications (along with or other than insulin) to help control their blood glucose level. They would take this medication either in conjunction with other diabetes medicines or singularly. (These injectable medications are not for people with type 1 diabetes.) For example, a class of injectable drugs called glucagon-like peptide-1 (GLP-1) agonists are often prescribed, along with a healthful diet and exercise. (These drugs are also associated with a low rate of developing hypoglycemia in people with diabetes.) They include such drugs as Victoza (generic name liraglutide; it is similar to the body's naturally occurring hormone to help control blood glucose, insulin levels, and digestion), Byetta (exenatide; it helps control blood glucose levels by helping the pancreas produce insulin more efficiently), and Tanzeum (albiglutide; it improves blood glucose levels when used in conjunction with a good diet and exercise). In general, it is thought that the GLP-1 agonists work by stimulating the pancreas's insulin-producing beta cells in order to release insulin in response to a person's high blood glucose levels.

## Are there any experimental drugs that treat or may eventually treat diabetes?

Yes, there are many experimental drugs and medications that are—and may eventually be—used to treat diabetes or complications from the disease. For example, a drug called Herberprot-B, developed in Cuba, has been used around the world to treat diabetic foot ulcers. (This medicine was not available in the United States because of an embargo on trade with Cuba. In late 2016, it was reported that clinical trials on Herberprot-B were being conducted in the United States, but it is not known when the drug will become available.)

There are also experimental drugs that may or may not help people with diabetes and its complications, with one of the more controversial—and research-contrary—ones being medical marijuana. The reason for the controversy is the profusion of opposing studies about medical marijuana and diabetes. For example, several studies indicated that marijuana users had lower fasting insulin levels and less insulin resistance than non-users. In a different study, it appeared that there was a 30 percent lower risk of developing diabetes for those who used marijuana. But other studies disagreed, including one from the National Institutes of Health that warned that marijuana users had more abdominal fat, along with more insulin-resistant fat cells. Still other studies indicated that former marijuana users had higher glucose and insulin levels in their blood than those who had never used the drug. No one to date can actually say that marijuana can help or hinder a person with diabetes.

# MONITORING FOR HYPOGLYCEMIA, HYPERGLYCEMIA, AND DIABETIC KETOACIDOSIS

## Why is hypoglycemia a concern for a person with diabetes?

Hypoglycemia—or low blood sugar—is one of the most common, and often dangerous, side effects of any medication for lowering blood glucose. The goal of a person with diabetes should be to keep blood glucose levels as close to normal as possible. If a person with diabetes has a blood glucose level below 70 mg/dl (milligrams per deciliter), he or she can begin to experience a hypoglycemic low. Some causes may be missing or postponing a meal or even eating less than the right amount of carbohydrates; exercising more than usual; emotional upset or stress; injecting the wrong dose of insulin; or consuming too much alcohol for that person. Often, these lows occur for no apparent reason. That is why many health care professionals—and sometimes people with diabetes who have had hypoglycemic episodes—recommend that a person with diabetes always carry some form of quickly absorbed glucose.

## What are some symptoms of hypoglycemia?

When people with diabetes become hypoglycemic, they are often extremely confused. At first, the brain sends out signals to raise the glucose level, and the alpha cells in the pancreas release glucagon. This tells the liver and muscles to release the stored glycogen and then change it back to glucose to raise the blood sugar back to normal. In the meantime, the body releases epinephrine, a hormone that increases hunger, causes a re-

## Why is it important not to become hypoglycemic?

It is important for a person with diabetes not to become hypoglycemic. Not only does it cause the body to lose control—and, if a person is in the later stages of hypoglycemia, to hurt him- or herself—but it also can take a toll on the body as a whole (especially if it happens many times in a short period). The best way to treat hypoglycemia is to recognize the first symptoms and take action right away. For many people with diabetes, it usually means ingesting something that will get into their system quickly, such as glucose tablets, fruit juice (around 4 to 6 ounces), 2 tablespoons of raisins, or sugary candies. (Do not reach for foods containing chocolate, peanut butter, nuts, or fats unless it is the only sugary food available. The fat can actually delay the rise in blood glucose levels.) Most of these foods will be absorbed into the system quickly and begin to raise blood glucose within five to ten minutes.

sistance to the insulin's action, and further stimulates the breakdown of the liver's glycogen into glucose. Other hormones are released, including cortisol, to counteract the insulin and raise the blood glucose levels. The result is that a person can experience dizziness, a pale or flushed face, often dilated pupils, irritability, hunger, sweating, a rapid heartbeat, weakness, nervousness or anxiousness, and shakiness.

The symptoms do not stop there. Later symptoms are caused by the decreasing availability of glucose to help the brain and nervous system. These symptoms include headache, blurred vision, slurred speech, confusion, euphoria, hostility, lack of coordination, drowsiness, possible convulsions and seizures, and loss of consciousness. At this point, emergency help should be called and the person should be taken to the hospital.

## What is a glucagon kit?

Although it may never have to be used, a glucagon kit is for a diabetes emergency—in particular for severe hypoglycemia, especially for people with type 1 diabetes. The glucagon (to be injected into the person having a hypoglycemic episode) in the kit will raise the blood glucose levels when a person with diabetes is unconscious or uncooperative while having a severe hypoglycemic attack caused by low blood glucose. The kit contains a liquid and a powder to produce glucagon; the powder must be mixed with the liquid in the kit right before it is injected. The dosing is different for children and adults. In general, if a child weighs less than 50 pounds (22.7 kilograms), half of the dose should be given; if more than 50 pounds, a full dose should be given. But overall, the amount of the dose should be understood by the person administering it, whether family, a friend, or emergency medical technicians.

It is important that people with diabetes help their family and/or friends understand not only where the glucagon kit is located in the person's home but also how to ad-

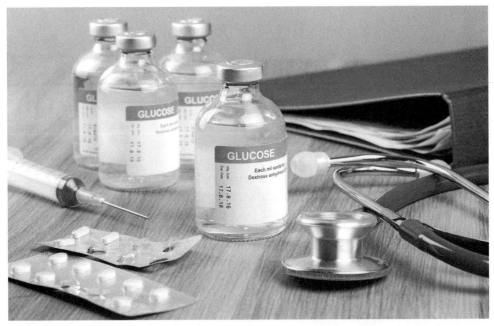

Hypoglycemic patients might experience low blood glucose levels without warning—and sometimes without apparent reason. Having a glucagon kit can bring levels back to a normal range quickly.

minister the glucagon. In most cases, if emergency personnel are called when a person with diabetes has severe hypoglycemia, the emergency medical technicians will have such a kit. (Note: Also be aware that glucagon can induce vomiting. If the person having a hypoglycemic episode has eaten recently, then it is best to keep his or her head turned, especially if the person is unconscious.)

### Is the glucagon in a kit the same as glucagon naturally produced by the body?

Yes, the glucagon (also known as glucagen) in a kit is similar to the glucagon naturally produced by the body. Like the natural hormone, it raises the blood glucose level by releasing glucose stored in the liver. The glucagon in the kit is injected intramuscularly or subcutaneously and takes about ten to 15 minutes to work. But there is one caveat: If the stores in the person's liver are low, then the injected glucagon may not be effective. In addition, if the person has been drinking alcohol to excess, has a very poor appetite (or has eaten a small amount of food recently), or had a hypoglycemic episode the day before, the glucagon may not work.

### Is it possible to overdose injected insulin?

Yes, it is possible to get an overdose of insulin, although it is very rare if a person keeps careful tabs on his or her insulin injections. In this case, an overdose of insulin causes hypoglycemia, or a very low blood glucose level, or glucose levels lower than 4 mmol/l (micromoles per liter). In general, the symptoms of hypoglycemia include anxiety, confusion, sweating or clammy skin, trembling hands, extreme hunger, fatigue, or extreme irritability. If levels continue to fall after an overdose, other more serious conditions can occur, such as seizures or unconsciousness. Not everyone with diabetes experiences these symptoms with low blood sugar. (Although no one knows why at this writing, some people—most often with type 1 diabetes—have few symptoms as their blood sugar drops. This is also why most health care professionals advocate that people with type 1 and 2 diabetes keep tabs on their blood glucose levels periodically throughout the day.)

Overdoses of insulin can occur in people with type 1 diabetes, as they have to inject the hormone into their system. It can also happen to the people with type 2 diabetes who inject insulin (usually because the blood glucose levels cannot be controlled by oral medication or there are changes in lifestyle, diet, or exercise). The following lists several ways in which a person with diabetes can get too much injected insulin:

- A person with diabetes injects the insulin but does not eat afterward. Blood glucose rises after a meal, and the injected insulin helps to lower it to a healthy level. If the person does not eat, the insulin can lower the blood glucose to a potentially dangerous level. This is why it is important to time insulin injections with meals.

- The person injects too much insulin. This may be because the person is not paying attention, is having difficulty reading the syringe or vials, or is not familiar with a new product for insulin injections. Once again, the extra insulin in the system will lower the blood glucose levels.

- The person injects the right amount of insulin but the wrong type. For example, short-acting insulin differs from long-acting insulin. If the person mixing the

## What is GlucoGel™ (or Gluco Gel or glucogel)?

GlucoGel™ is the brand-name gel used by many people—including emergency medical technicians—to raise blood glucose levels quickly. It also provides a fast-acting energy boost to a person with diabetes. One of the reasons it was developed is that many diabetics having a hypoglycemic episode are irritable, hostile, and unreasonable. Many refuse to eat anything. The gel is easier to administer than food.

Formerly known as Hypostop, GlucoGel™ is a "sugar" gel (around 40 percent dextrose) that is mostly used for hypoglycemia and can be prescribed by a general practitioner or purchased over the counter. It should be used only if the person who is having a hypoglycemic attack can swallow (there is the risk that an unconscious person will choke). The gel must be squeezed from the tube into the mouth and between the teeth and cheek. This is because the gel is absorbed by the lining of the mouth. The person's blood glucose levels should rise within 15 minutes. After this treatment, it is advised that the person eat a starchy carbohydrate snack such as toast or a sandwich—then check blood glucose levels to see whether they have normalized. If not, the above steps can be repeated as necessary.

dosage usually takes ten units of short-acting insulin and 20 units of long-acting insulin but switches the amounts, the incorrect dosage can put too much insulin into the system. (For more about short- and long-acting insulin, see this chapter.)

### How should a person treat an overdose of injected insulin?

There are several ways to handle a *minor* insulin overdose. If the person has injected a great amount of insulin, seek medical help immediately by calling emergency (911 in the United States). But in most cases, if a person is at home (and conscious), the following are some suggestions from several diabetes organizations in case of a *minor* overdose:

- Don't panic.
- Check blood glucose level. (If it is very low, call emergency.)
- Drink a half cup of sweetened fruit juice and/or eat a sweet or glucose tablet. If a meal has been skipped, eat something now. For most people, eating 15 to 20 grams of carbohydrates should raise their blood glucose level.
- Rest—don't walk or exercise. It will affect glucose levels.
- Recheck blood glucose level after 15 (some say ten) to 20 minutes after taking in the sugar or carbohydrates. Seek medical help if the level is unaffected by what was eaten.
- Pay attention to how the body feels for the next few hours. If the symptoms don't improve or if other symptoms begin to occur, then seek medical help.

# ANIMAL HELP AND DIABETES

### What is the role of animals in the lives of humans, including some people with diabetes?

The role of animals is obvious to most people. In particular, domesticated animals—from cats and dogs to hamsters, horses, and goldfish—give emotional support, help to lower blood pressure, and offer companionship. Some special animals even help people with diabetes. For example, there are specially trained dogs that help detect when people are experiencing high and low blood glucose levels. Dogs can also be good for a person with diabetes to help promote exercise and provide social contact. And because most dogs are "creatures of habit," they can help a person with diabetes maintain a routine to monitor blood glucose and take medications.

### What are Diabetic Alert Dogs?

A Diabetic Alert Dog (DAD) is trained to detect a hypoglycemic or hyperglycemic attack in a person with diabetes. During either episode—low or high levels of glucose in the blood—the body releases certain chemicals. The chemical scents are not detectable by humans but can be noticed by specially trained DADs.

## How do specially trained Diabetic Alert Dogs help some people with diabetes?

Although not all people with diabetes can benefit from Diabetic Alert Dogs (and not all dogs can be alert-trained), the people who do benefit do so greatly. Because one-eighth of a dog's brain is composed of the olfactory bulb (tissue located at the front of the dog's brain that processes scents detected by cells in their nose), dogs can be trained to recognize a single, distinct scent (this is why dogs are also used in such activities as police or forensic work). These dogs do not take the place of monitoring blood glucose levels. But they can detect and alert a person to changes in blood glu-

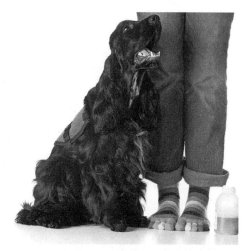

A trained Diabetic Alert Dog can detect, through its acute sense of smell, whether a person's blood glucose is getting too high or low, often even before the patient can tell.

cose levels or even alert others if the person with diabetes becomes incapacitated. (For resources on these dogs, including organizations such as the Diabetic Alert Dogs of America and Dogs 4 Diabetes, see the resources section at the end of this book.)

## Who may need a specially trained dog to alert him or her to a high or low blood glucose level?

Not everyone with diabetes is a candidate for a dog trained to detect high and low glucose levels in the blood. Therefore, people working with these dogs usually suggest that certain conditions be met to determine whether a person with diabetes is a good fit for such an animal. For example, for people with diabetes using insulin or sulfonylureas (a group of medications used to treat diabetes), very low blood glucose levels can often be a major problem. They need to be paired with dogs that can prevent such events as high and low blood sugar, warning the person if an episode is imminent. This is done by exposing the dog to the smell of sweat or saliva from the person when his or her blood glucose levels are either high or low. The dog is trained to alert a person to high or low blood glucose levels by a recognizable method, such as by nudging or touching the person with its paw.

## Are all alert dogs specially trained?

Although most dogs are specifically trained to alert people with diabetes to high and low blood glucose levels, some other dogs seem to do the task naturally. Stories about dogs adopted from a shelter that have helped their owners detect hypoglycemia or hyperglycemic episodes have been reported, but it often takes a special type of dog to take

## Why do dogs have such a keen sense of smell, especially in comparison with humans?

They have much better scent receptors. It is estimated that a dog's sense of smell is about a thousand times more sensitive than a human's. The reason is the receptors—a dog has more than 220 million scent receptors (44 times the number humans have) in its nose, covering an area about the size of a normal handkerchief. Most humans have just over 5 million scent receptors in their nose, which is about the size of a postage stamp. Another way of looking at it is that the dog's olfactory bulb is 40 times larger than a human's relative to brain size. And for people who have had certain problems with their sense of smell, such as chronic sinus infections, damaging chemicals, or even medicines that lessen the sense of smell, there are even fewer scent receptors available to smell. (For more about the senses and diabetes, see the chapter "Diabetes and Inside the Human Body.")

on such a task. This is why, if a person with diabetes wants a diabetes alert dog and already owns a dog, he or she may want to enroll in a workshop in which the person can learn whether the dog is suitable. Most diabetes alert dog trainers also note that although a puppy can be trained as an alert dog, it probably will not be a reliable one until it is at least a year old.

# DIABETES AND EXERCISE

## GENERAL EXERCISE AND DIABETES

### Do people with diabetes benefit from exercise?

Yes, people with diabetes benefit from exercise in many ways. In particular, exercise—or any activity that keeps a person moving—helps with blood glucose control. This is because when muscles are used, fatty acids and glucose are burned. Thus, during and after exercise or activity, the body's glucose decreases, which means the pancreas's beta cells decrease the release of insulin, reducing the workload of the pancreas. The lower amount of insulin signals the liver to empty its glucose reserves (glycogen) into the bloodstream for the muscles to use as energy. Unless a person is on diabetes medication that can cause hypoglycemia, physical activity can help keep blood glucose levels in control. It also can improve insulin sensitivity, lower blood pressure and fats, and help with cardiovascular (heart in particular) wellness.

### When does a person with diabetes not benefit from exercise?

Some exercises are not considered appropriate for a person with diabetes under certain conditions. For example, certain activities that include straining, such as weightlifting, can increase a person's blood pressure during the activity. If an individual already has hypertension (high blood pressure), such activities can aggravate the condition. In addition, if a person has diabetic retinopathy, it also may be aggravated by straining exercises—and even those activities that include jarring or rapid head motions. If a person has peripheral neuropathy in the feet, he or she can still usually exercise but must conscientiously check his or her feet as nerve damage may cause the person not to feel an injury. Overall, the best course of action for a person with diabetes who wants to do any type of physical activity is to discuss it with a health care provider.

## What is more important for a person's health—losing weight or exercise?

Both losing weight and exercise are important for many people with and without diabetes. But there is an interesting bias toward losing weight and exercise: when some people exercise and notice that their weight does not change, they stop, thinking it does no good. In reality, people who exercise are reducing their risk of heart disease and stroke. In fact, most experts agree that exercising may be more important to a person's health than losing weight. They think of it as exercising for health, not for becoming thin.

In one study, more than 25,000 men and 7,000 women were tracked for eight years, with the researchers testing in particular body weight and fitness level. They found that for most people, an active lifestyle—which can include walking, biking, weight-bearing exercises, and so on— actually overrides certain risk factors for heart disease, such as genetics, high cho-

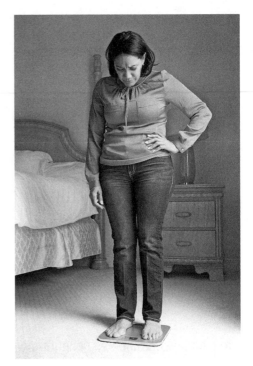

Don't be discouraged if you are trying to lose weight but the scale shows the same result. You are still boosting heart health, and if you gain muscle and lose fat, the total weight might seem the same.

lesterol, smoking, or even being overweight. Men and women who were moderately to highly fit, no matter what their risk factor(s), had the lowest death rates from all causes. This is not to say that being overweight or obese is all right for a person's health. (For more about obesity, see the chapter "Diabetes and Obesity.") Almost all health care professionals agree that being overweight or obese increases a person's chances of developing heart disease, diabetes, and other ailments. In fact, the more extra pounds a person carries, the greater the chance of illness, especially if the person is sedentary.

## Is there a double benefit to exercise for diabetes and the heart?

Yes, there is apparently a double benefit to exercise, especially if a person has diabetes and has (or has a potential for) heart disease. For example, in a recent study, 4,000 nurses between ages 40 and 65—all with diabetes—reduced their chances of developing heart disease by 28 percent just by having a regular walking regime. If someone exercised more vigorously, then the risk went down by another 5 percent.

# WEATHER, EXERCISE, AND DIABETES

## What should a person with diabetes be aware of when exercising in hot or cold weather?

If a person with diabetes exercises in hot or cold weather, depending on the situation and level of physical activity, low blood glucose levels can result. For example, if people with diabetes exercise in the heat, causing them to sweat profusely, then they may become dehydrated. This will cause a rise in their blood glucose levels and, in turn, make them urinate frequently, producing even higher glucose levels. In addition, if people use insulin injections to treat their glucose levels at this time, their dehydration causes a reduction of blood supply to the skin, resulting in less of the injected insulin being absorbed. (For more about weather and the outdoors, see the chapter "Coping With Diabetes.")

## What are some temperatures considered safe for exercise by a person with diabetes?

There are some general guidelines when it comes to walking and exercising in the great outdoors, depending on where you live, especially during the hottest and coldest times of the year. For example, when it comes to walking, for most people (with or without diabetes) the following applies: 90°F (32°C) and below, most people can walk (as long as the humidity is not high); 91–104°F (33–40°C), proceed with caution; 105–129°F (40–54°C), consider walking indoors in air conditioning, such as in a mall; 130°F, stay inside. Of course, not all of these numbers are definitive. Many times, with a temperature of 90°F (32°C), the humidity is around 75 percent, which makes it very difficult to walk or do most any exercise (unless the person is used to the conditions and as long as he or she consumes fluids, takes many breaks, and dresses to fit the weather). As with any exercise, a bit of common sense goes a long way.

## Is it safe for a person with diabetes to walk (or exercise) in the warmer weather?

In most cases, yes, it is fine for a person with diabetes to walk in the warmer weather. But there are some caveats. First, bring a water bottle on the walk, as dehydration is especially dangerous for people with diabetes because it can increase the blood sugar levels. Some snacks may also serve to prevent low blood sugar if needed or whatever a person knows works for him or her in treating low blood sugar. For example, some people with diabetes carry glucose tablets or gels with them, especially if they are prone to low blood sugar levels whether they exercise or not. (For some people with diabetes, it is always necessary to carry a glucagon kit; for more information about glucagon kits, see the chapter "Taking Charge of Diabetes.") Another suggestion is to make insulin adjustments as needed; people with diabetes can ask their health care provider or diabetes educator for the best way to adjust their insulin according to their specific needs. Probably the best practice when exercising in warmer weather is to test blood glucose levels more frequently, which will help a person with diabetes take appropriate action—immediately, if necessary—to keep glucose levels stable.

### What are some of the best times for a person with diabetes to walk or exercise when it's hot?

Most people agree—even those who do not have diabetes—that there are better times to walk than when it's too hot. Some people exercise early or late in the day, when the temperatures are cooler. Still others get their physical activity in air-conditioned places, such as a gym or their own home.

### Is it safe for a person with diabetes to walk (or exercise) in colder weather?

There are many precautions to take before venturing out to walk for exercise in the lower temperatures. In particular, cold-weather workouts can be risky for people with diabetes. This is because walking in the cold burns more calories to increase the body's warmth, so it increases the demands for blood sugar (glucose). This increased demand may be fine for people without diabetes, but for a person with diabetes it can lead to hypoglycemia, meaning too-low blood sugar.

Another concern is frostbite. This is because people with diabetes have poor circulation in their extremities, making it easy not to feel too cold—and frostbite can affect the feet and hands. A person with diabetes who loses feeling in the hands or feet should get indoors as soon as possible. Another possible condition is cyanosis—when skin looks blue—which is the first sign of frostbite. If this occurs, the person with diabetes should see a doctor immediately.

# BLOOD GLUCOSE AND EXERCISE

### What blood glucose goals should a person with diabetes have when exercising?

The biggest goal for people who exercise and have diabetes is to maintain their blood glucose levels during the activity. In particular, they should avoid becoming hypoglycemic (low blood glucose) before, during, and after exercise. The best way is to check blood glucose levels often. According to the Joslin Diabetes Center, this means checking blood glucose before, halfway through, and after exercise. For someone just beginning a certain exercise activity, this data becomes important, as it will help him or her learn the impact of that exercise on blood glucose levels. Overall, the person's health care professional or diabetes educator can make suggestions to keep blood glucose better balanced during physical activity.

### What are some suggestions to maintain blood glucose levels before exercising?

According to the Joslin Diabetes Center, if a person with type 2 diabetes is on oral medications, his or her blood glucose level should be 90 milligrams per deciliter (mg/dl), or slightly above, before exercising. (Note: A person with type 2 diabetes with a blood glucose level of 400 mg/dl or higher should avoid all exercise and contact a health care provider for ways to lower the blood glucose.) Another suggestion is to contact the health care professional before starting any exercise program to make sure the medication being taken will not lead to hypoglycemia (some diabetes medications can increase the risk of hypoglycemia). Someone with type 1 diabetes who is taking medication and insulin is more at risk for hypoglycemia—so it is suggested that the blood glucose target level be 110 to 140 mg/dl or above before starting exercise. And people with either type 1 or type 2 diabetes should also pay attention to how various exercises affect their glucose levels: for example, how aerobic exercise will result in different glucose levels than resistance training.

## What should a person with type 1 diabetes know about ketones and exercise?

If possible, a person who has type 1 diabetes should talk to a health care professional about how to check for ketones in the blood before physical activity, especially if it is rigorous activity. If there are ketones, it is best to avoid the exercise and ask the health care provider how to lower ketone levels in order to do any physical activity. If there are no ketones, it is suggested that the person perform low-to-moderate physical activity.

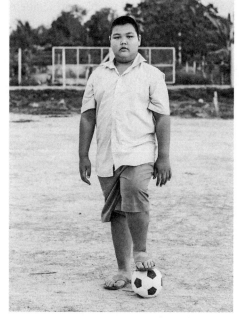

Exercise is vital in controlling diabetes, and monitoring blood sugar becomes even more important when establishing a routine. Check your glucose before, during, and after exercising, just in case.

## Do muscle-strengthening exercises help women prevent type 2 diabetes?

Yes, according to a study conducted in 2014, women who do exercises that strengthen muscles seem to have a lower risk of developing type 2 diabetes. The study included 100,000 women between ages 36 and 81. The researchers found that women who practiced yoga, lifted weights, or did stretching or toning exercises had a lower risk of developing the disease than participants who did not perform muscle-strengthening exercises. They also found that 60 minutes of muscle-strengthening exercises per week, along with 150 minutes of aerobic exercise such as running, walking, or cycling, had an even greater benefit.

# EXERCISE WEAR AND DIABETES

## Why should people with diabetes be careful when they buy shoes and sneakers?

It *does* pay, so to speak, for a person with diabetes to pay attention when shopping for shoes and sneakers. This is because the feet are one of the weakest points in anyone    263 with diabetes. Many people with diabetes walk for exercise, so here are some shopping tips that may help. For example, people can shop at the end of the day, when their feet are largest (the foot can be almost a half size larger by afternoon than in the morning). If possible, they should have their feet measured in order to obtain the best shoe size and fit. They should wear the socks they wear while exercising or walking, and when trying on a shoe, make sure there is plenty of room (experts say at least a finger's width) beyond the end of the toes (and measure while standing, not sitting). Not all shoes that are good for a person with diabetes will be stylish or trendy. But footwear that fits usually means fewer problems with the person's feet. That is why most health care professionals—especially those who deal with foot care—agree that when it comes to diabetes and a person's feet, it is better to have function over style.

### When should a person replace his or her walking shoes?

In general, it is recommended to replace walking shoes every 500 to 700 miles (although this number varies depending on the organization recommending shoe replacements) in order to keep a person's feet, ankles, knees, and lower back healthy and free of injury. Of course, most people don't count how many miles they travel in a pair of walking shoes or sneakers. So the rule of thumb is that if the heel shows wear, or the upper part of the shoe looks as if it has been pushed to one side, or if, of course, the shoe's seam is ripped or the upper part of the shoe is falling apart, then it is time to get new walking shoes. People with diabetes should look for two pairs of walking shoes to keep on hand, not just one. That way, if the shoes become wet, they can use the dry shoes. Wet shoes often cause blisters and can promote or exacerbate athlete's foot, both of which are dangerous for a person who has diabetes. (For more about feet, blisters, and athlete's foot and the diabetic, see the chapters "How Diabetes Affects Bones, Joints, Muscles, Teeth, and Skin" and "How Diabetes Affects the Nervous System.")

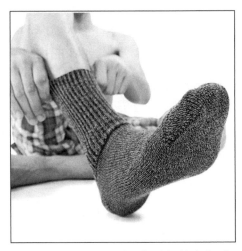

### Why are socks so important to a person with diabetes who exercises?

For most people with diabetes—type 1, type 2, and other types—exercise is an important part of their daily routine, especially to help manage weight and control glucose levels. Whether it is walking, hiking, or lifting weights at a gym, finding the right socks for exercise is especially important for people with diabetes. The major reason is that the feet can experience nerve damage (neuropathy), a problem for an estimated 50 percent of all people with diabetes. This causes a loss of

Believe it or not, even getting the right kind of socks can be important when you are exercising. Padded, good-fitting socks made for diabetics are the best choice.

sensation in the feet, meaning that a blister or wound will not be noticed until it worsens. Thus, health care professionals offer the following tips for socks for people with diabetes (see below for shoe recommendations):

- Get a fitted pair, not shapeless tube socks that can bunch up and cause chafing and blisters. The best fabric for socks is acrylic; the fibers wick sweat away from the feet and keep them drier than do cotton socks. This means the person will have fewer blisters and foot infections.

- Find socks that are specifically for people who have diabetes. Some hints about the best types of socks can be found on the American Podiatric Medical Association website at www.apma.org.

- Try to get padded socks but not so padded that there is little room for the foot. A too-tight fit in the shoe can cause foot blisters and infections. And make sure the tops of the socks are not too tight, as they may restrict the blood flow to the legs and feet.

## Why are shoes so important to a person with diabetes who exercises?

Because exercise is an important part of the daily routine for most people with diabetes, having the right shoes becomes very important. Whether it is walking, hiking, or lifting weights at a gym, finding the right shoes can be the most important part of the exercise. This is because the feet can experience nerve damage (neuropathy), causing a loss of sensation in the feet. If the shoes do not fit, then a blister may not be noticed. Thus, many health care professionals offer the following tips for finding the best shoes for people with diabetes (see above for sock recommendations):

- Try visiting a local, more personal, specialty shoe store where the staff would know more about the best shoes (including for a person with diabetes) and would offer more personal attention.

- The best time to shop for shoes is at the end of the day. This is because a person's feet swell throughout the day and are the largest toward evening. Shopping toward day's end will help one choose the correct size.

- Many people's feet are not the same size. If so, see whether the shoe store staff can suggest ways to make both shoes fit correctly, without chafing or causing blisters.

- Look for shoes that are comfortable almost immediately, with no pinching or pressure. The shoes should also be well padded and should not rub the foot. Also look for a large toe box, or the front of the shoe, so the toes can wiggle easily but without so much room that the foot slips around (that can cause chafing).

- Unfortunately, not all of the best shoes for a person with diabetes will be trendy or showy. High heels, for instance, can injure women's feet.

- Finally, don't be afraid to replace walking/exercise shoes regularly. It is suggested that most walkers buy new shoes every 500 to 700 miles, which translates to about every six months to a year if a person walks two miles five times a week.

# DIABETES AND NUTRITION

## DIABETES AND NUTRITION

### Why is nutrition important?

The nutrients that people take into their body (what they eat) have a major effect on how much they weigh, their health, and their likelihood of developing a chronic disease or not. Overall, there is no one set of nutritional requirements for human health. Such requirements vary from person to person and depend on many factors, including age, size, gender, and health conditions. For example, the nutritional requirements of a person with type 1 diabetes versus a person without diabetes can be very different.

### Why are nutrients important to humans?

Nutrients are so important to humans because they are the compounds that help the body to survive and remain healthy. Not all nutrients are the same, either, and they range from vitamins and minerals to non-nutrients, such as water, with each one affecting the body in certain ways. Foods contain these chemical substances that provide the body with heat and energy, help to grow and repair the body's cells and tissues, and aid in regulating the body's overall processes.

### Does any single food supply all the nutrients humans need?

Although there are claims to the contrary, no single food can supply all the nutrients in the amounts humans need to survive. For example, lemons may supply vitamin C, but they have no calcium. This is why dietitians recommend a balanced diet of foods that contain most of the body's daily nutrient needs. Or if a person has diabetes, the dietitian would recommend foods that would help keep the person's blood glucose levels more stable.

### What are the six essential nutrients that cannot be synthesized by the human body?

The six important nutrients are familiar to most people. They are carbohydrates, fats (lipids), proteins, vitamins, minerals, and water. Each has a specific function and relationship to the body, and not one of these nutrients can act independently of the others. In addition, scientists now know that each nutrient is equally valuable for human health. Thus, although factors can alter the amounts of nutrients people ingest (depending on such things as age, body volume, gender, health, and lifestyle), deficiencies in any of these nutrients can lead to an imbalance in the body.

### Is there a connection between nutrition and diabetes?

Yes, there is a connection between diabetes and nutrition, especially in that a person should pay close attention to nutrition if he or she has diabetes! Although the tendency to develop diabetes (type 1, but especially type 2) seems to be associated with heredity, pregnancy (gestational diabetes, which often disappears after the baby is born), surgery, or physical and emotional stress, one of the biggest reasons (especially for type 2 diabetes) is obesity. In the majority of cases, prediabetes (and eventually diabetes) occurs when a person is overweight or obese due to bad eating habits, including too many foods rich in fats, salts, and sugars. In fact, many people who are prediabetic—or who are at a higher risk of developing type 2 diabetes—have been known to reverse or slow down the development of the disease by weight control, proper nutrition, and exercise. (For more about connections between obesity and diabetes, see the chapter "Diabetes and Obesity.")

# NUTRITION HELP
# FOR PEOPLE WITH DIABETES

### What is the difference between a dietitian and a nutritionist?

People often mistakenly use the terms dietitian and nutritionist interchangeably, and although they are related in some ways, it is the level of education and qualifications that separate the two professions. Dietitians must have a certain level of education and registration. A nutritionist is free from government regulations, although some states require nutritionists to obtain an occupational license from a Board of Nutrition. Other states require no qualifications, and a person can practice without any previous education, training, or work experience.

### What are the qualifications to become a registered dietitian?

In general, a dietitian helps people (including those with diabetes) determine the right number of daily calories and distribution of food throughout the day. This health care professional has to have university qualifications consisting of a four-year college degree (bachelor's) in nutrition and dietetics or a three-year science degree followed by a master's degree in nutrition and dietetics. Whichever program the dietitian takes, it must be approved by the Accreditation Council for Education in Nutrition and Dietetics (ACEND) and include a practical component. This can include a period of practical training in a hospital or community setting (in some areas, it includes about 1,200 hours of supervised practice). Dieticians can also have specialty skills, such as a clinical dietitian.

To become a certified registered dietitian (who most often has "RD" after his or her name, and is usually found in a professional health care facility), the person must: earn a degree from an ACEND program; complete a supervised clinical program; pass the CDR (Commission on Dietetic Registration) examination; and complete continuing professional education credits that are needed to maintain CDR registration.

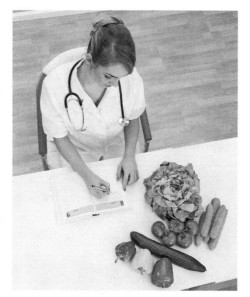

Dieticians are licensed professionals with bachelor's or master's degrees in dietetics. They need some medical background in order to write diets suitable for people suffering from various diseases.

## Where do you find a dietitian?

A dietitian can be found in various employment settings, including the following:

- Health care, such as in hospitals or other health care facilities, and schools or daycare centers
- Business and industry, such as in corporate wellness programs or public relations
- Communities and public-health facilities that offer education to the public about better eating habits
- Education, at places that teach physician's assistants, nurses, and dietetics students about the science of food and nutrition
- Research groups, such as those found in food and pharmaceutical companies or in university and hospital settings
- Government agencies that offer information based on up-to-date research or education to professionals and the public
- Private practice groups, such as those working under contract with health care groups or food companies or running their own businesses

## How can a dietitian help a person with diabetes?

It is difficult for people with diabetes to balance their blood glucose levels, which is often tied to the foods they eat. Thus, dietitians can help people make better food choices, as     269 they are often involved in the diagnoses and dietary treatment of many diseases, including diabetes.

## What are the qualifications for becoming a nutritionist?

At this writing, there are no true qualifications for becoming a nutritionist, except that in some states, a nutritionist must obtain a license. The term "nutritionist" is not protected by law in almost all countries, so people with varying levels of food expertise can use the term without any degree or license all over the world. Thus, if a person with diabetes is looking for someone to help him or her maneuver through the intricacies of eating with the disease, then it is best to be careful in choosing a qualified nutritional professional.

## How can a nutritionist help a person with diabetes?

Although there are people who call themselves "nutritionists" and have no credentials, there are some qualified nutritionists who have completed university degrees in food science, human nutrition, food and nutrition, or food technology (some also call themselves food scientists). In most cases, a nutritionist is concerned with the nutritional value of certain foods, such as the calories, carbohydrates, fiber, protein, total fat, saturated fats, sodium, and cholesterol per serving. Suggestions from a nutritionist can be helpful to people with diabetes who want to limit and improve their food choices in order to control their blood glucose levels. The best way to find a qualified nutritionist (or dietitian) is to ask a health care professional for recommendations. And some hospitals have qualified people to help a person with diabetes eat better.

## What is a dietetic technician, registered?

A dietetic technician, registered (DTR) is a person who is educated at the technical level of nutrition and dietetics. According to the Academy of Nutrition and Dietetics, a DTR plays a part in the health care and food-management services and knows about food safety and quality. The DTR works under the supervision of a registered dietitian nutritionist (RDN) in such places as hospitals, clinics, nursing homes, hospices, home health care programs, research institutions, and retirement centers. Or the DTR can work independently, providing general nutrition education in such places as schools, daycare centers, restaurants, health care facilities, corporations, hospitals, programs for the public (such as Meals on Wheels), health clubs, and food companies.

In addition, DTRs are credentialed food and nutrition technical practitioners who have met certain criteria, both educational and professional. One route to this goal includes completing an accredited dietetic-technician program, 450 hours of

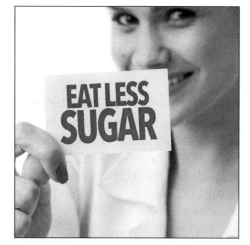

Diabetes educators help those with the disease understand and manage it better by teaching them how diabetes affects their bodies and what they can do about it.

supervised practice in various community-based programs, health care and food-service facilities, and completing at least a two-year associate's degree at a regionally accredited college or university. Another route to becoming a DTR involves earning a bachelor's degree from a regionally accredited college or university or foreign equivalent. The candidate must also complete an Accreditation Council for Education in Nutrition and Dietetics (part of the Academy of Nutrition and Dietetics, with the acronym ACEND) Didactic Program in Dietetics and an ACEND-accredited Dietetic Technician-supervised practice program.

## What does being a diabetes educator mean?

A diabetes educator is a health care professional who focuses on all aspects of diabetic care, including knowledge of prediabetes, diabetes prevention, and management of the disease. The educator aids and educates people with diabetes, helping them to understand how blood glucose levels work and how food affects blood sugar. They also give guidance to people with diabetes, such as to how to take medications properly and how to lower the risk of developing complications from the disease.

## Does a diabetes educator need to be certified?

Most diabetes educators become certified as certified diabetes educators (CDE) and must go through certain certification examinations to become health professionals. Many are members of the American Association of Diabetes Educators in Chicago.

## What was a nurse educator?

"Nurse educator" is an older term used to describe a person who worked in clinical practice and in hospital teams to improve the quality of a patient's diabetes education. The    271 role was developed mainly because a physician's contact time with a patient with diabetes was limited. The nurse educator—similar to what is referred to now as a diabetes educator—would be the liaison between the physician and the patient, evaluating and educating the patient and interpreting how the person was managing his or her diabetes.

## What is a diabetes health care team?

A diabetes health care team is a group of people whose goal is to help people with diabetes manage and maintain their health with the disease. Although the most important aspect of treating diabetes is self-management, many hospitals and health care facilities offer a team of people to help people with diabetes understand and manage the disease. The team usually includes a person's primary-care physician or an endocrinologist who specializes in diabetes, a diabetes educator (often a nurse or nurse practitioner), and a dietitian.

For long-term care through the disease, other professionals may be called to help the team, including an ophthalmologist (as the eyes are often affected); a podiatrist (for foot problems, mainly from neuropathy); a wound-care specialist (for foot-related wounds and other wounds that don't heal as well when the person has diabetes); a nephrologist (kidney specialist); a cardiologist (for heart problems); and/or a nerve specialist (for problems with neuropathy).

# DIABETES AND VITAMINS

## What are vitamins?

A vitamin is an organic, non-protein substance that is necessary for an organism—plant or animal—to maintain normal metabolic function but that cannot be synthesized by that organism. In other words, vitamins are crucial molecules that must be acquired from outside sources. While most vitamins are present in food, vitamin D is produced as a precursor in our skin and converted to its active form by sunlight.

## What is the difference between fat- and water-soluble vitamins?

Vitamins are often classified as fat-soluble or water-soluble. Fat-soluble means the vitamin is stored in the body and can accumulate if too much is ingested (which is why it's best to use any vitamin supplement under medical supervision). Water-soluble vitamins are not as readily absorbed or stored in the body. For example, vitamins A, D, E, and K are soluble only in fats; vitamins C and the B vitamins are soluble only in water. In addition, if foods that have fat-soluble vitamins are cooled, the vitamins will not be lost. But more often than not, water-soluble vitamins lose their potency from heat when cooked.

## What vitamins are essential for human health?

The following lists the fat- and water-soluble vitamins that are essential for human health (the ones associated with glucose and diabetes are italicized):

## Essential Vitamins

| Vitamin | Essential for Health |
| --- | --- |
| *Fat-soluble Vitamins* | |
| Vitamin A | Beta carotene, retinols: Needed for growth and cell development; prevents night blindness; helps fight some cancers; helps the cardiovascular system; needed to maintain healthy gums, glands, bones, teeth, nails, skin, and hair; beta carotene is also considered to be an antioxidant |
| Vitamin D | Calciferol: Needed for calcium absorption and helps build strong bones and teeth; helps maintain the brain, *pancreas (responsible for insulin balance),* and reproductive organs; also targets the kidneys and intestines; *some studies show it may help reverse insulin resistance* |
| Vitamin E | Tocopherols: Helps maintain muscles and red blood cells; it's also a major antioxidant |
| Vitamin K | Necessary for efficient blood clotting; *may help eliminate inflammation and improve insulin sensitivity and blood glucose levels* |
| *Water-Soluble Vitamins* | |
| Biotin | Needed for energy and metabolism |
| Folate | Folic acid, folacin (some call this vitamin F; it is more often thought of as $B_9$): Necessary to make DNA, RNA, red blood cells, and to synthesize certain amino acids |
| Niacin | Vitamin $B_3$, nicotinic acid, nicotinamide: Necessary to metabolize energy and to promote normal growth; for some people, larger doses often help lower cholesterol |
| Pantothenic acid | Vitamin $B_5$: Helps to metabolize energy; *normalizes blood sugar levels,* and helps the body to synthesize antibodies, some hormones, cholesterol, and hemoglobin (in the blood) |
| Riboflavin | Vitamin $B_2$: Necessary to metabolize energy and helps the body's adrenal function |
| Thiamine (thiamin) | Vitamin $B_1$: Necessary to metabolize energy; needed for proper nerve function, normal digestion, and appetite |
| Vitamin $B_6$ | Pyridoxine, pyridoxamine, pyridoxal: Helps to metabolize proteins and carbohydrates (for energy) in the body; good for proper nerve function and helps synthesize red blood cells |
| Vitamin $B_{12}$ | Cyanocobalamin: Necessary to make DNA, RNA, red blood cells, and myelin (for the body's nerve fibers); may help prevent heart disease in some people |
| Vitamin C | Ascorbic acid: Helps to build blood vessel walls and promote wound healing; necessary for iron absorption; said to help prevent atherosclerosis; considered to be an antioxidant |

## What are some health problems caused by vitamin deficiencies, especially for people with type 2 diabetes?

For people with diabetes (especially type 2), certain vitamin deficiencies can cause additional health problems. The following lists a few of the problems with vitamin deficiency:

*Vitamin D*—According to some studies, people with the lowest levels of vitamin D in their blood seem more likely to have insulin resistance. In some people, adding vitamin D to their diet—or even as supplements (taken under a doctor's care, of course)—may help reverse insulin resistance. (But there is still a major quandary about vitamin D and diabetes: No one knows whether vitamin D causes lower levels of glucose in the blood or having diabetes lowers vitamin D.) This deficiency also causes muscle weakness and an increase in infections, something that people with diabetes have to watch carefully since higher blood glucose levels can compromise their immune system.

*Vitamin E*—One study indicated a deficiency in vitamin E, an antioxidant, is often seen in people with type 2 diabetes. It also found that people with diabetes had a lower amount of antioxidants in their systems.

*Vitamin A*—A study conducted in 2015 indicated that a deficiency in vitamin A— which boosts beta-cell activity—may play a role in the development of type 2 diabetes.

## What oral medication for type 2 diabetes increases the risk for vitamin $B_2$ deficiency?

According to several studies, the commonly prescribed oral medication for type 2 diabetes called metformin is thought to increase the risk for vitamin $B_2$ deficiency—but the reason is still unknown. (There are several symptoms, including impaired memory, fatigue, and nerve problems in the hands and feet.) One study found that 10 to 30 percent of the participants who took the drug on a regular basis had problems with vitamin $B_2$

---

### What is vitamin K?

**V**itamin K, discovered in the 1930s, is a fat-soluble vitamin linked to heart, bone, and brain health. It is also thought that vitamin K has a relationship with calcium and vitamin D, all of which are thought to be necessary for maintaining healthy bones. Good food sources are spinach, salad greens, broccoli, Brussels sprouts, and cabbage, along with some vegetable oils, including olive and canola. As supplements, vitamin K, as $K_1$, can be from green plants (called phylioquinone). $K_2$ is a form that is more readily absorbed and lasts longer in the body than $K_1$. It is synthesized from bacteria (for supplements) and is found in some types of cheese. Most important, it is also synthesized in the digestive tract, which is why most people do not have to eat more foods rich in vitamin K or take supplements to get enough of the vitamin.

absorption. Another study indicated that the problems with B$_2$ levels increased for those who took a higher dose of the drug and who were on metformin for a long time. Thus, most researchers suggest that people who take metformin have their vitamin B$_2$ levels checked periodically.

## Does vitamin K affect glucose levels in the body?

Although more studies need to be conducted, it is thought that vitamin K may help eliminate inflammation in the body. It may also help to improve insulin sensitivity and thus help to balance blood glucose levels.

## Is it possible to take too many vitamins?

Yes, it is very possible to take excessive amounts of vitamins; the practice may cause health complications as serious as vitamin deficiencies. The clinical term for excessive intake of vitamins is hypervita-

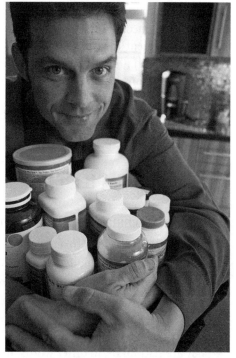

It is, indeed, possible to take too many vitamins, especially when it comes to fat-soluble ones, which can accumulate in the body over time.

minosis. It occurs when the dietary intake of a vitamin exceeds the body's ability to store, use, or excrete the vitamin. Hypervitaminosis is most common among the fat-soluble vitamins (vitamins A, D, E, and K) because the excessive quantities of the vitamins are usually stored in fat (lipid) tissues. In comparison, excessive amounts of water-soluble vitamins do not accumulate in the body since they are most often excreted in urine.

## Are vitamin supplements necessary for a person with diabetes?

Vitamin supplements may be useful for individuals who do not receive all of the nutrients they need from their diet. These individuals either cannot or do not eat enough or do not eat enough of a variety of healthful foods; thus, they need extra vitamins and often minerals (see below). But for most people who eat a balanced, healthful diet, vitamin and mineral supplements are not necessary. If a person has—or does not have—diabetes, the best way to determine whether supplements are needed is to ask a health care provider or, in the case of a person with diabetes, a diabetes educator.

## What unusual supplement has been suggested to control blood glucose?

The unusual supplement that has been suggested to control blood glucose levels is made from the native northern African plant aloe vera. Researchers gathered several clinical trials on this succulent plant and found that, taken as an oral supplement, it may reduce fasting blood glucose and HbA1c levels. But as with all unregulated supplements, the use of any supplement (or medicine, for that matter) that has not gone through rigorous clinical trials is highly debated. This is because there is no government regulation controlling such items. Even the researchers suggested that many more studies should be conducted to understand just how aloe vera affects the overall control of blood glucose—and even how it compares with treatments already available to people who have diabetes.

# DIABETES AND MINERALS

## What are macrominerals and microminerals?

The body contains or uses three types of minerals: macrominerals, microminerals, and electrolytes. The following lists the characteristics of each:

*Macrominerals*—Three to five percent of the average human body is composed of minerals. The macrominerals make up the majority—calcium, magnesium, and phosphorus. Most of the macrominerals are stored in the bones, but they also circulate in the blood. And as with vitamins, the best sources of macrominerals for the human body are natural or, in other words, ingested foods and not supplements, if possible.

*Microminerals*—Also called trace minerals, microminerals are found in lesser quantities in the human body, but all are necessary for health in varying quantities.

*Electrolytes*—The minerals dissolved in the body's fluids are called electrolytes, all of which create electrically charged ions. The most important ones in terms of eating and health include sodium, potassium, and phosphate.

## What are the most necessary minerals for our health?

The body needs a good amount of minerals—a combination of macrominerals, trace minerals, and electrolytes. The following lists these major minerals (not all are listed) and their role in human health (those associated with glucose and diabetes are italicized):

### Essential Minerals

| Mineral | Essential for Health |
| --- | --- |
| *Macrominerals* | |
| Calcium | Best for building bones and teeth and vital to muscle and nerve function; helps in blood clotting; helps to maintain stable blood pressure; *helps the body's cells use insulin* |
| Magnesium | Helps to stimulate bone growth; helps with metabolism and muscle function |
| Phosphorus | Found in some body enzymes; helps keep bones and teeth strong; necessary for metabolism |

| Mineral | Essential for Health |
|---------|---------------------|
| *Trace Minerals (Microminerals)* | |
| Chromium | *Helps insulin to metabolize glucose in the body* |
| Copper | Needed for iron absorption in the body; helps with connective tissues, nerve fibers, and red blood cells, along with being a component of several of the body's enzymes |
| Fluoride | Helps the body maintain strong bones and teeth |
| Iodine | Helps the body make thyroid hormones |
| Iron | Necessary to produce hemoglobin, by which the body transports oxygen |
| Manganese | Necessary for metabolism since it is a component of many body enzymes; helps in the formation of bones and tendons |
| Molybdenum | Necessary for the storage of iron in the body; necessary for metabolism since it is a component of many body enzymes |
| Selenium | Works with vitamin E to protect cell membranes from oxidation |
| Zinc | Helps certain enzymes in metabolism; necessary for growth and reproduction, along with supporting the body's immune system |
| *Electrolytes* | |
| Chloride | Helps to keep our body's chemistry stable; used to make our digestive juices; seawater has almost the same concentration of chloride ion as human body fluids |
| Potassium | Necessary to maintain our body's fluid balance; helps our metabolism and muscle function |
| Sodium | Along with potassium, helps to maintain the body's fluid balance; also helps with muscle function |
| Bicarbonate | Listed in some research as an electrolyte; acts as a buffer to maintain the body's normal levels of acidity in the blood and other fluids |

## Is there a connection between type 2 diabetes and the mineral magnesium?

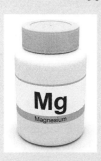

Yes, in a study conducted in 2013, researchers found that there may be a connection between the amount of magnesium ingested and the risk of developing type 2 diabetes. About half of all Americans get enough magnesium, the mineral that helps bone growth and muscles. In the study of 2,500 adults without diabetes, the researchers found that the highest magnesium intake was associated with a 37 percent lower risk of developing prediabetes. Those with prediabetes and a higher magnesium intake showed a 32 percent lower risk for developing type 2 diabetes. But there is a caution: Diabetics with kidney disease (or anyone with kidney disease) should check with his or her doctor before increasing the intake of magnesium, whether by supplements or with foods.

## Why do we need trace minerals for our health?

The trace minerals—chromium, copper, fluoride, iodine, iron, manganese, molybdenum, selenium, and zinc—all have their places in terms of a person's health (see above for more information). For example, chromium acts like a key to unlock insulin, and without it, insulin would have a difficult time controlling blood sugar. It also helps to build proteins. Copper is needed to make red blood cells, skin pigment, connective tissues, and nerve fibers. It also helps the body to absorb iron. And iron is necessary for the pigment (color) in our blood, specifically the red blood cells that carry oxygen throughout the body.

## What are symptoms of deficiencies of certain minerals?

There are several symptoms of macromineral, trace mineral, and electrolyte deficiencies. The following lists minerals (not all are listed) and symptoms if there is a major deficiency (the minerals associated with glucose and diabetes are italicized):

### Mineral Deficiency Symptoms

| Mineral | Result of Deficiency |
| --- | --- |
| *Macrominerals* | |
| Calcium | In children, rickets; in at-risk adults, it can lead to osteoporosis (brittle, porous bones); may also indicate a lack of vitamin D, which helps the body to absorb calcium |
| Magnesium | Deficiency is rare but can be depleted by alcoholism, long-term diarrhea, liver or kidney disease, and *severe diabetes; a deficiency is also often tied to high insulin levels and glucose intolerance that can lead to type 2 diabetes* |
| Phosphorus | Lack of appetite, weight loss, or even obesity; it may cause irregular breathing, mental and physical fatigue, and nervous disorders |
| *Trace Minerals (Microminerals)* | |
| Chromium | *Even slight deficiencies can lead to problems with metabolizing glucose and upset the function of insulin levels* |
| Copper | Although rare, deficiencies include low blood levels in children with edema or iron deficiency anemia; in adults, it may lead to general weakness, impaired respiration, and skin sores |
| Fluoride | Poor tooth development and dental caries (cavities) |
| Iodine | Enlarged thyroid (goiter) and hypothyroidism (low secretion of thyroid hormones); can lead to hardening of the arteries, obesity, sluggish metabolism, dry hair, slow mental reactions, rapid pulse, heart palpitations, tremors, nervousness, and irritability |
| Iron | Most common is iron-deficiency anemia; can lead to constipation, brittle nails or ridges in nails, lethargy, apathy, pallor, reduced brain function, headaches, and heart enlargement; can cause unusual food cravings (such as for ice, clay, and other non-food items; see sidebar) |
| Manganese | *Mostly affects glucose tolerance, resulting in the inability to remove excess sugar from the blood by oxidation and/or storage, causing diabetes;* can cause atherosclerosis; severe deficiencies can cause paralysis, convulsions, blindness, and deafness in infants; in adults, can cause dizziness, ear noises, and hearing loss |

| Mineral | Result of Deficiency |
| --- | --- |
| Molybdenum | Excessive deficiencies may cause fast heartbeat, increased rate of breathing, and visual problems |
| Selenium | May cause premature aging; major deficiencies may cause cataracts, liver necrosis, and growth retardation; low levels have been associated with several types of cancers, including bladder and colon cancers |
| Zinc | May show up in a diet high in grains and cereals and low in animal protein; it can cause retarded growth, delayed sexual maturity, and cause wounds to take longer to heal; it can cause brittle nails, and white spots on the nail may be a sign; it can also cause irregular menstrual cycles in teenage women and painful knee and hip joints in teens of both genders |
| *Electrolytes* | |
| Chloride | A deficiency can cause hair and tooth loss, poor muscular contractions, and impaired digestion; it also usually means there is a deficiency of sodium in the body |
| Potassium | An abnormal decrease (hypokalemia) or increase (hyperkalemia) affects the nervous system, and both can increase the chance for arrhythmias (irregular heartbeats); both can also affect the kidneys |
| Sodium | A major deficiency can cause intestinal gas, weight loss, poor memory, short attention span, difficulty in concentrating, muscle weakness, *low blood sugar*, and heart palpitations |
| Bicarbonate | Listed in most research as an electrolyte; difficult to determine a deficiency in some cases, and deficiencies are often connected to other conditions, such as kidney disease, respiratory function, and metabolic conditions |

## What is iron-deficiency anemia?

Iron-deficiency anemia is also called hypochromic anemia. It occurs when the amount of hemoglobin in the red blood cells is reduced and, as a result, the cells become smaller. Because of this, the oxygen-carrying capacity of the blood is reduced. Those at risk are usually women of child-bearing years (especially pregnant or lactating), older infants, children, and people with certain dietary restrictions, such as those with diabetes, the elderly, low-income people, and minorities. It is also estimated that one in four college women is deficient in iron, most often from menstruation and not eating as healthfully while in school.

## Can a person with diabetes become anemic?

Yes, just as with non-diabetics, the lack of iron in people with diabetes can lead to anemia. In fact, it is estimated that 25 percent of people with diabetes are anemic. It is thought that anemia occurs in people with diabetes because the erythropoietin, the hormone that controls the production of red blood cells, is produced in the kidneys. Since one complication of diabetes is kidney damage, the two conditions are often found together. In addition, if a person with diabetes has anemia, his or her blood glucose levels can be affected, with some reports of blood glucose test results being 20 percent too high. This is why it is important—especially for people with type 1 diabetes and their health care providers—to be aware of this combination.

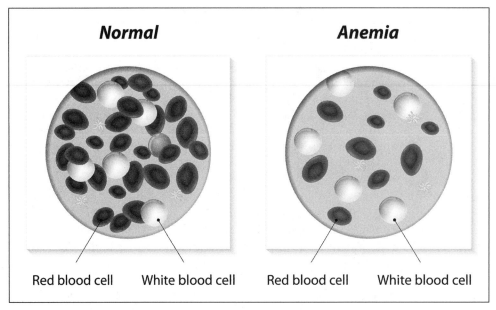

| Normal | | Anemia | |
|---|---|---|---|
| Red blood cell | White blood cell | Red blood cell | White blood cell |

Anemia occurs when one's blood is deficient in red cells. Since diabetics often have damaged kidneys, leading to lower amounts of erythropoietin, they may produce fewer red blood cells and become anemic.

### What is potassium and its connection to glucose in the body?

Potassium, along with sodium, is a very necessary mineral that helps to regulate the body's balance of fluids. It is also necessary for our metabolism, helps in the transmission of nerve impulses, and is needed for muscle function. Further, it regulates the transfer of nutrients to the cells and functions in the chemical reactions within the cells. It is important to our bodies' sugar levels, helping to convert glucose into glycogen so it can be stored in the liver. Potassium also helps stimulate the kidneys to eliminate our toxic body wastes and acts with sodium to help normalize our heartbeats.

# DIABETES AND FOOD

## MAJOR FOOD COMPONENTS
## AND DIABETES

### What are some targets recommended by the American Diabetes Association in terms of food components?

According to the American Diabetes Association's nutritional guidelines, targets are suggested for the many food components. The following lists those food components and the amounts that are recommended daily:

**Recommended Amounts of Food Components**

| Component | Daily Recommended Amount |
| --- | --- |
| Saturated fat | Less than 7 percent of total daily calories |
| Trans fat | Very minimal amounts, if any |
| Cholesterol | Less than 200 milligrams per day |
| Protein | Around 15 to 20 percent of total daily calories |
| Fiber | At least 14 grams per 1,000 calories a day |
| Sodium | No more than 2,300 milligrams per day* |

*This amount is highly debated; for more about the controversy surrounding the intake of sodium, see this chapter.

### Do some foods fight diabetes?

Yes, some foods—too many to mention in this text—seem to help fight diabetes, although the "help" from these foods is often controversial. Although many health care professionals do not advocate its constant use, vinegar has been shown to improve insulin sensitivity, and it may stop the after-meal spikes in a person's blood glucose levels, too. In one study, participants with type 1 diabetes drank a vinegar-water solution or plain water five minutes before eating a carbohydrate-heavy meal. Participants who drank the vinegar mixture cut their rise in blood glucose levels by almost 20 percent in comparison with those who drank only water. Even as little as 2 tablespoons of vinegar with a meal helped to stop spikes in blood glucose levels. In addition, lemon juice may have the same effect. It is thought that both vinegar and lemon juice have acid, which slows down a person's digestion, so the body absorbs

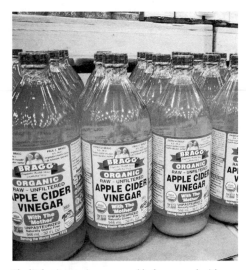

If a little vinegar is consumed before a meal with carbs in it, blood glucose will rise less.

sugar in the food more slowly. Another possible food contender to help diabetes is the white button mushroom. Found commonly in most grocery stores, these mushrooms are funguses filled with nutrients (vitamins C, D, $B_2$ [riboflavin], and folate), fiber, and many antioxidants—all of which are thought to help lower blood glucose levels in people with diabetes.

# WHAT ARE FOOD EXCHANGES?

### What are "food exchanges" in the context of food and diabetes?

Food exchanges put together groups of foods that have a similar combination of carbohydrates, fat, protein, and calories. The "exchange" comes from the idea that a person can exchange one food serving for another, depending on the carbohydrate amount. According to the Diabetes Teaching Center in San Francisco, foods with a similar amount of carbohydrates per serving size are grouped together (remember, serving size is different from portion size; for more, see this chapter). This way, people can manage the amount of carbohydrates they eat in a meal.

### How does a person use the exchange list?

To use the exchange list, a person chooses various foods based on their carbohydrate, fat, protein, or calorie content. This is a good way to keep blood glucose levels more stable and make meal planning easier. There are also exchanges for fats and proteins, although most people with diabetes concentrate on counting carbohydrates to manage their condition. For example, one carbohydrate exchange is equal to 12 to 15 grams of carbohydrate. This group is generally broken down into bread/starch, meats and meat substitutes, fruit, milk, fats, and vegetables. When a meal plan reads "2½ carbohydrate exchanges" (equal to 1 bread/starch, 1 fruit, ½ milk), it means a person can have, for instance, a slice of bread, a fresh peach, and a half cup of nonfat yogurt—or the equivalent carbohydrate exchanges if the other food sources (bread/starch, fruit, and milk) are also equivalent to 2½ carbohydrate exchanges. (For a short list of food exchanges, see Appendix A.)

# DIABETES AND GLYCEMIC NUMBERS

## What is a glycemic index?

The glycemic index (GI) is an important tool for diabetics as it gives a numerical ranking to foods based on the rate of their conversion to glucose in the body. The scale is from one to 100, with pure glucose (sugar) being the standard at 100. The lower numbers represent a low rise in blood sugar after a certain food is consumed; the higher numbers represent a more rapid rise in blood sugar after a certain food is consumed.

## Why do some health care professionals not agree with using the glycemic index?

Although the glycemic index (GI) does prove to be a useful tool, it is not a perfect system. One reason is that the GI ranking applies only when you eat something on an empty stomach—and most people eat many foods together at a meal. Another reason is that the GI doesn't take into consideration how much a person actually consumes. It is based on a serving of food that contains 50 grams of carbohydrates minus the fiber, then measuring the person's blood glucose levels over two hours. Because of these inherent problems, the glycemic load was developed.

## What is a glycemic load?

Not all foods will immediately give you a boost—even if the item has a high glycemic index. What also becomes important to a person with diabetes is the glycemic load, or the body's response based on the glycemic index and the amount of whatever carbohydrate is consumed. For example, even though a piece of candy has a high glycemic index, if it is small, it will have a relatively small glycemic response. According to the Harvard School of Public Health, where the idea of the glycemic load was developed, the glycemic load is equal to the glycemic index over 100, then multiplied by the net carbohydrates (that is, equal to the total carbohydrates minus the dietary fiber). Thus, people with diabetes eat both low-glycemic-index foods and restrict their carbohydrates in order to control their diabetes. (For information about foods and their glycemic index and load, see Appendix B.)

# DIABETES AND CARBOHYDRATES

## What are carbohydrates?

Carbohydrates are a major source of energy for cells and activities within the cells, which means they provide energy for the entire body. They are commonly known as sugars and starches and are organic compounds made up of carbon, hydrogen, and oxygen. They are also the major source of energy for cells and cellular activities and for providing energy for a person's entire system. In terms of foods, some of the best sources of carbohydrates are legumes, grains, potatoes, and many vegetables and fruits.

## Why are carbohydrates a major part of the human diet?

All human cells have evolved so that carbohydrates are the body's primary energy source. In fact, the body's entire metabolic system begins with glucose. In general, the digestive system changes carbohydrates into glucose, which is then used for energy for cells, tissues, and all the body's organs.

## Which is a better source of energy for the body—carbohydrates or fat?

In general, fats contain nine kilocalories (indirectly, a form of energy) per gram, while carbohydrates average about four kilocalories per gram. Thus, fats are useful for storing energy, but sugars are easier to break down during metabolism. But no one truly agrees which source of energy is "better." Perhaps the answer lies in individual situa-

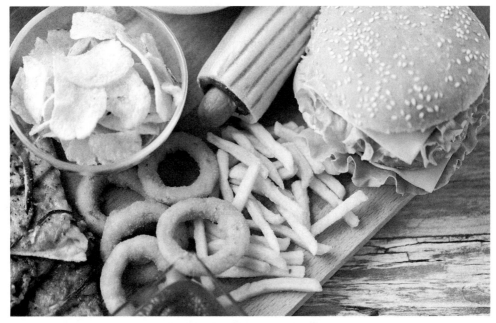

Foods rich in carbohydrates are a staple of people's diets because glucose is a main source of energy.

## Why is the role of carbohydrates in the human diet so highly debated?

The role of carbohydrates in our diet is a hotly debated subject, and the reason why is clear: Many popular diets, especially a low-carbohydrate diet, propose that the only way to lose weight is to eliminate carbohydrates. Because of such "trend" diets, for many people, the word "carbohydrate" has become inherently bad. But there seems to be more of a case for the other side. Carbohydrates are fuel for the brain, nervous system, muscles, and various organs. In fact, they are more high-quality fuels than fats and proteins, mainly because it takes little for the body to break them down and release their energy. Thus, the body metabolizes these simple carbohydrates (sugar) and starches into glucose (blood sugar), which becomes the body's primary fuel source—as long as carbohydrates are eaten in moderation.

tions. For example, babies require fat in their diets for both energy and to build a healthy nervous system, whereas many middle-aged adults often consume too much fat for their body's metabolic requirements—often leading to their becoming overweight.

## Is fiber a form of carbohydrate?

Yes, fiber is another form of carbohydrate, one that has many major health benefits. For example, whole grains are important for reducing the risk of colon cancer and keeping the body's digestive tract in good working order. Many long-term studies have shown that a diet with the most whole grains and cereal fibers—especially nutrient-rich grains and fibers that are less milled or processed—can provide protection from certain cancers, heart disease, and even type 2 diabetes.

## How were carbohydrates once classified, and why was the classification changed?

In the past, carbohydrates were classified as being simple or complex. The simple carbohydrates were considered to be those composed of sugar, such as glucose and fructose. They were the carbohydrates that because of their simple structure were easily and quickly used in the body for energy, increasing blood glucose and insulin secretions. They were also known as carbohydrates that could have negative health effects. The complex carbohydrates were those with the more complex chemical structures, with three or more sugars linked together. They were considered to be foods that contained fiber, vitamins, and minerals and took longer to digest, thus causing blood glucose to rise more slowly. Not all the complex carbohydrates were nutritious, either, especially such foods as white bread and potatoes, which contain mostly starch.

The reason for the change in classification was that these two divisions did not account for the effect of carbohydrates on blood glucose levels and chronic diseases. Therefore, more minute divisions of carbohydrates have been developed to indicate how these organic compounds affect the body. The glycemic index, and later the glycemic load, were developed to better represent carbohydrates, foods, and the body.

## How are carbohydrates currently classified?

In recent years, carbohydrates have been classified in several different ways. For example, they are classified by their overall length (monosaccharide, disaccharide, and polysaccharide), and often these classifications are broken down into smaller units. Thus, monosaccharides (single-unit sugars) are further grouped by the number of carbon molecules they contain, including triose (three carbon molecules), pentose (five), and hexose (six). Carbohydrates are also classified by function. For example, storage polysaccharides (glycogen and starch), which store energy, and structural polysaccharides (cellulose and chitin) are both categorized based on function.

## What are some of the uses of carbohydrates by the body?

Various carbohydrates have different functions in the human body. The following chart identifies some common carbohydrates—some associated with diabetes, others not—and their general functions:

| Carbohydrate Name | Type | General Function in the Body |
|---|---|---|
| Deoxyribose | monosaccharide | DNA (deoxyribonucleic acid) is a major constituent of hereditary material |
| Ribose | monosaccharide | Constituent of RNA (ribonucleic acid) |
| Fructose | monosaccharide | Important in cellular metabolism |
| Galactose | simple monosaccharide | Found in brain and nerve tissue |
| Glucose | monosaccharide | Main energy source for the body's cells |
| Lactose | simple disaccharide | Milk sugar; helps the absorption of calcium |
| Sucrose | simple disaccharide | Produces glucose and fructose |
| Cellulose | polysaccharide | Not digestible but is an important fiber that provides bulk for the proper movement of food through the intestines |
| Glycogen | polysaccharide | Stored in the liver and muscles until needed as an energy source and is then converted to glucose |
| Heparin | polysaccharide | Prevents excessive blood clotting |

## What are some sources of the various carbohydrates and their effect on blood glucose levels?

There are numerous sources for the various carbohydrates, some that raise a person's blood sugar rapidly and others that do so slowly. The following lists the name of the carbohydrate, type of carbohydrate, how fast it raises blood glucose levels, and which foods contain the carbohydrate (note: two starches in this list have a different response in the body, depending on whether it is a straight- or branched-chain type of starch):

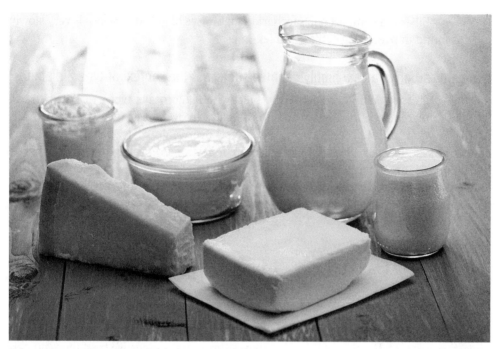

Dairy products such as milks and cheeses contain the sugar lactose, which will raise blood sugar, but it will do it more slowly than maltose or fructose.

*Maltose*—Maltose, or malt sugar, is a simple disaccharide made up of two glucose units; thus, it raises blood glucose levels extremely fast. It is produced during the breakdown of starches.

*Dextrose*—Dextrose is a simple disaccharide that raises the blood glucose levels very rapidly; it is found in many candies and in diabetic products, such as those meant to treat hypoglycemic events (also known as glucose tablets).

*Sucrose*—Sucrose is a simple disaccharide that raises blood glucose levels quickly; it is found in simple table sugar and in fruits, vegetables, and grains.

*Starch*—Starch is a straight chain and is made up of long chains of glucose; it raises the blood glucose levels swiftly and is found in potatoes, rice, bread, and cereals.

*Fructose*—Fructose is a simple monosaccharide that raises the blood glucose levels moderately quickly; it is found in such foods as table sugar, fruit, molasses, and honey.

*Lactose*—Lactose, also called milk sugar, is a simple disaccharide; it raises blood glucose levels slowly. It is found in milk and dairy products.

*Galactose*—Galactose is a simple monosaccharide that raises blood glucose levels slowly; it is found in milk and dairy products.

*Starch*—Starch (a different one than listed above) is a branched chain that raises blood glucose levels very slowly; it is found in legumes and pastas.

*Fiber*—Fiber is a complex polysaccharide that raises blood glucose levels very slowly; it is found in fruits, vegetables, and legumes.

### Why are carbohydrates a highly debated subject in the context of type 2 diabetes?

Carbohydrates are definitely a debated subject when it comes to type 2 diabetes. In particular, some researchers suggest that it is actually an overabundance of carbohydrates in the diet that leads to people's being excessively overweight. They believe that the ups and downs of glucose levels after carbohydrate ingestion eventually cause the pancreas to "wear out," or stop functioning well, leading to type 2 diabetes. (For more about this controversy, see the chapter "Diabetes and Obesity.") But overall, recent research has shown that people develop type 2 diabetes for many reasons.

# DIABETES, FIBER, AND FATS

### What is fiber?

Fiber (also called dietary fiber) is a type of carbohydrate that cannot be broken down by digestive enzymes. Because of this, fiber passes through the digestive tract more quickly, aiding in elimination. There are two basic types of fiber: insoluble and soluble. The insoluble fibers help to move food through the digestive tract, while the soluble fibers help to slow down food in the digestive tract. Because both types of fiber absorb water, in most cases, they help treat and prevent constipation. The soluble fibers dissolve in water and stick together. Fibers include such foods as oatmeal, oat bran, lentils, barley, and even pectin-rich fruits such as apples and strawberries. Insoluble fiber does not dissolve in water; it passes through the digestive system chewed but otherwise unchanged. Insoluble fibers include such foods as the edible skins of many fruits (such as apples, pears, and peaches), wheat bran, brown rice, and whole-wheat products.

### What are fibrous carbohydrates?

Fibrous carbohydrates are not like sugar or starch carbohydrates, as the body cannot use them for energy, but they are still important for the body's overall health. In fact, "fibrous carbohydrate" is merely another name for "fiber." (For more about carbohydrates, see this chapter.)

### What is the difference between a lipid and a fat?

These two terms are often confused. In reality, "fats" are a category of lipids, but everyone uses the terms interchangeably. Lipids are bio-organic molecules that are hydrophobic (they do not mix with or dissolve in water), but they can be dissolved in certain organic solvents such as ether, alcohol, and chloroform. Besides fats, lipids include oils, phospholipids, steroids, and prostaglandins.

## Why are fats important to the human body?

Fats are energy-rich molecules that are used as an internal source of energy for the body. They are stored in the form of triacylglycerols, or what are commonly known as triglycerides (for more about triglycerides, see the chapter "How Diabetes Affects the Circulatory System"). Fats also provide the body with insulation, protection, and cushioning (especially of the body's organs) and help the body absorb certain vitamins, including vitamins A, D, E, and K.

## What is the difference between saturated and unsaturated fats?

Saturated fats are solid at room temperatures (except palm, palm kernel, and some

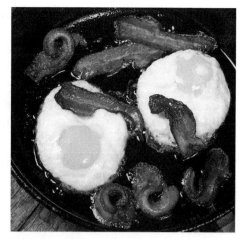

Bacon, eggs, and grease all contain lots of saturated fats, increasing the bad LDL cholesterols in the blood when consumed. This, in turn, can lead to insulin resistance and glucose intolerance.

coconut oils) and include most animal fats (meat, poultry, eggs, and dairy, such as beef, butter, and cheeses). Saturated fats are often associated with raising blood cholesterol. This usually occurs because saturated fats interfere with the removal of cholesterol from the blood.

Unsaturated fats (or the polyunsaturated and monounsaturated fats) have been known either to lower or to have no effect on blood cholesterol. But when polyunsaturated fats are hydrogenated, they become them firmer and more like saturated fats. They can then affect the body's blood cholesterol in the same way that saturated fats do. Monounsaturated fats are liquid at room temperature; they include olive, canola, and peanut oils, along with some nuts, seeds, and avocados. These fats are also considered helpful to human health (when eaten in moderation), as they are often associated with lowering the bad LDL cholesterol levels in the blood.

## Can excessive amounts of saturated fats increase the risk of diabetes?

Many foods can increase the risk of developing type 2 diabetes, including saturated fats, such as those found in high amounts in desserts like cheesecake and ice cream. The saturated fats definitely affect a person's immune system. The immune cells believe the saturated fats are foreign invaders and start pumping out inflammation-causing compounds, which are linked to diabetes. In fact, in one study, mice that had healthy immune systems and were fed a high-fat diet eventually developed glucose intolerance and insulin resistance, both precursors to type 2 diabetes.

## Can a high-fat meal raise blood glucose levels?

Yes, although they are not as "efficient" at raising blood glucose, fats can contribute to a rise in glucose levels. In general, a high-fat meal can cause an increase in what are called free fatty acids (FFAs) in the bloodstream. Higher levels of FFAs in a person's blood usually indicate more ingestion of high-fat meals, especially including highly saturated fats. Higher FFAs, along with obesity, are often found in people with liver insulin resistance. (For more about the liver and insulin, see the chapter "How Diabetes Affects the Digestive System.")

Liver insulin resistance caused by higher consumption of FFAs means that a person will need more insulin in his or her system. The insulin can come naturally from the pancreas for a person without diabetes or from insulin injections for a person with type 1 diabetes. (Some research also suggests that FFAs may reduce the amount of insulin that the pancreas's beta cells produce, but more studies are needed.) In addition, fats can also affect the timing of a person's blood glucose rise after a meal. This is because fats take a long time to go through the digestive tract—unlike carbohydrates, which are digested quickly—sometimes four to six hours after a meal. Thus, if a person with type 1 is taking insulin, FFAs may change the type of insulin (for example, fast- or slow-acting) and/or times the person injects himself after a high-fat meal.

### What should a person with diabetes be aware of after eating a fatty meal?

Even though fatty meals have been associated with changes in insulin, there is no reason for staying away from fats. In fact, an occasional fatty meal is usually fine, as long as it does not have more than 40 grams of fat (especially saturated fats found in meat, butter, etc.). If a person with diabetes eats a fatty meal, he or she should pay more attention to blood glucose levels, especially after the meal. In addition, if a person with type 1 diabetes knows he will be eating such a fatty meal, he may want to adjust the timing, amount, and/or type of insulin. If someone has type 2 diabetes and is taking oral medications, research has shown that doing some type of moderate physical activity (such as walking) after eating a high-fat meal will often help lower blood glucose levels—and some say help with digestion, too.

### What are omega-3 and omega-6 fatty acids?

There are two types of polyunsaturated fats—or polyunsaturated fatty acids, or PUFAs—the two essential fatty acids called omega-3 and omega-6. They are considered essential fats. In other words, the body cannot make them, so they must be obtained from the diet. Both are thought to play an important role in brain function, as well as in aiding normal growth and development of the brain and eyes in infants. The omega-3 fats are also thought to help prevent blood clotting, which is often known to trigger strokes or heart attacks. They are also thought to lower triglycerides, thus decreasing the risk of a heart attack (thus, they are often called "heart-healthy" fats). In addition, omega-6s are thought to lower LDL (the "bad" cholesterol) and to improve insulin sensitivity. But they have a "bad" side, too, as they are thought to increase inflammation in the body. Still another study points to a possible connection between the rise in inflammatory diseases—such as those associated with obesity and metabolic syndrome—and the increase in omega-6 fatty-acid consumption. This connection is suspected because omega-6 is called "pro-inflammatory," whereas omega-3 is considered to be neutral.

## Are fat calories the same as protein or carbohydrate calories?

No. Therefore, it is a myth that all calories from food are the same. In fact, the body's ancestral makeup is to blame—as it protects itself from starvation by using up carbohydrate stores before it dips into the fat reserves. Overall, calories from fat are more fattening than those from proteins or carbohydrates, and the body has a tendency to store more excess calories from fat intake than from excess calories from proteins or carbohydrates. The body not only stores more fat calories, but it also burns them less readily than those from proteins or carbohydrates. And because the stomach takes cues that the person is full based on food volume, not calories, calorie-for-calorie fat is less satisfying.

## Are various PUFAs associated with different risks for type 2 diabetes?

Yes, various types of polyunsaturated fatty acids (PUFAs) are associated with an increased and decreased risk of type 2 diabetes. In a study conducted in 2016, researchers measured circulating PUFAs in the blood samples of individuals from eight European countries (this was part of EPIC-Interact, the world's largest study of onset type 2 diabetes; for more about EPIC-Interact, see the chapter "Resources, Websites, and Apps"). They compared different PUFAs—both omega-3 and omega-6—and adjusted for various factors that contribute to the risk of type 2 diabetes (such as smoking, body mass index, age, and sex). The researchers found that higher amounts of omega-6 linoleic acid (from a variety of foods, such as vegetable oils) were associated with a lower risk of future type 2 diabetes. But higher levels of four other omega-6 fatty acids were associated with a higher risk of developing type 2 diabetes. Overall, the omega-3 fatty acids—most often associated with fish or seafood—were not associated with future type 2 diabetes, and a plant-origin omega-3 fatty acid called alpha linolenic acid was associated with a lower risk of developing type 2 diabetes.

The researchers know that more studies need to be done, as their work was limited by their inability to distinguish dietary and metabolic influence on PUFAs circulating in the blood. But what this study does show is that the emphasis in the research on PUFAs and diabetes should not be just on the entire class of polyunsaturated fats but on the individual types of PUFAs.

## What are trans-fatty acids?

Trans-fatty acids, or trans fats, are made when manufacturers add hydrogen to liquid vegetable oil—in a process called hydrogenation—creating solid fats like shortening and hard margarine. Hydrogenation increases the shelf life and flavor stability of foods containing these fats. Diets high in trans fats raise the LDL (low density lipoprotein) or "bad" cholesterol, increasing the risk for coronary heart disease. Cakes, crackers, cookies, snack foods, and other foods made with or fried in partially hydrogenated oils are the

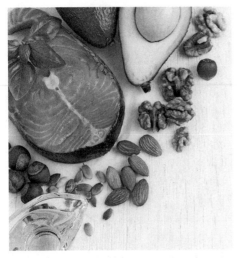

Healthy omega-3 fatty acids are found in foods such as fatty fish (salmon, mackerel, sardines), nuts, and avocados.

largest source (40 percent) of trans fats in the American diet. Animal products and margarine are also major sources of trans fats. Since January 2006, the U.S. government has directed that the amount of trans fat in a product must be included in the "Nutrition Facts" panel on food labels.

## Can excessive amounts of trans fats (trans-fatty acids) increase the risk of type 2 diabetes?

Yes, most health care professionals agree that excessive amounts of trans fats increase the risk of type 2 diabetes in many people. For example, foods such as french fries contain trans fat, and like saturated fat, trans fats seem to boost the inflammation response in the body. In several studies, the more trans fats people consumed, the more likely they were to develop diabetes.

## How do refined grains increase the risk of developing type 2 diabetes?

It is thought that a diet heavy in refined grains—such as white bread—boosts a person's insulin resistance and causes problems with blood glucose levels. In one study, older adults who ate the most refined grains had the highest fasting blood glucose levels. This is because refined grains are actually carbohydrates that are easily digested and absorbed into the bloodstream. Overall, this means more of a rise—and quicker, too—of insulin in the body after eating, which can cause the insulin-making cells in the pancreas to "burn out" faster. It is also why so many health care professionals advise patients to eat foods that contain 100 percent whole grains, including products with whole wheat, whole rye, oatmeal, barley, wheat berries, or brown rice as the first ingredient.

# MANAGING EATING HABITS

### Is there one diet for a person with diabetes?

No! Everyone on the planet has different conditions and various needs when it comes to eating, and people with diabetes should also be treated individually when it comes to what to eat. Even though working out the best eating plan for a person with diabetes seems complicated at first, with education and experimentation, a person's way of eating can be a good diabetes-management tool. This is because what a person eats definitely affects his or her blood glucose levels.

## Why is it often thought that eating five small meals versus three big meals a day is better for most people?

For a person with diabetes, eating several small meals during the day—along with keeping tabs on blood glucose levels and eating wisely—will help keep blood glucose levels more balanced. According to many dietitians and nutritionists, one of the major problems with eating three big meals a day is that the foods eaten can put stress on the pancreas's insulin-producing mechanism.

In particular, as sugars from the foods enter the bloodstream, the pancreas secretes a dose of insulin at levels high enough to help get sugar into the muscles' and other organs' cells, where it is used for energy. If a large amount of sugar enters the bloodstream—for example, after a bigger meal—then the pancreas releases a great deal of insulin. For some people, this release often creates a problem in the cells, causing them to resist the insulin from the pancreas (called insulin resistance). If this occurs, then the glucose levels don't drop, and the body secretes even more insulin. This can cause the pancreas to literally wear out, which, in turn, can eventually lead to diabetes. In addition, the excess insulin promotes more fat storage, causing an overweight problem that can also contribute to diabetes.

## Why does more research need to be conducted concerning diet and diabetes?

How people eat—whether they have diabetes or not—has always been a difficult subject to research. Dietary guidelines for a long time have recommended eating a variety of foods, but researchers are not truly sure why a varied diet can promote health. Although there has been plenty of research about how various foods relate to nutrition (such as which foods contain certain vitamins and minerals), little is known about whether or not eating a diversity of foods is related to lowering the risk of diseases such as type 2 dia-

### Is it possible to be overweight from producing more insulin as opposed to overeating?

According to some research, producing too much insulin in the body (as per the way in the above question) is why some people who cut down on calories still gain, or cannot lose, weight. They just take in too many carbohydrates for their particular system. Taking in too many carbohydrates causes an excess of insulin. This, in turn, can cause the metabolism to develop cells that begin to resist the insulin (called insulin resistance). The body's glucose levels don't drop, and it starts producing more insulin. This can result in two major problems: more insulin can overwork the pancreas, resulting in diabetes, and/or it can promote more fat storage. Thus, in this instance, being overweight may be more from producing more insulin than from overeating.

betes. Overall, little research is conducted about whether a diet consisting of the five major food groups reduces the risk of such diseases as diabetes or whether the variety of foods within each of the five food groups is what is important to stave off such diseases. One study suggested that people who ate from all five food groups had a 30 percent lower risk of type 2 diabetes than people who ate only from three food groups. But more studies need to be conducted to truly determine the role of diet and diabetes.

## Why are some herbs and spices usually good for people with diabetes?

Some herbs and spices are usually good for people with diabetes to consume (but as always, people should check with a health care professional if they have any questions about an herb or spice they want to eat). One reason for eating herbs and spices is that they contain antioxidants, which are compounds that inhibit tissue damage and inflammation caused by high blood glucose levels. The main antioxidants found in herbs and spices (mainly fresh herbs and some spices) are called polyphenolic compounds, compounds also derived from coffee and tea. These compounds have anti-inflammatory capabilities that are thought to help reduce not only the risk of some cancers, cardiovascular disease, and osteoporosis, but also of type 2 diabetes.

Also owing to their high polyphenolic concentrations, certain herbs and spices help block formation of what are called AGE compounds, or advanced glycation end products. AGE compounds form during a process caused when blood sugar levels are high and are part of the reason for tissue damage caused by diabetes. According to a study conducted at the University of Georgia, it is thought that some herbs and many spices have a relatively high polyphenolic content. For example, marjoram, garam masala, ground oregano, and cinnamon all seem to inhibit AGE compounds even when ingested in smaller quantities.

## What are some spices and herbs that can affect blood glucose levels?

People with diabetes should talk with their health care professional if they consume any of the following herbs (one reason is that according to some research, some of these herbs do affect blood glucose levels, albeit not significantly unless the herb is eaten in large quantities):

*True cinnamon and cinnamon extracts*—True cinnamon (*Cinnamomum burmannii*)—native to Sri Lanka—has been around for centuries and was prized by King Solomon, known by Aristotle, and used by the ancient Greeks and Romans to boost appetite and relieve indigestion. Some research indicates that cinnamon not only can help balance cholesterol and relieve bloating and gas after a meal, but it may help control blood glucose levels of people with type 2 diabetes. In particular, in one study done at the Beltsville Human Nutrition Research Center, people with diabetes who took one capsule of cinnamon daily for 40 days saw a marked decrease not only in cholesterol but also in blood sugar just after 20 days. Researchers believe the compounds in cinnamon can make insulin more efficient and especially improve the hormone's ability to regulate the way glucose enters the cells in the body. And it didn't matter if the cinnamon was in supplement form—it is thought to be beneficial if it is cooked, baked, put in a liquid, or even steeped as a cinnamon stick in tea or cider.

*Coriander*—Often used in Indian cooking, coriander (as seeds or ground) may help lower blood glucose levels in people with type 2 diabetes. The extract made from coriander seeds is especially effective. Also for some people with type 2 diabetes, coriander may help the few working beta cells left in the pancreas to produce more insulin.

## What are some of the best fruits to lower the risk of type 2 diabetes?

According to several studies, some fruits are best to consume to lower the risk of developing type 2 diabetes. In particular, those who ate at least three servings per week of apples, blueberries, or grapes were at a lower risk for developing the disease than those who ate less of these fruits per week. Some fruits in studies actually

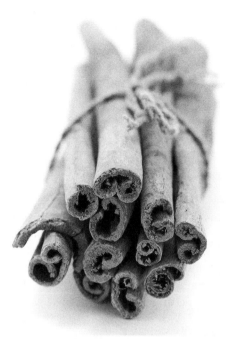

Cinnamon—*real* Sri Lankan cinnamon—helps balance cholesterol, as well as having other healthful effects.

raised the risk for developing type 2 diabetes—especially cantaloupe or fruit juices. More research is definitely needed to understand just what components in these fruits are responsible for helping fight or cause diabetes.

## Does grapefruit affect blood glucose?

Yes, some studies show that grapefruit has many attributes, including improving insulin sensitivity and blood glucose tolerance. In addition, eating grapefruit before a meal seems to stimulate weight loss in some people, which can help if a person is trying to lose weight and not develop type 2 diabetes. It also is thought to keep the liver from pumping out very low density (VLDL) cholesterol, thought to be the "bad" cholesterol in the body. The main ingredient responsible for such responses is called naringenin, a nutrient that tells the body to stop storing fat in the liver and to burn it instead. But eating grapefruit in abundance is not the answer, which is why the once popular "grapefruit diet" has been abandoned by most people. In addition, for some people, grapefruit may be harmful, especially if they take medications such as statin drugs—so they should check with their doctor if they want to consume the fruit.

## What is juicing of fruits and vegetables?

Juicing—besides being a trend of non-health care-professional celebrities such as Gwyneth Paltrow and Megan Fox—is a way of "drinking" various fresh fruits and veg-

The carob tree has fruit called carob pods. Within the pods are the seeds most people know as carob, which is often used as a uncaffeinated substitute for chocolate. The pods also contain pinitol, a naturally occurring substance thought to act like insulin by making cells more receptive to taking in glycogen. Although sometimes debated, some research claims that pinitol may help people who are insulin resistant by increasing the ability of muscles to use glycogen.

etables by pressing them through a juicer. This extracts the liquid from the foods (sometimes referred to as nectar) and leaves the pulp, seeds, and skins. Many juicing advocates say the intake of juice from juicing is a good way to get a person's recommended servings of vegetables and fruits, along with necessary vitamins and minerals. Although juicing is extremely controversial, people who rely on it believe that the body absorbs nutrients from juices better than it does from the foods themselves; they believe it is a way of getting more carotenoids and flavonoids (which fight major diseases such as cancer and heart disease), and they believe that juicing cleans the body of toxins and boosts the immune system. Though juicing is a way of easily ingesting vegetables and fruits, these "scientific" claims have yet to be proven.

### Why do some health care professionals caution people with diabetes about juicing?

Most health care professionals see nothing wrong with diabetics' choosing to juice fresh fruits and vegetables once in a while, but the practice should not be used as a steady, consistent diet. One reason is that our bodies are designed to eat and absorb nutrients from solid foods, such as vegetables and fruits. Another reason is that eating the entire fruit or vegetable is much better at lowering the risk of heart disease and cancer, helping with weight loss, and improving overall health—all things that juicing advocates claim but that remain unproven.

Overall, there are many health and body reasons that eating the entire fruit or vegetable is better than juicing. Too much juicing results in a low amount of protein—and no protein in the diet can lead to muscle-mass loss, even in a few days. In addition, much of the fiber from the food is lost, and lack of fiber can lead to problems with the digestive tract.

### What if a person with diabetes still wants to juice fresh fruits and vegetables?

If people with type 1 or type 2 diabetes—or even those who are prediabetic—do want to add fruit and vegetable juicing to their diet, then there are some things they can try, especially under the supervision of a doctor or other health care professional. One is to test how certain juiced foods affect them. For example, juicing cabbage may not spike a person's blood sugar as much as juicing carrots. While trial and error works for some peo-

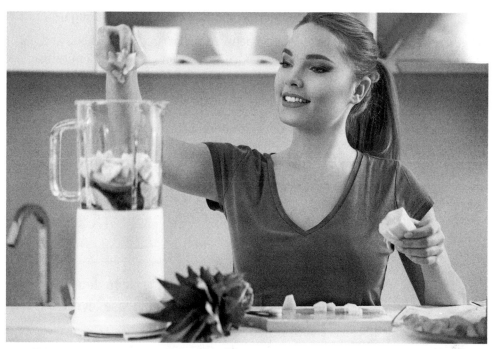

Juicing of fruits and vegetables has become a popular trend in cooking these days, but diabetics are warned not to make juices a regular part of their diet. It's important to eat solid foods, as well.

ple with diabetes, overall, doctors and nutritionists usually recommend that a person eat regular, whole, unjuiced foods for the best nutritional value. This is because many foods that are juiced are high in carbohydrates. For example, an 8-ounce glass of fruit juice can contain 30 grams of carbohydrates, a number that can cause blood glucose levels to rise too fast and too much.

# SUGAR, ARTIFICIAL SWEETENERS, AND DIABETES

### Is it all right to consume sugar if a person has diabetes?

There is a misconception that a diabetic should stay away from all refined sugars, such as white or brown sugar, honey, or syrup, no matter what the source (whether in manufactured foods or from the pantry in recipes). No health care professional would advocate that a person with diabetes eat unlimited amounts of these sugars. This is because whether a person has diabetes or not, these sugars provide carbohydrates and calories but don't offer any fiber, vitamins, or minerals found in other carbohydrate-containing foods such as whole fruits and vegetables. Thus, most people with diabetes can eat refined sugar in moderation.

## Should a person with diabetes cut back on fruit because it contains sugar?

Whether to eat fruit should be a decision between the person with diabetes and his or her health care professional. In general, it is a good idea for everyone to limit sugar (see the chapter "Diabetes and Obesity") because it is often one of the causes of excess weight gain. But eating fruit can be advantageous to everyone, including many people who have diabetes (they should check with their health care professional if there are any doubts). This is because whole fruits have plenty of healthful antioxidants, along with other nutrients, and are high in fiber. Fruits also have sugars, and the body's digestive enzymes must break down the fruit cells, releasing the sugars slowly into the bloodstream. This is why it is much better to eat the actual whole fruit than to drink fruit juice, in which the crushed fruit juice squeezes the cells, releasing the sugars. This puts the sugar into the bloodstream much faster than when the whole fruit is eaten and may even make a person hungry sooner.

## What sweetener is known to be potentially toxic to dogs— especially in terms of affecting their blood glucose levels?

Recently, the U.S. Food and Drug Administration (FDA) issued a stronger warning about a common sweetener and its effect on dogs: xylitol, which tastes similar to sugar and is found in such products as chewing gum, mints, baked goods, cough syrup, children's chewable vitamins, mouthwash, toothpaste, and other products. The warning is based on the effects of the sweetener on dogs. In particular, if a dog ingests xylitol, then the sweetener is quickly absorbed into its bloodstream, causing a dramatic release of insulin in the pancreas. (Xylitol does not stimulate the release of insulin from the pancreas in humans.) This causes a drop in blood sugar, causing the dog to become hypoglycemic (the reaction can occur within ten minutes to an hour after ingestion). If the ingestion is caught in time, then the dog may recover; others less fortunate can often experience too-low blood sugar, seizures, coma, liver damage, and sometimes death.

A prior warning was issued in 2011 by the FDA's Center for Veterinary Medicine, mentioning how the sweetener can affect not only dogs but also ferrets. The stronger warning in 2016 came because of an increase in xylitol-related illnesses reported by pet poison control centers, with one report noting that xylitol is estimated to be 100 times as toxic as chocolate to dogs. The biggest concern is how many xylitol-containing products dogs can ingest. The most common source is sugar-free gum. Other sources include specialty nut butters that owners often give their pets as a treat or to administer medications. The FDA reports that ingesting a few pieces of gum can poison even a large dog. So far, the FDA notes that xylitol toxicity in cats has not been well documented. One suggestion is that a cat is less apt to eat sweets left out on a table than is a dog.

## What is the difference between fructose and glucose?

Glucose and fructose are both considered sugars, but glucose tends to dampen a person's appetite, whereas fructose increases the appetite. In addition, a person's body turns more fructose than glucose into fat—and does it faster. If a person is already overweight or obese, then fructose tends to speed up the sugar's fattening process. These facts are also why there is so much controversy—and concern—about high-fructose corn syrup found in many foods including fruit juices, ketchup, high-fiber cereals, salad dressings, baked beans, canned goods, regular soda, and salad dressings. (For more about the controversy surrounding high-fructose corn syrup, see below.)

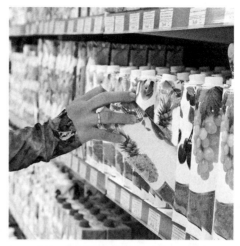

Canned, boxed, and otherwise processed foods often have high-fructose corn syrup added to them. The additive is cheaper than regular sugar, but some people believe high levels of it can promote diabetes.

## Why is high-fructose corn syrup so controversial?

High-fructose corn syrup is formed by changing the simple sugar glucose into another simple sugar called fructose. Fructose is cheap to produce and acts as a preservative to extend the shelf life of many sweets and baked goods. Unfortunately, it is high in calories and low in nutrition. And because it is in so many beverages and processed foods, it is linked to obesity. But not everyone agrees. For example, the Mayo Clinic notes that there is "insufficient evidence to say that high-fructose corn syrup is less healthy than any other type of sweetener." But Mayo does add that any added sugar, not just high-fructose corn syrup, can contribute many unnecessary calories. Those calories are linked to health problems such as weight gain, type 2 diabetes, and metabolic syndrome—all of which increase the risk of heart disease, too.

## How can sugar affect the body's immune system?

Ingesting too much sugar can have a negative effect on the body, especially in terms of suppressing the immune system. In particular, eating or drinking around eight tablespoons (100 grams) of sugar—equivalent to about two and a half 12-ounce cans or bottles of soda—can reduce the ability of white blood cells to kill germs in the body by almost 40 percent. This weakening of the immune system occurs less than 30 minutes after a person ingests the sugar-laden foods or drinks; the effects on the immune system last close to five hours. This is important to a person with diabetes, as he or she already has a compromised immune system from high blood glucose levels.

## How much sugar is too much?

Sugar consumption—no matter what the type—is yet another one of those hotly debated subjects when it comes to overall health. One study conducted by the Food and Nutrition Board of the National Academy of Medicine concluded that there is no scientific evidence that any level of sugars increases the risk of dental cavities, changes in behavior, cancer, the risk of obesity, or high cholesterol. This finding was, of course, countered by the World Health Organization and the Food and Agriculture Organization of the United Nations. They stated that sugar leads to obesity—and eventually type 2 diabetes in many people—especially when it replaces other, more nutritious foods in the diet and that sugar definitely does cause dental problems. More recent studies seem to agree. For most people, the intake of sugar affects them on an individual basis. What is a good intake for one person may lead to obesity in another. And thus the debate continues.

### What sweetener name should already be removed from ingredient lists?

In 2009, the FDA stopped the food industry from using many names on a label's ingredient list. For example, they asked that the term "evaporated cane juice" be removed from all food labels, as it is a misleading name. After all, it is merely sugar syrup dried into crystals, not something special and "wholesome" as many companies tried to make the public believe. But to date, there are still manufacturers who use the term, and several consumer advocacy groups are bringing lawsuits against these food producers, calling the term deceptive. If a food shopper sees this label, then he or she should understand that evaporated cane juice is just another name for sugar.

### Why are artificial sweeteners of concern to many health care professionals—and people with diabetes, too?

Artificial sweeteners are added to many foods and usually give the food a sweet taste without the calories. For most people with diabetes, artificial sweeteners are the answer to eating less or no sugar in their diet. But there are concerns, especially for people who consume large quantities of artificial sweeteners or have allergies or severe reactions after ingesting certain sweeteners. For example, the artificial sweetener aspartame often gives susceptible people a headache about ten to 20 minutes after it is consumed. It also may be a problem for the part of the brain that senses when a person is full, thus causing some people to gain weight. In one study, people who drank artificially sweetened beverages also began to ingest more fat (especially saturated fats) as part of their daily calorie intake. And for people with diabetes who need to keep their weight in check, artificial sweeteners can lead to an inability to control their blood glucose levels.

# DIABETES AND SODIUM (SALT)

## Does salt affect a person's blood pressure, especially if he or she has diabetes?

Most health care professionals agree that, for most people, ingesting too much salt can cause the body to develop high blood pressure over time. In fact, when a person eats too much salt, it causes the body to hold extra water in order to eliminate the salt from the system. For some people, this causes extra pressure in the blood, which results in a rise in blood pressure and stress on the blood vessels and heart. Thus, the American Heart Association suggests that people with high blood pressure, or a tendency toward developing it, should eat foods lower in fat, salt, and calories. And in general, for people with diabetes, most research indicates that salt intake should be low since diabetics are more likely to have high blood pressure than people without diabetes. (For more about blood pressure, see the chapter "How Diabetes Affects the Circulatory System.")

## Why is there a controversy over how much salt should be eaten daily?

The average daily intake of salt, in terms of milligrams, has recently become a much-debated subject. For example, the recommendation for daily sodium intake given by the government (Food and Drug Administration, or FDA) for the general population is a maximum of 2,300 milligrams (mg) per day (or about 1 teaspoon of salt). The American Heart Association number is lower; the group recommends a daily sodium intake of no more than 1,500 milligrams for most people. For comparison, the average American diet contains around 4,000 milligrams of sodium a day.

There is good reason for the discrepancies in recommendations. One of the major problems lies in scientific methods. Determining with finality just how much sodium should be consumed daily would require conducting a randomized, controlled trial. In this case, half of a large population would have to consume a high-sodium diet and half a low-sodium diet for a long period. (If some participants ended up with high-sodium diets and were susceptible to sodium in terms of blood pressure, heart problems, and strokes, then few people would want to participate—or even should participate.) In addition, every meal, piece of food, and beverage would have to be measured for sodium content over the entire study period—and for such a study, that would mean following the participants for months or even years. Thus, instead of conducting that somewhat impossible trial, scientists have had to make recommendations based on other "indirect" studies. The majority of them show that an excessive sodium intake is associated with high blood pressure, heart attacks, and strokes, all of which people with diabetes often develop.

## Where do most people get their daily intake of sodium?

The most familiar source of sodium is table salt that is added in cooking and/or at the table. But in reality, it is estimated that most people consume around 25 percent of their daily sodium from this source. The other 75 percent commonly comes from processed grocery items and fast foods.

### How can a person with diabetes reduce sodium intake?

If a person with diabetes is told to cut back on salt for health reasons, here are some suggestions:

- Pack a homemade meal for lunch instead of eating fast-food takeout.
- Always taste cooking food before adding any salt, and if it needs salt, add it sparingly.
- Use other no-salt-added seasonings in place of salt from the salt shaker, and eliminate (or use less of) those seasonings that contain salt. Look into salt substitutes, or use fresh herbs and spices instead of salt in cooking.

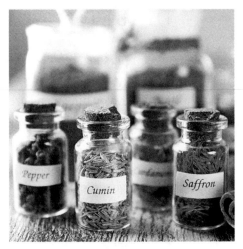

Instead of adding salt to food, try a mix of other spices to make your dish savory without the sodium.

- Don't add salt to cooking water for vegetables, rice, or pasta—it really isn't necessary.
- Buy canned goods with low or no sodium on the label. For example, for canned foods such as tuna, buy water-packed, no-salt-added foods.
- Be cautious when buying reduced- or fat-free salad dressings or any pre-packaged sauces as they often are higher in sodium than the regular salad dressings. Also be cautious about other "fat-free"—and even some sugar-free—foods, which often contain excessive amounts of salt.
- Read the nutrition label on any food, and pay attention to the suggested daily sodium percent. Since the labels are currently for people taking in 2,000 calories per day, for those who are lowering their calorie intake (or normally do not take in as many daily calories), choose foods that have a lower amount of sodium listed on the label.
- Avoid processed foods whenever possible (for more about processed foods and diabetes, see the chapter "Shopping for Food and Eating Out"). Such foods as salted meats or such processed meats as bologna usually have a great deal of salt. Some sauces also contain a great deal of salt. Use them sparingly, or cut down on the amount of salt by adding water to a sauce (it can be thickened with flour or cornstarch, if desired).

# DIABETES AND BEVERAGES

### Do people with diabetes need to drink more water daily than people without diabetes?

Yes, people with diabetes, if possible, should drink more water daily than people without diabetes. According to a study published in 2016, people with diabetes who drank more than 34 ounces of water a day were less likely to develop hyperglycemia (high blood glucose levels) than those who drank only 16 ounces of water or less. One reason water helps control blood sugar is a hormone known as vasopressin, which is released when a person is too dry. This hormone tells the kidneys to hang on to water and tells the liver to release stored blood sugar, and it also raises the blood pressure. If the person doesn't drink enough water and there is too much vasopressin in his or her system, then the kidneys don't make urine, and any extra blood sugar will not pass out of the body—a perfect scenario for developing hyperglycemia.

## How much water should a person with diabetes drink per day?

Overall, it often depends on certain conditions. Research varies, and suggestions range from eight to 15 cups per day (the best amount may be somewhere in between). This is because there are water losses for various other reasons during the day, such as physical activity, hot or dry weather, or even high altitudes. Illnesses can also mean more water is needed, including if a person has a fever, high fiber intake, diarrhea, or high blood sugar. And, for a person with diabetes, higher than normal blood glucose means the blood is thicker and stickier, which can cause an increase in insulin resistance (which means glucose has a harder time moving through the small blood vessels to the cells). Drinking more water each day may help with this condition.

## Why are some fruit drinks thought to increase the risk of developing type 2 diabetes?

Although not all fruit drinks are in this category, when it comes to fruit drinks, health care professionals and nutritionists advocate reading the bottle's label. This is because many of these drinks are filled with added fructose, another name for sugar. Studies have shown that large amounts of fructose can lead to insulin resistance, obesity, type 2 diabetes, and even high blood pressure. Fructose is not only found in fruit and soft drinks but also in baked goods, condiments such as ketchup, syrups (even in what is often called "pancake syrup" presented as replacing real maple syrup), and candies. In addition, in the process of making fruit juice, the fruit is squeezed, breaking open the cells and releasing the sugars faster. This means the fructose in the juice goes into a person's system faster, and he or she is more likely to feel hungry—and thus eat more—not long after drinking the juice.

## What are the so-called "energy drinks"?

Energy drinks are beverages that boast of boosting energy levels, improving mental performance, and even aiding weight loss. They are high in caffeine, sugars (the types of sweeteners vary), and herbal compounds (presented as supplements). Because they claim to be dietary supplements, the FDA does not regulate the safety of the ingredients, meaning the manufacturers are responsible, which is often a major controversy involving such beverages.

## How do "energy drinks" affect blood glucose levels?

Energy drinks are known to cause insulin levels to spike, which can often make it difficult to bring blood glucose levels down to normal. In a recent study, the caffeine in en-

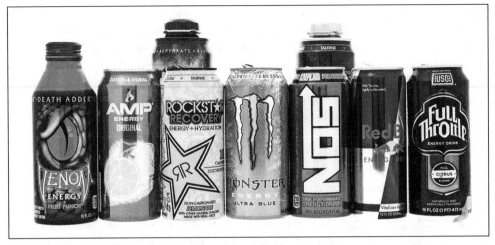
Energy drinks are filled with caffeine and sweeteners that can affect blood glucose levels.

ergy drinks resulted in a 20 to 30 percent decline in the body's ability to deal with the high sugar load. In addition, they found that because the caffeine stays in the body for four to six hours after the beverage is drunk, the resulting insulin resistance may eventually lead to problems with glucose metabolism. This can especially affect adolescents who are consuming so many of these drinks. As they grow older, and if they are susceptible, they may be more at risk of developing such problems as heart disease and diabetes.

### Is there a connection between drinking coffee and lowering the risk of developing type 2 diabetes?

Several studies have shown a possible connection between drinking coffee and lowering the risk of developing type 2 diabetes. For example, in 2015, a report in the American Chemical Society's *Journal of Natural Products* suggested that two compounds may help decrease the risk of type 2 diabetes. Initially, when scientists found that drinking coffee—regular or decaffeinated, up to three to four cups per day—helped to prevent the onset of type 2 diabetes, they believed that the coffee's caffeine was responsible. Eventually, they showed that caffeine had only a short-term effect on glucose and insulin in the body. Investigators then isolated several bioactive compounds responsible for diabetes prevention, and, using rat cells, tested the effects of different coffee substances on those compounds. Two were found to increase insulin secretion when glucose was added: cafestol and caffeic acid. Cafestol also increased the glucose uptake in muscle cells, an increase that the scientists believe may contribute to the preventive effects on type 2 coffee drinkers. They hope this knowledge will soon help researchers to develop new medications not only to prevent but also to treat the disease.

Another study reported in the *Journal of Agricultural and Food Chemistry* indicated that coffee drinkers were at a lower risk for developing type 2 diabetes for yet another reason: compounds in the coffee that affect a polypeptide called hIAPP, or human islet amyloid polypeptide, were thought to be one of the causative factors of type 2 diabetes. The researchers believed that certain coffee compounds such as caffeine, caffeic acid, and chlorogenic acid help lower the risk of type 2 diabetes (especially caffeic acid) by suppressing the formation and thus the toxic effects of hIAPP.

## Can even one cup of coffee affect the risk of developing type 2 diabetes?

According to a Harvard University study published in 2014 in the *Diabetologia* journal, researchers followed over 100,000 people for about 20 years, concentrating on a four-year period. They discovered that if a person increased his or her daily intake of coffee by one cup, then the risk of developing type 2 diabetes dropped by 11 percent. People who *reduced* their daily intake of coffee by one cup actually increased their risk of developing diabetes by 17 percent. As most researchers and doctors agree, this is not a recommendation to drink an overabundance of coffee each day, but it is yet another step toward understanding just why coffee has such an effect on diabetes.

## How does the caffeine in coffee affect glucose and insulin in diabetics?

A study in 2004 showed that a dose of caffeine consumed by a person with type 2 diabetes before eating caused a higher blood glucose level and an increase in insulin resistance after eating. This is why the effects of consuming coffee are so confusing: Drinking coffee may help lower the risk of developing type 2 diabetes, but for a person with type 2 diabetes, it may pose an immediate risk after the drink is consumed!

More studies are needed concerning coffee and diabetes. For example, some researchers suggest that other compounds in coffee may have a different effect on insulin and/or glucose levels. In addition, no one knows whether drinking caffeinated coffee over a long period of time (and how much) may change the body's glucose and insulin sensitivity. And there is always the problem of what a person chooses to put into coffee—especially creamers that contain an overabundance of saturated fats, carbohydrates, and calories. The best suggestion, as always, is for a person with diabetes to discuss coffee intake with the primary-care physician, diabetes educator, and/or nutritionist.

## How do other compounds in coffee affect a person with diabetes?

Caffeine is not the only compound found in coffee. For example, a person with diabetes may receive more benefits from drinking decaffeinated coffee. In particular, chlorogenic acid and other antioxidants in the decaffeinated coffee may have beneficial effects, and the magnesium found in coffee may also have a positive effect on insulin sensitivity.

But as with all recent coffee studies, the jury is still out concerning diabetes and coffee compounds. As of this writing, no one has yet discovered how much coffee a person with diabetes can consume, what compounds help or hinder glucose and insulin levels, which types of coffee are most beneficial (compounds in the coffee vary depending on where the beans are grown), or even the effects of how the coffee is prepared.

## Should a person with diabetes abstain from drinking alcohol?

Not necessarily, especially if the person has control of his or her blood glucose levels. But there are some caveats. For example, there is the question of healthful versus unhealthful drinking, so no matter whether a person has diabetes or not, he or she should drink responsibly. As for a person with diabetes, keep in mind that too much alcohol can lead to hypoglycemia, or low blood sugar, especially if the individual drinks on an empty stomach. (In addition, according to the American Diabetes Association, people who are on sulfonylureas or insulin should drink alcohol only with meals.) This is because the liver not only processes alcohol, it also stores and releases glucose. Thus, wine, beer, and liquor hinders the liver's ability to release the necessary glucose, causing hypoglycemia. (Because symptoms of hypoglycemia and inebriation are similar, many law enforcement officials may not be able to tell the difference—which may mean people with diabetes will not get the help they need quickly.) Alcohol provides no nutrition but does contain fat, which can lead to weight gain. And if a person with diabetes is taking any medication, then he or she may want to abstain from drinking any alcohol. If a person with diabetes who is in control of his or her blood glucose levels does want to drink, then some health care professionals suggest having only one drink (or two) a day at the most, eating something to slow the absorption of alcohol into the bloodstream, and nursing a drink over a few hours to lessen the burden on the liver.

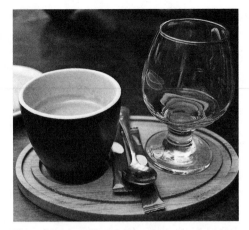

The caffeine in coffee can raise glucose levels and increase insulin resistence, while alcohol, if not consumed carefully, can lead to hypoglycemia.

# DIABETES AND FASTING

## What is fasting?

Most people with diabetes are familiar with the term "fasting" in reference to "fasting blood glucose levels." This usually means a period after a person fasts (usually while sleeping), with blood glucose levels checked upon awakening. But fasting can also mean not eating for a certain amount of time for various reasons, including for religious, medical, or health reasons, or an unintended fast. For example, certain religions fast for a day or several days, usually in observance of holy days; certain surgeries or medical procedures may include a fast for a day or so; some people fast for a day to "detoxify" the body (although more long-term studies are needed to understand whether there are truly benefits of such practices); and sometimes a person unintentionally misses a meal for various reasons.

## How does the body respond to fasting?

Depending on how long a person fasts, changes take place in the body. In most healthy adults, the body usually enters a fasting state about eight hours after the person's last meal. At first, the body will use stored sources of glucose, such as in the muscles. Later, if the fast is prolonged, then the body breaks down fat stores as an energy source. This has been seen historically, especially in people who used fasting as a means of protest and lost a great deal of weight. But all health care professionals agree that fasting should not be used as means of losing weight in the long term, as it can cause major imbalances in various body systems and reactions—including problems with digestion, blood glucose levels, and dehydration.

## How can a person with diabetes cope with fasting for religious purposes?

Depending on the religion, fasting lasts for different periods of time. For example, people who follow Hinduism and Judaism tend to fast only for individual days during religious holidays. Other religious observances, such as the Islamic observance of Ramadan, often include longer periods of fasting. During Ramadan, it is necessary for all healthy Muslims to fast each day between sunrise and sunset for an entire month (the often-heard phrase is "the Islamic month of Ramadan"). In some cases, depending on the religious leader's ideology and/or the religion or culture, certain groups of people in different circumstances are exempt from fasting. These may include children (under puberty), the elderly, pregnant women (and those who are breastfeeding or menstruating), people who have an illness, those who are traveling, or anyone who would be putting him- or herself at serious health risk by fasting.

## How can a person with diabetes observe religious practices that include fasting?

For a person who has diabetes and is in relatively good health (meaning his or her blood glucose levels are balanced), fasting for religious purposes is often possible—but also can be quite a challenge. According to several diabetes organizations, the first and best thing to do is consult a health care professional to see whether it makes sense for the person to fast. In many cases, the medical recommendation will be not to fast if the person has diabetes, especially with a history of ketoacidosis, is pregnant, or has poor blood glucose control. People who do

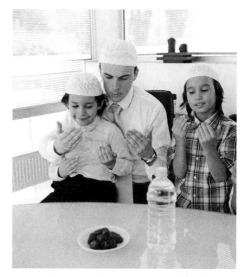

Some religious people practice periods of fasting, which can be problematic for a person with diabetes, but it can still be done safely if precautions are taken.

307

heavy manual labor or have certain illnesses—and diabetes—probably will also be advised against fasting.

But if someone with diabetes is in relatively good health and still decides to fast, then it is best to consult a health care professional to help prepare for potential problems. For example, according to organizations such as Diabetes UK, for a person observing a fast such as Ramadan:

- People with type 1 or type 2 diabetes should speak to their health care team before fasting, especially to better understand how to control possible blood glucose problems before, during, and after the fast. The goal is to prevent blood glucose levels from dropping too low (hypoglycemia, which is usually defined as a blood glucose level less than 70 mg/dl; possible symptoms include feeling shaky, sweaty, and/or disoriented), especially if the person is taking insulin or other diabetes medication. In addition, for people with type 1 diabetes, there is a danger of blood glucose levels measuring too high (hyperglycemia), resulting in the buildup of ketones, creating ketoacidosis (symptoms include excessive thirst, passing copious amounts of urine, and tiredness). Understand that people taking insulin may need less of it before the start of the fast or more—depending on their condition.

- People may need a different type of insulin from their usual type because of fasting during the day.

- Before a fast, include more foods in the diet that are absorbed slowly, such as basmati rice, pita bread, and dhal, along with fruits, salads, and vegetables.

- Check blood glucose more than usual over the course of the day.

- If a person has any sign of hypoglycemia (low blood glucose levels), then it is better to break the fast and immediately start such treatments as taking glucose tablets, or GlucoGel. (For more about treating hypoglycemia, see the chapter "Taking Charge of Diabetes.")

- Know when to break a fast. Both extremely high and low blood glucose levels are dangerous to a person with diabetes. Religious leaders tend to agree that fasts are truly not meant to create life-threatening situations.

- After fasting for the day, eat only small amounts of food and avoid eating sweet or fatty foods (or just have very small amounts). Too many sweets and fatty food will cause weight gain.

- In the case of such observances as Ramadan, try to eat just before sunrise (before the fast starts), and regulate insulin or diabetes medication to fit.

- At the end of fasting, drink plenty of sugar-free and decaffeinated liquids to avoid becoming dehydrated.

### What is juice fasting—and is it good for people with diabetes?

Juice fasting means abstaining from solid foods for a couple of days and getting nutrients from juices through juicing. Many people advocate this to allegedly cleanse the body of toxins, such as pesticides, pollution, artificial colors, and preservatives, but cleansing claims have not been proven. And for people with diabetes, especially type 2, juice fasting can aggravate their condition. In particular, ingesting just vegetable and fruit from juicing can cause excessive highs or lows in blood glucose levels. If a person with diabetes does want to try juice fasting, then it is best to be supervised by a health care professional or a dietitian familiar with diabetes and nutrition.

# DIABETES, DIETING, AND EATING DISORDERS

## Why are some "fad" diets so controversial, including for people with diabetes?

There are plenty of controversial "fad" diets that should be viewed cautiously. Most fad diets are thought to be more harmful than helpful, mainly because they do not provide all the nutrients the body needs to stay healthy. In fact, most studies have shown that many fad diets do not help people really lose weight. For example, because people lose water weight fast, especially at the beginning of many diets, the fad diet can give the illusion of losing weight. Most fad diets do not teach anyone how to eat well and keep the weight off but are just a "quick fix." And when the dieters go back to their usual eating routine (often because the fad diet becomes boring or too hard to follow), they usually regain any weight lost.

For people with diabetes, eating a lower amount or different types of foods advocated by the fad diet may not be what they need to maintain healthy blood glucose levels. According to the National Institutes of Health, low-calorie diets—such as those based on less than 800 calories a day—can affect the heart and other organs and, indirectly, may even contribute to people's becoming overweight (as the body thinks it is starving, thus it stores more fat). This type of diet can also increase the risk of diabetes for many people. For those who have diabetes, it may contribute to such problems as hypoglycemia.

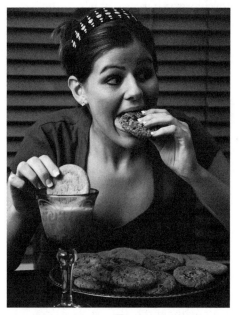

## What is an eating disorder?

According to the American Diabetes Association, eating disorders are considered an illness with a biological basis that is mod-

Binge eating—as well as other disorders such as bulimia and anorexia—can wreak havoc with one's blood glucose levels.

## What is diabulimia?

According to several recent studies, a somewhat new eating disorder—especially for young people with type 1 diabetes—is diabulimia, an alarming way to lose weight. Although it is not a recognized medical condition, diabulimia has recently been showing up in alarming numbers in teens and young adults who have type 1 diabetes. People with type 1 diabetes need to have continuous treatments with the insulin hormone in order to get glucose from their bloodstream into the cells. But people with diabulimia try to manipulate blood glucose levels through what they eat, along with withholding their normal insulin injections or manipulating their insulin pumps. This makes their glucose levels rise, causing the sugars to spill into the urine. And this, in turn, causes rapid weight loss. But diabulima is dangerous. It can lead to hyperglycemia (high blood glucose levels) from insulin deficiency and/or damage small blood vessels, leading to peripheral neuropathy, causing eye problems and trouble in the extremities. If a person is diabulimic for a long time, then it can lead to other more serious health problems, including diabetic ketoacidosis, and the increased risk of kidney disease, nerve damage, amputations, and heart disease.

ified and influenced by emotional and/or cultural factors. The disorders include anorexia (or anorexia nervosa, in which the person has an obsessive fear of gaining weight, so he or she starves or eats very little in order to lose and keep off weight); binge-eating disorder (compulsive overeating, in which a person has periods of uncontrolled, impulsive, or continuous eating despite feeling full); and bulimia (in which a person rapidly consumes a great amount of food, then purges the food).

### Are people with diabetes immune to eating disorders?

No, people with diabetes can have eating disorders, and many of the eating problems can compromise the ability to manage blood glucose levels. For example, in many women with type 1 diabetes, bulimia is the most common eating disorder. There is also a relatively new term, diabulimia, meaning when people with type 1 diabetes try to control their glucose levels by reducing or not taking their insulin injections in order to lose weight (see sidebar). In many women with type 2 diabetes, binge eating is the most common eating disorder.

### What can happen to a person with diabetes if an eating disorder is not controlled?

If a person with diabetes has an eating disorder, then it can lead to several health problems, with most of the problems precipitated by uncontrolled blood glucose levels. These include a higher risk of developing infections; higher A1c levels (that don't go down unless the eating disorder ends); more trips to the hospital and emergency room (usually because of hypoglycemic episodes); possible episodes of diabetic ketoacidosis (or DKA, a dangerous kidney problem); and more frequent occurrences of—and more rapidly developing—diabetic complications, such as heart and kidney disease, nerve damage, and eye problems.

### What are some ways to recognize an eating disorder in a person with type 1 diabetes?

People with type 1 diabetes are known to develop certain eating disorders. In fact, it is thought that women with type 1 diabetes are more than twice as likely to develop an eating disorder than women of the same age who do not have diabetes. Some researchers suggest that there are signs that a person with diabetes has an eating disorder. They include an unexplained rise in the person's A1c values; the person's expressing extreme concerns about his or her weight and body shape; a change in eating habits; unusual patterns of intense exercise (this often occurs with bouts of hypoglycemia; for more about hypoglycemia, see the chapter "Type 1 Diabetes"); and for women, skipping their monthly periods (called amenorrhea).

# SHOPPING FOR FOOD AND EATING OUT

## SHOPPING AND READING LABELS

### Is there a difference between a serving and a portion on a food label?

Yes, a serving is an amount of food determined to be appropriate by the U.S. Food and Drug Administration (FDA). On nutrition labels that appear on most packaged foods, the serving size is noted, along with how many calories per serving, total fat, cholesterol, sodium, total carbohydrates, protein, and any relevant vitamins and minerals. A portion is how much food you decide to eat at one time, whether at a restaurant or at home. In many cases, our food portions do not match the serving size because many people eat a larger portion than the serving size—which is one of the possible reasons for weight gain.

### How should people interpret food label claims, especially people with diabetes?

There are differences in the terms on labels, and people with diabetes who want to maintain a healthy weight and have less sugar in their diet need to understand certain label terms. The Food and Drug Administration has strict guidelines on how these food label terms can be used. Here are some of the most common claims seen on food packages—and there are many—and what they mean, as per the FDA and the American Heart Association:

*Low calorie*—Must have 40 calories or fewer per serving.

*Low in saturated fat*—Must have one gram of saturated fat or less, with not more than 15 percent of the calories from saturated fat.

*Low fat*—Must contain less than three grams of fat per serving.

*Reduced fat*—Must contain at least 25 percent less of the specified nutrient or calories than the usual product; for example, a reduced-fat mayonnaise must contain at least 25 percent less fat than regular mayonnaise.

*Less*—A food must contain 25 percent less of a nutrient than a certain other food; for example, a pretzel label can claim that pretzels contain 25 percent less fat than potato chips.

*Good source of*—Must provide at least 10 to 19 percent of the Daily Value of a particular vitamin or nutrient per serving; for example, to be a good source of calcium, the food must contain 10 to 19 percent of the daily value for calcium.

*Light (or lite)*—A food must have a third fewer calories or half the fat of a certain other food, or the sodium in a low-fat, low-calorie food must be reduced by 50 percent; for example, light mayonnaise must contain at least 50 percent less fat than regular mayonnaise.

*Calorie-free*—Must contain less than five calories per serving.

*Fat-free/sugar-free*—Must have less than ½ gram of fat/sugar per serving.

*High in*—Provides 20 percent or more of the Daily Value of a specified nutrient per serving.

*High fiber*—Must contain five or more grams of fiber per serving.

*Good source of fiber*—Must contain 2.5 to 4.9 grams of fiber per serving.

*Lean meat*—Must contain less than ten grams of total fat, 4.5 grams of saturated fat or less, and less than 95 milligrams of cholesterol per serving.

*Extra lean*—Must have less than five grams of fat, two grams of saturated fat, and 95 milligrams of cholesterol.

*High protein*—Must contain 20 percent (or more) of the Daily Value for protein.

*Natural flavoring*—The FDA standard states that foods with this label must be extracts from nonsynthetic foods, such as essential oils, spices, and so on; its function in the food is flavoring, not nutrition.

*Fresh*—Although this term has been misused over the years, it originally meant unprocessed, uncooked, and unfrozen foods (with washing and coating [usually wax] of fruits and vegetables allowed). Fresh-frozen is also included, meaning food that is quickly frozen; the term is usually seen in association with fresh fish.

*Good source*—This means a serving must contain between 10 and 19 percent of the recommended Daily Value of a certain nutrient, such as vitamin A or D.

*Fortified*—A fortified food must have 10 percent or more of a Daily Value per serving, but it can be used only to represent vitamins, protein, minerals, dietary fiber, and potassium; for example, most milk in the United States is fortified; thus, one cup has to have about 30 percent of the Daily Value for vitamin D.

The FDA also sets standards for health-related claims on food labels to help consumers identify foods that are rich in nutrients and may help to reduce their risk for certain diseases. For example, the manufacturers can make health claims that highlight the link between calcium and osteoporosis, heart disease and fat, and high blood pressure and sodium.

## What are some other labels to be aware of if a person has diabetes?

Even though it is estimated that close to 50 percent of consumers read food labels before buying, sometimes labels can be misleading. Here are some of the more common confusing labels:

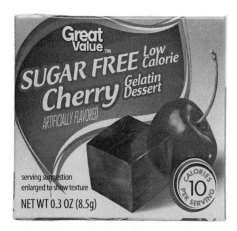

It's important to understand what labels such as "low fat," "low sugar," and "sugar free" really mean, and one needs to also consider portion size.

*Low fat*—Many people on a diet look for the low-fat label. This may mean that, as per regulations, the product has three grams of fat or less. But often, when one ingredient is missing, food manufacturers add something to make up for it. In the case of "less" or "low fat," it usually means more sugar, sodium, and calories that can cause weight gain that may lead to diabetes.

*Low sugar versus reduced sugar*—Many people want less sugar in their diet but should be aware of two phrases: "Reduced sugar" means that the product has 25 percent less sugar than the regular version, but "low sugar" has no standard definition.

*Sugar-free*—This means that the food has to have less than a half gram of sugar per serving, but the serving size may be very small. A serving size can range from a tablespoon to a cup! Sugar-free products may also cause gastrointestinal problems in people, especially those sensitive to other sugar substitutes, such as sorbitol. Overall, instead of looking at the "sugar-free" label on a package, a person with diabetes should pay more attention to the product's total carbohydrate count.

## What are the main parts of a nutrition label on most foods?

There are standard food-nutrition labels that are based on government recommendations. The numbers, listings, and percentages are based on a 2,000-calorie diet for the "average" person, but there is a major debate about what is truly "average." (It also means that changes are coming in the government's recommendations; see sidebar). The following are some of the major items listed on food-nutrition labels:

*Serving size*—This is the number used to determine one serving of food. It is also often written in terms of grams.

*Total carbohydrates*—This is an important percentage for people who have diabetes (and for those who wish to limit their intake of carbohydrates). It represents the total percentage of carbohydrates in one serving, in terms of a percentage of the "average" diet.

*Dietary fiber*—This is also an important percentage listed under carbohydrates, usually in two forms—grams and percentage of the total in one serving.

## Why and how will the government change food labels?

There has been a major problem with the government-recommended numbers and percentages on food labels that has created a great debate. In particular, the information on a label is based on an "average" person who eats 2,000 calories a day. But a great deal has changed since the Food and Drug Administration sent out guidelines for nutrition labels in 1993—especially with the American diet. The FDA label's serving-size standards were based on the "reference amounts customarily consumed" (RACCs)—numbers based on consuming in the late 1970s and 1980s. But Americans eat more now—as evidenced by the increase in heart diseases and obesity—and instead of a third of an English muffin (the "serving size"), a person eats the entire muffin (which means more calories consumed). Now the FDA wants to emphasize this difference in serving size and give more realistic numbers; it also wants the food manufacturers to be more realistic and if most people eat the entire muffin to label the package as "one serving," not many. These changes will not only help consumers make better decisions about how much they truly want to eat but also make more healthful choices. But when these changes will occur is another matter.

*Sugars*—The amount of sugar is also part of the total carbohydrate listing and can refer to both natural and added sugars. It will not list the types of sugar but only the amount (the types of sugar are often listed under the ingredients on a package).

*Sugar alcohol*—If applicable, the sugar alcohol may be listed or the sweeteners in the form of sugar alcohols, such as sorbitol, mannitol, and xylitol. These sugars are not listed individually on the nutrition label but may be listed in the ingredients.

*Vitamins*—Vitamin percentages may also be listed on nutrition labels, although they usually represent only the more "common" vitamins, such as C, A, or D. In addition, the more "common" minerals are often listed as percentages, including calcium and iron.

### What are the names for sugar that a person with diabetes should understand when reading a food label?

Sugars are listed on food labels in various ways, but as most dietitians and nutritionists will tell you, sugar is sugar. The most obvious word on a label is "sugar," but there are other words to pay attention to, including the following:

- Brown sugar: refined sugar coated with molasses (the molasses is taken out, then added back in, or it can even have an artificial caramel coloring)
- Corn syrup: manufactured from corn and containing various amounts of glucose, maltose, and dextrose

- Dextrose: pure glucose or a sugar made of only one molecule
- Fructose: sugar from fruit and maple sap
- Glucose: known as dextrose, or grape sugar (it is also used in reference to a person's blood glucose levels)
- High-fructose corn syrup: concentrated corn syrup that is made mostly of fructose
- Lactose: natural milk sugar
- Maltodextrin: made from maltose and dextrose
- Maltose: a sugar from starch, most often grains
- Raw sugar: less refined white sugar with a minute amount of molasses
- Sucrose: the refined, crystallized white sugar found in most sugar bowls
- White grape juice: a purified version of fructose

## What are some tips for people with diabetes when they go shopping for food?

Food shopping for a person with diabetes can be a challenge. Here are some tips from various organizations that specialize in helping those with diabetes:

- Expand your food options, and learn about new tastes and foods. There are excellent cookbooks, cooking websites, and apps for people with diabetes who want to learn to cook or experiment with various types of foods (several of which are mentioned in this book's "Resources, Websites, and Apps" section).
- Instead of eating the same thing every day, start experimenting with new foods from the grocery. Most foods have to be labeled, making it easier to keep track of fats, sugars, and other nutrition information.
- Take a list to the grocery store, and follow it. Most stores know humans can be impulsive buyers, especially when it comes to food, and stores are set up to entice people to buy things they don't truly need to eat. Try to stick to the list.
- Don't consider any food "good" or "bad." Even though a person has diabetes, most foods (unless the person is allergic or has an intolerance to certain foods, too) can fit into the person's healthful-eating plan, as long as the individual adjusts for any given food (for example, balancing insulin or substituting one food for another to keep blood glucose levels balanced).

# DIABETES, PROCESSED FOODS, AND ADDITIVES

## Why should processed foods be a concern, especially to a person with diabetes?

Although many processed foods are fortified with vitamins, minerals, and other nutrients, a diet that consists of all processed foods is a concern to many nutritionists. In     317 particular, the "replacement nutrients" are in the food artificially. And, in many cases, these nutrients are not as easily absorbed into our systems as the natural nutrients found in fresh meats, fruits, and vegetables. The consumption of processed foods can be balanced. According to the Academy of Nutrition and Dietetics (AND), "processed" foods can mean anything from what a person processes in her own food processor to a packaged frozen pizza. And although some processed foods are not too bad (such as canned beans, vegetables, etc.), the AND cautions against consuming too many of the more heavily processed foods. In particular, they warn consumers who do buy processed foods to be aware of what is listed on the food labels and especially how much—such as sugars, especially for people who have type 1 and type 2 diabetes. Sugars are hidden everywhere, including as added sweeteners to ice cream, pasta sauce, etc., and also for more "hidden" things such as sugars in breads. Other things to scan labels for include fats (for flavor and to make the food last longer

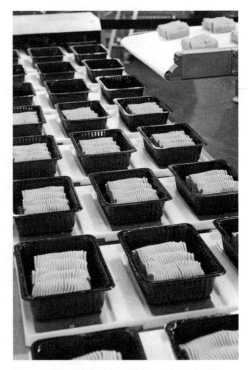

A couple issues with processed foods include: 1) chemical additives, such as preservatives, might not be healthy, and 2) the artificially added vitamins and minerals are not as easily absorbed into the body as natural vitamins and minerals.

on the shelf) and sodium (for almost all foods for enhanced flavor and as a preservative). Too much of any of these ingredients can add on the weight that can eventually lead to certain chronic diseases, such as diabetes.

### What recent studies connected diabetes to processed foods?

There have been many recent studies of people who eat processed foods and who have diabetes. In one study from Harvard Medical School, the researchers discovered that eating processed meat (but not unprocessed red meat) caused an increase in the risk for diabetes by 19 percent and heart disease by 42 percent. In another study conducted in Finland over a 12-year period, people who ate processed meats raised their type 2 diabetes risk by 37 percent, whereas eating red meat and poultry did not.

### Why should people with diabetes be aware of their intake of simulated foods?

Like processed foods, simulated (also referred to as fake) foods can be high in sugar, fats, sodium, gums, artificial flavors, dyes, and so on. For example, imitation crab meat may be cheaper than real crab, and to most people, it tastes as good. The fake crab meat is made with a type of fish called surimi. But it also has fillers, flavoring (sometimes including sugars and salt), and colored dyes, all of which make the fake crab mimic the taste, texture, and color of real crab. Although most fake crab meat is low in fat and calories, it can be extremely high in sodium, with some containing 800 milligrams of sodium or more in a three-ounce (very small) serving.

Other examples include fake cheeses, most of which contain fillers, oils, and emulsifiers (called "processed cheese" by most producers); frozen dairy desserts that only have to contain at least 10 percent milk fat but are also high in corn syrup, gums (like guar gum) and whey; and even fake, dehydrated potato flakes that also come with preservatives, emulsifiers, artificial flavorings, and trans fat. For a person with diabetes, adding such sugars and fats to the daily diet may add on weight and also cause blood glucose levels to fluctuate. Therefore, most health care professionals recommend that simulated foods be a small part of the person's daily diet.

## What are the most common food additives?

The most common modern food additives are sugar, corn syrup, other sweeteners, and salt. They are all used to enhance flavor and/or prevent the food from spoiling. Still other food additives are used as preservatives, colorings, antioxidants (to prevent foods from going rancid), flavor enhancers, emulsifiers, thickeners, and stabilizers.

## Which additives should a person with diabetes be aware of consuming?

According to several recent studies, people with diabetes should be aware of consuming certain additives. In particular, one study on a simulated human gut showed that emulsifiers found in most processed foods seem to be connected to obesity, inflammatory bowel disorders, and diabetes (mostly type 2). Another study warns of ingesting aspartame and monosodium glutamate (MSG). In the case of aspartame, not only does it often cause headaches in many people, but it can also cause an increase in fasting blood

### What are some of the more interesting additives used in foods?

One of the more interesting "scary-sounding" additives is carnauba wax, which is usually associated with polishing a car, not with food. This ingredient is listed first in the ubiquitous marshmallow treats most associated with the Easter holiday (used for the eyes of the candy animal). Another interesting ingredient is shellac. It is a secretion from the female lac bug in India, and in terms of food, it is called "confectioner's glaze." This additive is used to give the glossy covering to such foods as jelly beans and other candies and is mainly used to stop the food from drying out. According to research done on both additives, there seem to be no adverse effects. Thus, they are approved for use in foods by the Food and Drug Administration.

glucose levels. When aspartame and MSG are combined, they cause even more of an increase in glucose levels.

# EATING OUT

### What should a person with diabetes look for on a restaurant menu?

Eating out at any restaurant can be a challenge for people with diabetes. Depending on their eating habits to maintain their blood glucose levels, they may have to curb fatty and sugary foods. Doing so becomes difficult as many restaurants, diners, and dinner clubs offer large portions packed with calories, saturated fats, and sugar. And because people with diabetes have to pay more attention to their intake of carbohydrates, they must be more diligent when looking for something to eat on the restaurant menu. Below are some hints for ordering:

- Don't be afraid to ask how an entrée (or anything on the menu) is prepared. Try to avoid dishes served with heavy sauces or gravy, fried foods, and certain dairy products, such as heavy cream and thick cheeses. If everything on the menu includes such items, then eat only a reasonable proportion of the food and, if possible, take the rest home.

- Most restaurants are aware that many people have certain dietary restrictions and are thus used to dealing with special diets. Ask whether the foods can be prepared in a certain way, such as steaming vegetables, or ask for skinless chicken, fish, or lean meat that is broiled, poached, baked, or grilled.

- If a meat or vegetable is accompanied by a fattening sauce or butter, then ask whether that can be served on the side—and use it sparingly, if desired. Similarly, many restaurants will provide salad dressings on the side, allowing the customer to add as much of the dressing as desired.

- No rule states that a person has to clean his or her plate. If only a portion of the food is eaten, then ask for a container to take the remainder home.

- Get the server's advice as to low-fat or low-sugar meals. Usually servers will be more than happy to help with dietary requests.

- If the person with diabetes is on insulin and knows that a certain restaurant is usually slower than others when it comes to serving, then time the injection appropriately. If the service is slow, then some diabetics can slowly eat a roll or piece of fruit until the full meal is served. Some people always bring certain food items along with them—for example, crackers—just in case a meal is delayed.

- Not everyone with diabetes can or will have dessert. But if a person wants to have a dessert, then share one. That way, the person won't be tempted to eat the entire dessert, which may cause blood sugar to become unbalanced.

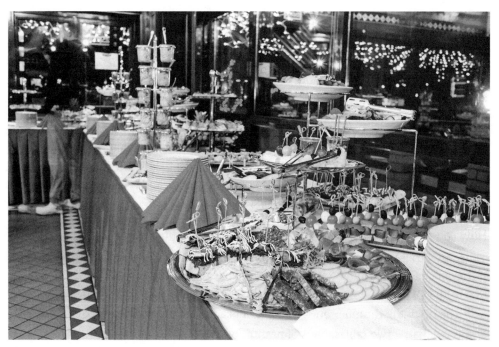

The temptations of eating out, whether at a restaurant or at a holiday or other party, can test anyone's self-control. Don't hesitate to talk to a dinner host about your special dietary needs.

## What are some ways to measure and count carbohydrates while eating out?

In most social situations, a person with diabetes cannot get out a scale and determine size and approximations of carbohydrates when eating out. But there are simple ways to estimate sizes of servings and count carbohydrates. The following list is one way of estimating the measure of a handful (large, medium, and small), and the index finger and thumb positions (not touching, just touching, and overlapping) to determine amounts:

*Large* (not touching)—This is approximately equal to two (30 grams) of non-sugar carbohydrate servings (for example, breads, potato, rice, barley, pasta, grits, oatmeal, non-sugary cereals, corn, peas, winter squash, pretzels, crackers, fruit, and popcorn); four servings (60 grams) of sugar-carbohydrate desserts (cake, pie, cookies, doughnuts, pastries, muffins, frozen yogurt, ice cream, pudding, sherbet, and custard); and eight servings (120 grams) of candy carbohydrates (chocolate, caramels, hard candy, marshmallows, honey, syrup, jams, and jellies).

*Medium* (just touching)—This is approximately equal to one (15 grams) of non-sugar carbohydrate servings; two servings (30 grams) of sugar-carbohydrate desserts, and four servings (60 grams) of candy carbohydrates.

*Small* (overlapping)—This is approximately equal to 1/2 (eight grams) of non-sugar carbohydrate servings; one serving (15 grams) of sugar-carbohydrate desserts, and two servings (30 grams) of candy carbohydrates.

### Why are holiday parties and special celebrations often a challenge for a person with diabetes?

Holiday parties and special celebrations are especially difficult if the host/hostess does not have diabetes, has never known anyone with the disease, and no other guests have diabetes. There are still many misconceptions about the disease, and as with many other conditions, many people don't understand it if they have never experienced some of the frustrations. This does not mean a person with diabetes should stop going to parties and celebrations. It means that the person may have to be more diligent about what he or she chooses to eat or drink. Attentive eating includes asking the host/hostess about the foods offered, being careful about food choices offered, and even bringing one's own food to the party. (See below for other suggestions.)

### How can people with diabetes measure smaller quantities when eating out?

There are other ways to estimate portions if people with diabetes are eating out or even if they need to know about a portion size while eating at home. The following is modified from Harvard Medical School and the Academy of Nutrition and Dietetics:

- The tip of the thumb = one teaspoon of peanut butter, sugar, or butter
- A golf ball = two tablespoons of peanut butter
- One finger length or a tube of lipstick = one ounce of cheese
- One fist = a cup of cereal, pasta, or vegetables
- One handful = one ounce of nuts or raisins
- One palm (woman's) or deck of playing cards = three ounces of cooked meat (any type), poultry, or fish
- Two handfuls = two ounces of pretzels

### How can a person with diabetes cope with eating at holiday parties?

There are some ways for people with diabetes to help themselves cope at a holiday—or any other—party. The following are some suggestions (note: not all suggestions can be fulfilled before or during a party, but most understanding hosts/hostesses will try to make the person with diabetes more comfortable):

- If the party or celebration will include a dinner at a certain time, a person with diabetes can call and ask when the meal will be served. This way, if the person is taking insulin, then he or she can plan on when to administer an injection before eating.
- Eat a regular meal before attending the party or grab a snack. This can include foods that are high in fiber and low in sugar and fat, such as crackers, soup, a vegetable salad, or yogurt. This way, the person with diabetes will not be hungry and/or tempted to eat snacks and sweets that may make the blood glucose levels fluctuate. It is also *not* a good idea to skip a meal the day of a party in order to "save up" for overeating at the party. This, too, will more often than not cause a dramatic fluctuation in blood glucose levels.

- Eat slowly in order to keep from consuming more than needed—or enough to make blood glucose levels become imbalanced.
- After eating a plate of food at a party, wait around 20 minutes before going back for more (or don't go back at all). This is because it takes at least 20 minutes for the brain to know that a person has eaten enough to make him or her feel full. If after 20 minutes a person is still hungry, then he or she could go back for one more serving of one type of food instead of filling the plate again.
- It may be a good idea to stand away from the food tables, especially the appetizers and desserts. That way, the temptation to graze or eat before a meal (or after) will not be as great. Depending on the party, a person with diabetes can keep far from the food table by engaging in conversations, sharing stories, watching movies, or participating in activities, such as badminton or lawn darts.
- Drink plenty of water before the party. It makes a person feel full and consequently eat less. (Drinking alcohol and sugary beverages will only add calories and can cause problems with blood sugar levels.)
- Don't be afraid to ask the host/hostess about the types of foods and drinks that will be served—and be sure to ask *before* the party. (Preferably ask days before, not the day before or day of the party!) After all, it is better to ask than to have a bad hypoglycemic or hyperglycemic episode.
- If, after asking the host/hostess what will be served, the person with diabetes finds nothing to eat, then he or she may want to suggest bringing some of his or her own food and drink to the party, especially low-fat and/or low-sugar dishes. Not only will it help to control portions, but the person will not be tempted to eat foods that may be unhealthful to consume.
- After eating, keep moving, if possible. Not only will it keep one's mind off food, but light physical activity, such as a stroll or playing games such as badminton, also speeds up metabolism, burns calories, helps with blood glucose, and is good for digestion.
- Know that not everyone understands what life with diabetes entails. Don't be tempted to eat something at a party that may send blood glucose levels too high (or low). If someone asks the person with diabetes to eat something that will cause a blood glucose problem, then the person should gently refuse and explain about blood sugar. It may be a chance for the person without diabetes to better understand the challenges faced by a person with diabetes!

## How can a party host help a person with diabetes, especially in terms of food and drinks?

If a host/hostess knows that someone with diabetes is attending the party, then he or she can help in several ways—and most of the foods and drinks won't be that much different from what is usually offered at parties. The following lists a few of the ways to help if a person with diabetes attends a celebration or special party:

- Ask whether the person with diabetes can bring some of his or her own foods, especially any low-fat foods and/or low-sugar desserts. Most parties include high-fat, high-sugar desserts that can wreak havoc with a diabetic's blood glucose levels. Also be sure to let other guests know which dishes do not have sugar if it is not obvious.
- Ask what foods would be best to offer the person who has diabetes. Most people with diabetes would be grateful to know that they won't have to guess at what to eat when they get to a party. It may also help if the host/hostess explains how some of the foods are prepared—for example, if they are steamed or fried—especially if the foods are high in fat or sugar.
- Be careful when showing people with diabetes the foods they can or cannot eat at the party. Some people do not believe it is anyone's business that they have diabetes, mainly because they do not want to be treated "differently." Others will be fine with its being known that they have diabetes and may even want to educate others as to the challenges of having diabetes.
- Have water, tea, and coffee—non-sugar drinks—available. Some people with diabetes also drink sugar-free beverages, so have some of those on hand, too (or ask the person what types of drinks he or she prefers).
- Offer low-fat and low-sugar foods such as fruits (grapes, apple wedges, or strawberries), vegetables (carrots, cauliflower, cherry tomatoes, celery, cucumbers, or summer squash sticks), some breads and starches (low-fat offerings are best, and if purchased, those with lower carbohydrates listed on the label), and dips (such as tomato salsas or black bean dips).
- The host/hostess may also want to ask the person with diabetes for meat preferences (low fat, such as turkey, lean roast beef, or chicken) if it will be offered.
- If the host/hostess's house is large enough, then have a nearby room or room extension away from food tables where people can gather.
- If a guest has diabetes and needs to take insulin before a meal, plan on telling the person when food will be served. This is important in order to keep the diabetic's blood glucose levels balanced. (In addition, the host/hostess may want to know whether the person with diabetes, especially someone taking insulin injections, has a glucagon kit in case of a hypoglycemic episode at the party.)

Cluster of islet cells
(produces insulin, amylin, and glucagon)

Encapsulated islet cells
(protected against auto-immune destruction)

# THE FUTURE
# OF DIABETES

Biocompatible outer layer
(implant will survive without a fibrotic response)

Semi-permeable material

## HEALTH CARE AND DIABETES

### Why is health care so costly for treating diabetes?

There are many reasons that health care for diabetes is so costly. Many experts cite the spending policies of the health care system. In particular, little is spent to keep people healthy through preventive care. Great sums are spent when a person becomes sick or disabled—which is truly necessary—but not for chronic diseases such as diabetes. In addition, other costs are associated with diabetes because it is not a disease that "goes away" as readily as some other ailments; these costs include purchases of needles for insulin, medications, test strips, etc. The prices of these necessities continue to rise, and as the number of people with diabetes rises (as most agree it will), demand for such items will rise. Instead of helping, most health care insurance plans choose to ignore the extra costs of living with diabetes. These extra costs may be one of the reasons that people often choose to ignore the fact that they have the disease.

### How can governments handle the number of people projected to have diabetes in the next decade?

The number of people projected to develop diabetes—both type 1 and type 2—will no doubt rise in the next decade, and some say beyond. Several organizations are addressing this problem. For example, the International Diabetes Federation launched the Global Diabetes Plan in 2011 after the world leaders met at the United Nations in New York to agree to actions concerning diabetes and other non-communicable diseases. Several countries, including Australia, have their own plans to help understand what needs to be accomplished in terms of helping people with diabetes or even trying to reduce the number of people who develop the disease. There are also programs using dig-

325

ital means to collect information and data from people with the disease as a step toward providing education and access to information to the public. (For more information about organizations helping the diabetes effort, see the chapter "Resources, Websites, and Apps.")

# MITIGATING DIABETES

## What is the ultimate goal for those who research diabetes—and, especially, for people who have diabetes?

Of course, the main goal not only for diabetes research, but also for people who have diabetes, is to restore the body's ability to manufacture its own insulin. For many people with diabetes, that also means eliminating the need for injections or diabetes medications.

## What recent research involves helping people with diabetes produce their own insulin?

In 2016, researchers at the Diabetes Research Institute (DRI, under the University of Miami in Florida) announced they were one step closer to the goal of enabling people with type 1 diabetes to produce their own insulin instead of relying on injections. The first person to receive the new method of transplanting insulin-producing cells was a woman who developed type 1 diabetes in her teens. She was a prime candidate, as she has what is called severe hypoglycemia unawareness, or the inability to sense that her blood glucose levels are dropping to a dangerously low level (for more about severe hypoglycemia unawareness, see the chapter "Type 1 Diabetes").

The researchers used what is called a "biodegradable scaffold" that was implanted on the surface of the omentum (the sheet of protective tissue that hangs down from the stomach and covers the abdominal organs). In a new technique, they implanted donor islet cells, those that produce insulin, into the scaffold. The old technique used islet cells infused into the liver, but because the liver is not an ideal site for transplantation—mainly because inflammation can develop—the researchers implanted the cells in the omentum. The results so far are promising: to date, the woman is no longer injecting insulin for her diabetes.

# NEW TESTS FOR DIABETES

## Why are so many people with diabetes undiagnosed?

According to recent research by the Centers for Disease Control and Prevention, nearly 28 percent of the people (or about eight million people) who have diabetes are undiagnosed. One of the major reasons is understandable to many people. The CDC found that

> ### Are researchers working on a device that uses light to measure glucose levels?
>
> One of the most sought-after devices for people with diabetes is one that would measure glucose levels without having to prick a finger to get blood. One such device that may be offered in the future uses light to measure glucose levels through the skin. The research is based on chemistry. The researchers shine light on different substances to determine which ones absorb light and how much is absorbed. In the case of glucose, researchers are trying to detect the sugar molecule's signature absorption of infrared light, but so far, the measurements only track the glucose levels closely—but not in as detailed a way as needed.

because the screening test for diabetes involves drawing blood with a needle, many people avoid the procedure. In addition, a person is required to fast before the test—usually for more than 12 hours—something that makes the procedure even more uncomfortable for many people.

## What device was recently developed that uses sweat to detect glucose?

Although the study is in its infancy, researchers are trying to develop a device that can detect glucose levels using sweat. In 2016, a team from the Hong Kong Polytechnic University and Zhejiang University in China developed such a device to help early diagnosis of diabetes. The technology is part of two fields, one called optofluidics, which melds the fields of photonics (using light to detect certain chemicals), and the other called microfluidics (controlling small amounts of fluid along microchannels). The researchers hope that this device will eventually be used to detect glucose levels in a person's body from droplets of sweat, but more tests on the "lab-on-a-chip" need to be made. In particular, the device uses a fiber-optic biosensor and a microfluidic chip, creating a way of monitoring glucose levels that promises to be not only cheap but also portable.

## What are some other ways glucose levels may be measured in the future?

Many research institutions are working hard to find a way for people with diabetes to measure glucose levels without having to prick fingers, thighs, or arms. For example, in 2015, the University of California at San Diego reported it had developed a temporary tattoo that used electrodes and sensors to measure blood glucose levels. Google (yes, the search-engine company) is also seeking better glucose monitoring through the use of contact lenses for people with diabetes. The computer company Apple is working on a smartwatch that can monitor and display health-sensor data including blood glucose levels (such a watch is available but so far without the blood glucose readings). And in 2014, a saliva test kit called the iQuickIt Saliva Analyzer went through clinical trials to measure blood glucose with a simple saliva test. It works by putting a one-time-use strip (called a

Draw Wick) into the person's mouth for a few seconds, obtaining a small sample of saliva. Although none of these devices or methods is currently available to the general public, it shows that there are institutions—and people—who are sensitive to the plight of people pricking their fingers day after day to monitor their blood glucose levels.

### Are there any devices that screen for prediabetes and type 2 diabetes without using needles?

Yes, in 2016, a device produced in Canada was developed that tests for prediabetes and type 2 diabetes without needles, blood, or fasting (currently, it is used only in Canada and the European Union and only as an investigational device in the United States). The Scout DS™ device uses technology that employs light to detect and measure specific biomarkers associated with prediabetes and type 2 diabetes. The patient lays his or her arm in the device's armrest, and in around 80 seconds, a number is displayed on the attached screen. If the score is high, then the patient is advised to see a health care professional for a follow-up evaluation. It is hoped that such a device can be used in other places, such as pharmacies, offices, etc., to allow quick screenings—to catch people who are at risk for diabetes or allow an easy check for people who have diabetes.

# FUTURE MEDICINES TO TREAT DIABETES

### Will there ever be a generic insulin?

As of this writing, there is no generic insulin on the market. In 2012, the Food and Drug Administration outlined many tough standards for the approval of biosimilars (generic versions of medications that are made by microorganisms), including insulin. As of this writing, there is no generic insulin being submitted or tested by the FDA, but that may change soon. The patents for several types of insulin will soon expire, meaning there may be more of an interest in developing generic insulin. But it will take a long time for testing and approval.

### What study is being conducted to determine whether metformin can help delay or prevent type 1 diabetes in at-risk children?

Although in its infancy, at this writing, a six-year study is being conducted in Scotland to determine whether the oral medication called metformin—the most commonly prescribed diabetes medicine in the world, taken by people with type 2 diabetes—can help prevent, or at least delay the onset of, type 1 diabetes in at-risk children. One of the reasons for the interest is that Scotland has the third-highest rate of type 1 diabetes in the world, and for reasons yet unknown, the numbers continue to rise.

For people with type 2 diabetes, metformin decreases the amount of glucose in the liver. It also improves the body's insulin sensitivity not only in the liver but also in mus-

## What drug more associated with the lungs is currently being tested on people with diabetes?

One drug associated with the lungs (in particular to treat emphysema) is currently being tested on people with type 1 diabetes, called by the general name alpha-1 antitrypsin (A1AT; several companies call the drug by specific names, but they are not mentioned here). In type 1 diabetes, the body's autoimmune system attacks the beta cells that are responsible for secreting insulin from the pancreas. As the disease progresses and more and more of the beta cells no longer function, the person with type 1 diabetes usually becomes completely dependent on insulin. It is thought that the A1AT drug may help those with type 1 diabetes if the clinical trials prove successful. In particular, researchers believe the A1AT may stop pancreatic inflammation and allow the survival of active and operating beta cells.

A form of A1AT was first tested on animals with diabetes, with promising results. Another smaller-sample test on humans who had type 1 diabetes was run around 2012, with results showing that many of the participants were able to take significantly less insulin than when they started the trial. The alpha-1 antitrypsin drug is currently being control-tested on many pediatric and young-adult patients with type 1 diabetes in several cities across the United States and in other countries, with most of the projected results expected by 2017. But there is one caveat: At this writing, the drug may be successful only with people with newly diagnosed diabetes or periods during which there may still be some existing functioning beta cells in the pancreas.

cles and fat cells. This process also helps protect beta cells in the pancreas from stress. Type 1 diabetes is an autoimmune condition in which the pancreas's insulin-producing beta cells are destroyed. The researchers believe that stress signals sent out by the beta cells is what starts the immune-system attack in type 1 diabetes, not a problem with the immune system itself. They hypothesize that relieving the stresses on the beta cells in at-risk children will stop the process of developing type 1 diabetes. And that relief may come from taking metformin.

## What other conditions have been treated with the anti-inflammatory drug alpha-1 antitrypsin (A1AT)?

Type 1 diabetes is currently the center of study for the anti-inflammatory drug known as alpha-1 antitrypsin (A1AT), but it has also been used in the past for other health conditions. For example, it has been used to treat people with severe lung diseases, such as emphysema. It is also hoped that besides type 1 diabetes, A1AT can eventually be used to treat other autoimmune diseases, such as rheumatoid arthritis and certain types of asthma.

# NEW WAYS OF TREATING DIABETES

## What is islet-cell transplantation?

Within the islets of Langerhans are the important alpha and beta cells. The alpha cells produce glucagon, while the beta cells secrete insulin—both important in keeping blood glucose levels balanced in the body (for more about the islets, see the chapter "How Diabetes Affects the Endocrine System"). Islet-cell transplantation involves the pancreas, specifically the islets of Langerhans. In particular, the beta cells are found in small clusters (islets) of the pancreas and are responsible for producing insulin. Researchers hope not to transplant the entire pancreas but to target, extract, and replace only those cellular components that are needed to restore the pancreas's normal function.

## What is an "artificial pancreas"?

At this writing, an artificial pancreas is not a physical unit that replaces a person's own pancreas but is a combination of two technologies—a unit that monitors a person's glucose levels and a pump that delivers the correct amount of diabetic medication to the person to balance their glucose levels. This mimics what a person's pancreas would do in terms of monitoring glucose levels and determining how much insulin or glucagon the body needs. For a person without diabetes, the body's pancreas naturally finds a

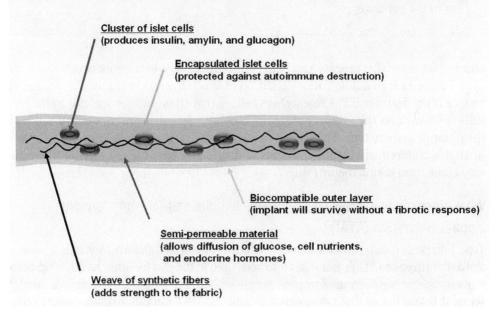

The "Bio-artificial Pancreas" using Islet Sheet technology

Cluster of islet cells
(produces insulin, amylin, and glucagon)

Encapsulated islet cells
(protected against autoimmune destruction)

Biocompatible outer layer
(implant will survive without a fibrotic response)

Semi-permeable material
(allows diffusion of glucose, cell nutrients, and endocrine hormones)

Weave of synthetic fibers
(adds strength to the fabric)

An artificial pancreas would function much like a real one, producing insulin, glucagon, and amylin.

good balance between glucose, insulin, and glucagon. But for a person with diabetes (especially type 1), insulin is needed several times a day to keep blood glucose levels in check. The artificial pancreas helps people with type 1 diabetes whose beta cells make little, if any, insulin by monitoring blood glucose levels and compensating for imbalances with insulin and glucagon pumps.

The melding of this type of technology is not new. These pieces of equipment have been around since the 1970s, but the larger devices were clumsy to use. Today's technology has allowed scientists to develop much smaller devices. People can use smartphone technology to keep balanced glucose levels no matter what activity they pursue or what they eat. For example, one version of an artificial pancreas has been tested many times and includes a smartphone that has an "artificial pancreas" app. A person's continuous glucose monitor takes measurements every few minutes and wirelessly sends the information to the smartphone that contains the artificial pancreas app, which uses the measurements to calculate how much insulin or glucagon to give the user. From there, the smartphone beams the information to two pumps the person is wearing to balance the glucose levels. In this case, the insulin pump delivers medication to lower the blood glucose level, or the other pump containing glucagon delivers medication to raise the level.

## Will there ever be a true artificial pancreas?

The ultimate goal for people who have diabetes and researchers who study the disease is to develop what is often termed a "bionic pancreas," one that could actually replace a person's non-functioning pancreas. In fact, there are laboratories working on melding the continuous glucose-monitoring units with insulin and glucagon pumps to create such an artificial pancreas.

But there are several difficulties so far, especially the size of such a unit. In addition, there are problems with the speed of the insulin delivery and with the shelf life of glucagon. Even with the current so-called "artificial pancreas" (see above), there are often problems with the lag time between the sensor reading and fluctuation in blood glucose levels. For example, one test showed that by the time the blood glucose started to rise after a person ate, there wasn't enough time for insulin measurements and sub-    331 sequent delivery to prevent blood glucose levels from rising too fast. In addition, glucagon usually comes in powdered form and needs to be dissolved in water before injected or infused. The problem with a glucagon pump is that the glucagon has a short shelf life—usually just a day—before it becomes unstable. Studies are continuing, and with advancements in technology, many researchers believe such a unit is possible. Some say as of this writing that the problems will be solved within the next half decade.

# THE FUTURE OF GENETICS AND DIABETES

### Do researchers believe a person's genetics is connected to developing type 1 diabetes?

Yes, some parts of a person's genetic makeup can be connected to type 1 diabetes, but for most people, genetics is only a part of what contributes to the disease. Research on type 1 diabetes has shown that dominant genes associated with diabetes can either protect against or cause a person to be more susceptible to the disease.

### Do researchers believe a person's genetics is connected to developing type 2 diabetes?

Some parts of a person's genetic makeup can be connected to type 2 diabetes, but like type 1 diabetes and genetics, it is not all that contributes to the condition. As with type 1 diabetes, research on type 2 diabetes has shown that dominant genes associated with diabetes can either protect against or cause a person to be more susceptible to the disease. But with type 2 diabetes, there appears to be a stronger connection between genetics and disease. In particular, scientists have discovered that a gene on chromosome 7 in the human body is linked to type 2 diabetes. It is thought that when the gene mutates, it creates a gene that releases a faulty enzyme, which is then unable to stimulate the pancreas to produce insulin. (For more about genetics, mutations, and type 2 diabetes, see the chapter "Prediabetes and Type 2 Diabetes.")

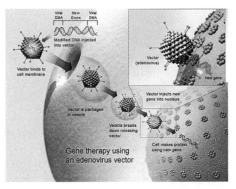

### Why is the study of genetics so difficult to interpret at this time, especially in terms of such diseases as diabetes?

One of the major reasons why the study of genetics is so difficult to understand in terms of certain diseases is that ge-

In gene therapy, a vector is used to carry a modified gene into cells, which then are able to use the gene to produce the desired proteins they couldn't produce before.

## Can genes affect other genes?

**Y**es, researchers have found that two or more genes not only can alter the effects of other genes but can also mask other genes. Technically termed epistasis, this phenomenon may be why people develop such diseases as diabetes and Alzheimer's. Researchers have also discovered that this gene interaction can be both negative and positive and vary from person to person. Currently, epistasis is one of the major reasons for the difficulty in interpreting the interrelationship between genetics and such diseases as diabetes.

netic mechanisms are so complex. For example, genetic diseases fall into three different types of categories: a single gene that is defective, mutations in multiple genes, and abnormalities in a person's chromosomes. In addition, whereas one person may show symptoms of a disease at birth, others may not show symptoms until many years later—sometimes for three to seven decades. And with most people living longer, especially in the Western cultures, the incidence of mutations, abnormalities, and defective genes becomes even more problematic. Thus, some diseases such as diabetes, cancer, and heart disease are also on the increase. But to find out a definitive cause and effect is often a matter of speculation, especially when it comes to a person's genetics.

The reason for the interest in genes and how they are involved in diseases, especially of the aging population, is obvious. If certain combinations, mutations, or degradations of certain genes can be identified in association with a disease such as diabetes, then there may be a way to mitigate or even slow down the progression of the disease, especially for at-risk people.

## Why are chromosomes important in the future study of genetics and diabetes?

Diabetes is a complex disease influenced by what is called epistasis and environmental factors. For example, some research has indicated that the interactions between loci (the plural form of the word; it is the location or position of a gene's DNA sequence on a chromosome) of chromosomes 2 and 15, along with loci on chromosomes 1 and 10, are found in most people with type 2 diabetes. Thus, research is currently being conducted on both type 1 and type 2 diabetes, loci, and chromosomes. Seven new loci were recently discovered, all linked to type 2 diabetes in the Japanese population. Researchers also discovered that four of the loci seemed to coincide with the risk of the disease in several other populations. More research needs to be conducted to determine all the connections and responsible genes for type 1 and type 2 diabetes, along with other epistasis-influenced diseases. And once these relationships are understood, it is hoped that the result will be better diagnosis and treatment of these diseases.

### Are there any organizations that are collecting data to determine the future of genetics and diabetes?

Yes, several organizations are collecting data for a database concerning genetics and diabetes. For example, the American Diabetes Association has a national database that contains information and genetic material from many families that have members with type 2 diabetes. This data is meant to help researchers conduct genetic links and locate the genes involved in type 2 diabetes. (For more about such organizations, see the chapter "Resources, Websites, and Apps.")

# A FUTURE WITHOUT DIABETES?

### Will type 1 diabetes ever go away?

Although many organizations are working to eradicate type 1 and type 2 diabetes, it will be much more difficult to get rid of type 1 diabetes than type 2. This is because type 1 diabetes is an autoimmune disease in which a person's body essentially attacks itself so the person makes no insulin. But there may be hope. In 2014, scientists from Harvard University engineered a way to make large quantities of insulin-producing cells. They did this by using embryonic stem cells that were prompted to turn into insulin-producing cells. By 2015, researchers at the Massachusetts Institute of Technology had planted into mice similar engineered cells that switched off the disease for six months (which is thought to translate to several years in humans). If this research comes to fruition (it is still being studied, with the first human tests in 2016), then it would mean people with type 1 diabetes would just need a transfusion of engineered cells every few years to keep their blood glucose levels stable.

### Is it true that once a person has type 2 diabetes, he or she will always have the disease?

This is an important question and one that researchers and those who have type 2 diabetes truly want answered. In the recent past, the fate of people with type 2 diabetes was usually sealed. In other words, they would have the disease for the rest of their lives and suffer the consequences of and complications from having diabetes. Most of the research shows that type 2 diabetes may be reversible but usually only a short time after the diagnosis. More recent studies show it may also be reversible in people who have had the disease for many years. But as always, more research is needed.

### What recent study tried to find a way to reverse type 2 diabetes?

A study reported in early 2016 was based on a small clinical trial in England. The trial studied the effects of a strict liquid diet on 30 people—ages 25 to 80—and who ranged from being overweight to extremely obese. Each participant had lived with type 2 diabetes for up to 23 years. They were to complete an eight-week, low-calorie milkshake diet (taking no diabetes medication and eating only 600 to 700 calories a day, all from three diet milkshakes at mealtimes and half a pound of non-starchy, liquified vegetables). After the trial, participants would return to normal eating. Overall, around half of the participants went into remission immediately after the trial and were still diabetes-free after six months. The researchers don't know why this worked, but there are a few speculations. One is that when a person goes on a low-calorie diet, the body may use up the fat from the liver, causing the fat levels to drop in the pancreas, too. This may cause the insulin-producing cells in the body to become active again, normalizing blood glucose levels. But the study was not for everyone. For instance, no one knows how long the effects will last or whether the regimen will work for the typical person with type 2 diabetes. And most of all, the biggest challenge at the end was returning to normal eating, especially after consuming a liquid diet.

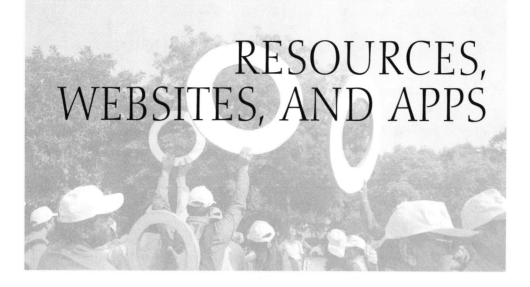

# RESOURCES, WEBSITES, AND APPS

## What is available on the Internet for me?

There is a wealth of information about diabetes on and off the Internet. Without such resources, the authors could not have done all the research necessary for this book. For people who don't own a computer or who don't want to gather their information from the Internet, we offer some contact information and other resources from books, magazines, and organizations about all facets of diabetes.

For Internet users, we list sites that help the general public manage the labyrinth of the what, where, and how of diabetes. Some sites include information about prediabetes, types 1 and 2, and gestational diabetes. There are sites that generously help parents cope with their child's diabetes diagnosis. There are scientific papers available from the government, universities, institutions, and organizations that go into more scientific details about diabetes. And more recently, there are sites that present studies that may eventually help eradicate diabetes—or at least lessen the number of people with the disease.

Below, you'll find some of these contacts and more "user-friendly" sites, but don't be afraid to check out other links. (Although some sites may seem to offer help, the authors generally get their information about diabetes from organizations that specialize in the disease. This is mainly because such groups are the most familiar with educating and helping the public and are up to date on the more recent scientific findings.)

(The authors have made every effort to verify the following sources, but websites, addresses, and phone numbers often change. We apologize for any inconvenience caused by such changes.)

# BOOKS AND MAGAZINES

## What are some general books that help people who have just been diagnosed with diabetes?

Many books help people who want to understand the nuances of diabetes, especially those who have just been diagnosed. And of course, the list should include this book! The following are other fine sources:

- *Cheating Destiny: Living with Diabetes,* James S. Hirsch, Mariner Books, 2006. Although this book is somewhat outdated in terms of technology, it is an excellent book that not only tells the story of Hirsch's own experiences with diabetes but also his young son's experiences after being diagnosed with type 1. In addition to his personal narrative, Hirsch brings in a great deal of history behind the introduction of insulin and the people who were and are affected by its discovery. He also writes about the realities of diabetes in America and some of the firsthand experiences of the trials and tribulations felt by those who have the disease.
- *Mayo Clinic: The Essential Diabetes Book,* second edition, Mayo Clinic, Oxmoor House, 2014. This is a comprehensive guide to diabetes by experts from the first and largest integrated, nonprofit group practice in the world.
- *American Diabetes Association Complete Guide to Diabetes,* American Diabetes Association, fifth revision, 2014. This complete guide to diabetes gives many of the basics behind diabetes, especially for those who have just been diagnosed.
- *Think Like a Pancreas: A Practical Guide to Managing Diabetes with Insulin,* Gary Scheiner, Da Capo Press, 2012. Written by a person who has had type 1 diabetes for over a quarter century, diabetes educator Scheiner interprets the ins and outs of having diabetes, along with his personal observations about having diabetes.

## What are some books that help parents who have children and/or teens with diabetes?

Several more recent books help parents understand and cope if their child has diabetes. These are only a few fine book sources:

- *American Diabetes Association Guide to Raising a Child with Diabetes,* Jean Betschart Roemer, American Diabetes Association, 2011. This book is written by a diabetes educator who has intimate contact with diabetes, as she has had type 1 diabetes for over 45 years. The book not only has basic information about diabetes and how to encourage children to take care of themselves with diabetes but also sections on how to cope—and help a child cope—with the diagnosis.
- *Raising Teens with Diabetes: A Survival Guide for Parents,* Moira McCarthy, Spry Publishing, 2013. A much-needed guidebook for parents—especially as teens and tweens go through not only a diagnosis of diabetes but also natural changes in hormones as they reach puberty. It explains how hormones versus blood glucose lev-

els vary and affect a young person with diabetes. In particular, it also looks at how diabetes can affect social situations, family dynamics, school safety, and even some tougher topics, such as drugs, alcohol, lying, depression, sex, and rebellion, especially in terms of having the disease.

## What are some children's books that explain diabetes?

There are so many books that help children understand what it is like to have diabetes—too many to mention here. The following lists only a few of the more favored ones, many of which are not only good for young children to read but their parents, friends, and teachers also:

- *Taking Diabetes to School,* Kim Gosselin, JayJo Books, 2004. This book is older, but still has some good information for preschoolers and up. It's not only informative to a child but also to his or her classmates (a read-aloud book).

- *Even Superheroes Get Diabetes,* Sue Ganz-Schmitt, Dog Ear Publishing, 2007. Again, an older book, but the concept is great for younger children, especially if they have diabetes or even know someone with diabetes.

- *The Great Katie Kate Discusses Diabetes,* M. Maitland DeLand, Greenleaf Book Group Press, 2010. This book is for ages six to nine and is a good resource to help children not only understand the disease but also help with their treatments.

- *Diabetes and Me: An Essential Guide for Kids and Parents,* Kim Chaloner and Nick Bertozzi, Hill and Wang, 2013. Although for kids age eight to twelve, it is also a great resource for parents who have a child with diabetes.

## What are some books that explain either type 1 or type 2 diabetes?

There are several recent books that explain some of the factors involved in having type 1 and type 2 diabetes. These are only a few sources:

- *The Mayo Clinic Diabetes Diet,* written by weight-loss experts from the Mayo Clinic, Da Capo Lifelong Books, 2014. This helpful book is from one of the major clinics in the nation, written for a person diagnosed with prediabetes or diabetes.

- *Type 1 Diabetes for People Who Don't Have It,* Lisa Powell, Lulu.com Publishing, 2010. As the book title implies, this is for people who don't have type 1 diabetes but want to know more—especially for friends, family, and others who want to know more about a friend's or family member's challenges with diabetes.

- *Taming the Tiger: Your First Year with Diabetes,* William Lee Dubois, Red Blood Cell Books, 2009. This is an older book, but it still has some good and valuable insight to a person's first year with the challenges of type 1 diabetes. Dubois also has type 1 diabetes and has written several other books, columns, and articles on the subject.

- *The First Year: Type 2 Diabetes: An Essential Guide for the Newly Diagnosed,* Gretchen Becker, Da Capo Press, 2006. Although this is an older book, it has some good tips. For example, it offers an in-depth discussion of type 2 diabetes, along with shorter chapters that are broken down into manageable sections.

- *Your Type 2 Action Plan,* American Diabetes Association, 2015. This book not only helps with diabetes education but also diet, exercise, and how people with type 2 diabetes can better manage their health.

### What are some books that help a person with diabetes eat more healthfully?

Not everyone with diabetes can eat the same foods. To help with dietary decisions and to understand the reasons for a diabetic diet, the following lists only a few of the specialized books available:

- *What Do I Eat Now?: A Step-by-Step Guide to Eating Right with Type 2 Diabetes,* Patti B. Geil and Tami A. Ross, American Diabetes Association, 2015. This is a good, recent guide to eating, especially for those who have just been diagnosed with prediabetes or have diabetes.
- *The Prediabetes Diet Plan: How to Reverse Prediabetes and Prevent Diabetes through Healthy Eating and Exercise,* Hillary Wright, Ten Speed Press, 2013. This informative book, as it says in the title, offers ways of eating healthfully, along with exercising, to help people diagnosed with prediabetes or who have the potential to develop diabetes.

### What are some books that explain the relationship between exercise and diabetes?

Although most exercise-and-diabetes books have much of the same information as an exercise book for people who don't have diabetes, there are some differences. The following lists a few of those books:

- *Diabetic Athlete's Handbook: Your Guide to Peak Performance,* Sheri Colberg, Human Kinetics, 2009. As the title promises, this handbook has a great deal of useful information about how exercise affects a person with diabetes and how to cope with the effects. The author is an exercise physiologist who has had type 1 diabetes since she was four years old. The book not only talks about blood glucose management and workouts but also focuses on special activities not often included in other exercise books, such as ballroom dancing and fencing.
- *The "I Hate to Exercise" Book for People with Diabetes,* third edition, Charlotte Hayes, American Diabetes Association, 2013. This book gives tips to people with diabetes who have a hard time fitting exercise into their daily routine.

### What are some books that explain diabetes in relation to gender?

Although there are not many books that explain diabetes in relation to gender, here are a few worth mentioning:

- *The Smart Woman's Guide to Diabetes: Authentic Advice on Everything from Eating to Dating and Motherhood,* Amy Stockwell Mercer, Demos Health, 2012. This book is written by a woman who was diagnosed with type 1 diabetes when she was 14. The book takes personal experiences with diabetes—what Mercer and other women she interviewed experienced—from adolescence to adulthood. She covers many female topics, too, including menstruation and pregnancy.

- *A Woman's Guide to Diabetes: A Path to Wellness,* Brandy Barnes and Natalie Strand, American Diabetes Association, 2015. This book helps a woman with diabetes with the day-to-day challenges, as well as how to cope physically, mentally, and emotionally.

- *Sex and Diabetes: For Him and for Her,* Janis Roszler and Donna Rice, American Diabetes Association, 2007. Although this book is not as new as some, it still carries some interesting topics, such as the physical and emotional ways diabetes can affect a person's sex life. For example, there is often a connection between erectile dysfunction in men and diabetes (for more about this, see the chapter "How Diabetes Affects the Reproductive System").

## What are some books that explain the technology available for people with diabetes?

Although these books often become a bit out of date—mainly because of new technology—they do give the reader insight as to what technology is available to those who have diabetes. The following are only a few examples:

- *Insulin Pumps and Continuous Glucose Monitoring: A User's Guide to Effective Diabetes Management,* Francine R. Kaufman with Emily Westfall, American Diabetes Association, 2012. This book, as the title promises, is a compendium of what is out there in terms of insulin pumps and continuous glucose monitors. It is a good resource for people with diabetes who may not know how or even why such machines are used, along with information about what to know about the technology before a purchase is made.

- *Pumping Insulin: Everything You Need to Succeed on an Insulin Pump,* John Walsh and Ruth Roberts, Torrey Pines Press, 2012. This book has everything about using insulin pumps from what they are to how to use them for children, while exercising, and when pregnant.

## What are some magazines for people who have diabetes?

Several magazines offer information and support for people who have diabetes. The following lists some of them:

- *Diabetes Self-Management*—This bimonthly magazine for people with diabetes is published by Madavor Media, LLC, 25 Braintree Hill Office Park, Suite 404, Braintree, MA 02184. The magazine can be reached for subscription information at 855-367-4813, or via online at http://www.diabetesselfmanagement.com/subscribe/.

- *Diabetes Forecast*—This monthly magazine is published through the American Diabetes Association. For subscriptions, call 800-806-7801, or subscribe online at http://www.diabetesforecast.org/about-forecast/subscribe.html.

• *Diabetic Living Magazine*—This periodic magazine is published as a Better Homes and Gardens Special Interest Publication, published by Meredith Corporation. For subscriptions, contact the magazine at 866-261-6866, or if ordering online, link to https://secure.diabeticlivingonline.com/order/?containerName=i63vuri57&psrc=MN_I63VURI57_R3.

# WHERE TO FIND DIABETES INFORMATION

## Where can a person with diabetes look for education and information about diabetes?

Several groups specialize in diabetes education. The following lists some suggestions, including phone numbers and addresses (along with email and websites)

• To find a Certified Diabetes Educator in a certain region and information about diabetes, contact the American Association of Certified Diabetes Educators at 200 W. Madison St., Suite 800, Chicago, IL 60606, phone: 800-338-3633, at https://www.diabeteseducator.org/.

• The Academy of Nutrition and Dietetics (formerly the American Dietetic Association) has a great deal of information about diabetes and can be reached at 120 South Riverside Plaza, Suite 2000, Chicago, IL 60606, phone: 800-877-600, at website: http://www.eatrightpro.org/.

• The American Diabetes Association also maintains a hotline for diabetes questions, including information and education, via phone number 703-549-500, or toll-free: 800-342-2383. The association can also be reached at 1701 N. Beauregard St., Alexandria, VA 22311, and at the website http://www.diabetes.org.

• NIH/National Institute of Diabetes and Digestive and Kidney Diseases has a great deal of information about diabetes. The offices are at Office of Communications & Public Liaison, Bldg. 31, Room 9A06, Bethesda, MD 20892-2560, phone: 301-496-3583, website: http://www2.niddk.nih.gov.

## How can a person with diabetes find information about diet?

Most health care professionals will have a person on staff, or at a local health care facility, to help diabetics determine the best diet. If the doctor cannot suggest someone on his or her staff, then try the local hospital, as many hospital dietitians are trained to educate not only people with such conditions as heart disease but also diabetes (which often goes hand in hand with heart disease).

Following the best diet for a person with diabetes can be difficult, but there are many groups that help with such a task. The following lists two places to learn about diabetes and diet:

- The Academy of Nutrition and Dietetics (formerly the American Dietetic Association) offers help to find a dietitian at 120 S. Riverside Plaza, Suite 2000, Chicago, IL 60606, phone: 800-877-600, at http://www.eatrightpro.org/.

- The American Diabetes Association has a good deal of information about eating and diabetes. The ADA can be contacted at 703-549-500, or toll-free: 800-342-2383. It can also be reached at 1701 N. Beauregard St., Alexandria, VA 22311, and at website http://www.diabetes.org.

# DIABETES ORGANIZATIONS AND FACILITIES

### What is the Joslin Diabetes Center?

The Joslin Diabetes Center in Boston is named after one of the researchers once at the forefront of diabetes research, Elliot Joslin (1869–1962; for more about Joslin, see the chapter "Introduction to Diabetes"). It is also considered the world's largest diabetes research center, as well as a diabetes clinic and provider of diabetes education. The center also notes that it has the world's largest team of board-certified physicians treating diabetes and its complications, along with the largest staff of certified diabetes educators in the world. It can be found at http://www.joslin.org/.

### What is the Latino Diabetes Association?

The Latino Diabetes Association offers education and diabetes-awareness information, especially for Latinos. It was organized in response to the increase in type 2 diabetes and

obesity within the Latino population—both in young people and adults. Although it is mostly aimed at Latinos in California, it offers some good educational material for everyone. It is found at http://lda.org/.

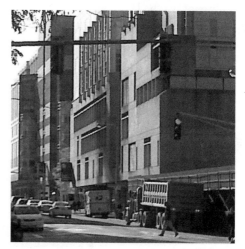

### What is the Barbara Davis Center for Childhood Diabetes?

The Barbara Davis Center for Childhood Diabetes is located at the University of Colorado's School of Medicine. It has one of the world's largest diabetes programs specializing in type 1 diabetes research and care. This is also one of the centers involved in clinical trials on how alpha-antitrypsin affects those with type 1 diabetes.

The Joslin Diabetes Center in Boston is the world's largest research center of its kind.

343

(For more about the studies involving alpha-antitrypsin, see the chapter "The Future and Diabetes.") It can be found at http://www.barbaradaviscenter.org/.

## What is the Diabetes Prevention Support Center?

The nonprofit Diabetes Prevention Support Center was established in 2006 at the University of Pittsburgh with the major goal of preventing diabetes and improving cardiovascular health. It was created through partnership with the military, and support from the Department of Defense, to supply such information to the military and the public. It also has a multimonth, group-based behavioral lifestyle-intervention program, called the Group Lifestyle Balance (GLB), which helps individuals 18 or older who are non-diabetic and overweight, prediabetic, or have metabolic syndrome. The GLB offers education, encouragement, and the tools necessary to help these people—and others, especially those at risk of developing diabetes—to reach and maintain a healthful lifestyle. It can be found at the website www.diabetesprevention.pitt.edu/index.php.

## What is the Diabetes Research Institute?

The Diabetes Research Institute (DRI) is located at the University of Miami in Miami, Florida. This group is very active in the its project DRI BioHub, in which researchers are developing a kind of mini-organ to mimic the pancreas and restore insulin production in people who have diabetes. (For more about the DRI BioHub, see the chapter "The Future and Diabetes.")

## What are some diabetes organizations in the United Kingdom?

The Independent Diabetes Trust (www.iddt.org) is an organization from Northampton, England, that specializes in helping those with diabetes. It has a hotline for questions and many publications to help people with diabetes understand the challenges of the disease. There is also the Diabetes Research & Wellness Foundation at https://www.drwf.org.uk/, a charity that raises awareness of diabetes, especially its complications, treatment, pre-

### What is the IDF Diabetes Atlas?

The International Diabetes Federation (IDF) Diabetes Atlas enables the Internet user to see where people with diabetes are distributed in different countries, with an emphasis on adults with diabetes ages 20 to 79. The first edition was published in 2000, and the seventh edition was published in 2015. It can be found at www.diabetesatlas.org/across-the-globe.html. There is one caveat that even the IDF mentions: Not all the data is known; for example, in Africa, the IDF estimates that more than two-thirds of the African people with diabetes are undiagnosed. (For more about international statistics and diabetes, see the chapter "Introduction to Diabetes.")

vention, and relief. Diabetes UK at https://www.diabetes.org.uk/ is the United Kingdom's largest diabetes charity that not only offers information and up-to-date research reports to those with diabetes but also lobbies the government for help to improve conditions for people with diabetes.

## Are there diabetes organizations in Canada?

There are a few diabetes organizations in Canada, many of them local. But the major organization is the Canadian Diabetes Association at http://www.diabetes.ca/. This group is similar to the American Diabetes Association, offering information and support to Canadians who have diabetes (and others, too—the website also has the basics of diabetes).

## What are some diabetes organizations in other countries?

There are a number of diabetes organizations around the world (not including the United States, Canada, or the United Kingdom). The following lists only a few of the most-followed websites of those groups (for a good list of many organizations in other countries, link to Diabetes Monitor's site at http://www.diabetesmonitor.com/resources/international-diabetes-organizations.htm):

*DiabetiCool*—This Spanish-language site is all about education and diabetes awareness. It can be found at http://www.diabeticool.com/.

*The International Society for Pediatric and Adolescent Diabetes*—This is an organization that often sets standards for people with diabetes, especially in terms of averages for such levels as HbA1C (or A1C). It can be found at https://www.ispad.org/.

*European Association for the Study of Diabetes*—This group's main goal is to encourage and support research in diabetes, along with disseminating the information in a timely fashion. (An offshoot of this group is the European Foundation for the Study of Diabetes, a nonprofit group supporting research in diabetes.) The association can be found at http://www.easd.org/index.php?option=com_content&view=featured&Itemid=435.

*World Diabetes Foundation*—This group seeks, in its own words, to "alleviate human suffering related to diabetes and its complications among those least able to withstand the burden of the disease." It can be reached at the website http://www.worlddiabetesfoundation.org/.

# KIDS AND DIABETES ON THE INTERNET

## What are some of the best websites to help children deal with diabetes?

Many websites offer information for children dealing with diabetes. For example, Children with Diabetes, at http://www.childrenwithdiabetes.com/, is a site that calls itself an "online community for kids, families, and adults with diabetes."

### Are there any digital books that help children who have diabetes?

Yes, there are many digital books that help children who have diabetes (including those in print form listed above). For example, the companies Lilly and Disney (http://www.lillydiabetes.com/lilly-disney.aspx) have collaborated on books that reach children and tweens living with type 1 diabetes. In one series for young children, familiar Disney characters such as Mickey Mouse have a friend Coco, a "fun-loving" monkey who has type 1 diabetes. In the tweens series, the books explore how diabetes can affect relationships with peers and adults at school, at home, and in sports.

### Is there a government publication that helps school personnel aid students who have diabetes?

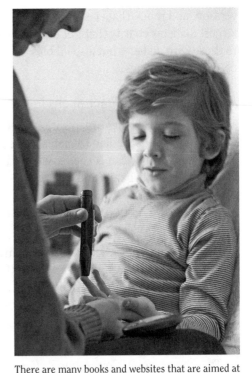

There are many books and websites that are aimed at helping children with diabetes.

Yes, the government publication *Helping the Student with Diabetes Succeed: A Guide for School Personnel,* by the National Diabetes Education Program, is a helpful reference not only for school personnel but also for parents and students in understanding diabetes and the law behind caring for students at school. (According to the website, "This comprehensive resource guide helps students with diabetes, their health care team, school staff, and parents work together to provide optimal diabetes management in the school setting.") The newest edition was published in late 2016 (online only; the print version is from 2012) and can be found at https://www.niddk.nih.gov/health-information/health-communication-programs/ndep/health care-professionals/school-guide/Pages/publicationdetail.aspx.

# LARGE–SCALE DIABETES STUDIES ON THE INTERNET

### What is EPIC-InterAct?

EPIC-InterAct is the world's largest study of onset type 2 diabetes. The InterAct consortium actually has a case study "nestled" within the existing large EPIC study; the EPIC study itself includes 350,000 participants across ten European countries. The

## What doll company is helping children cope with type 1 diabetes?

The doll company that is helping children with type 1 diabetes cope a little better is American Girl (http://play.www.americangirl.com/play), which has introduced a diabetes-care kit for dolls. The kit has ten make-believe items, including a blood-sugar monitor, lancing device, a vial of pretend glucose tablets, a medical bracelet, an ID card, logbook and stickers, a carrying case, and even an insulin pump that can be clipped to a doll's waistband with an adhesive to attach the infusion set. For dolls not using a pump, an insulin-injection pen needle is also supplied.

This was not just a company ploy. A young girl who had type 1 diabetes started an online petition asking American Girl to make the accessories for dolls. After she had gathered around 7,000 signatures, the company came out with the diabetes kit. Although some people still remain skeptical of the idea, it has helped more than hindered. And it is definitely a way for young people with diabetes to educate more people—young and adult—on the trials and challenges of having the disease.

biggest strength of the study is that the results represent standardized dietary and physical activity information collected across the countries and provide baseline data for participants. There are also DNA samples that have been extracted and genotypes, along with plasma samples analyzed for nutrition markers. Each participant was followed for an average of eight years, which is equivalent to four million "person years." Of the population during the time studied, about 12,403 individuals (in eight countries) were identified as having developed type 2 diabetes. This has been a boon for researchers, as the study data includes genetic and lifestyle observations, along with nutritional factors and physical activities of the participants, for comparison purposes in the study of the development of type 2 diabetes. The website is at www.inter-act.eu.

## What is the Diabetes Research Connection?

The Diabetes Research Connection (DRC) is a way of connecting young researchers with donors in order to fund research on the prevention and cure of type 1 diabetes. The DRC was established in 2012 by five people interested in type 1 diabetes—three are scientists with concentrations in diabetes and two are non-scientists who have had type 1 diabetes for years—so all of them have a more personal interest in the disease. As of this writing, the DRC grants up to $50,000 a year for each research project. The website is at https://diabetesresearchconnection.org/.

## What was the Diabetes Prevention Program, or DPP?

The DPP, or Diabetes Prevention Program, was a large, multiorganizational research study funded by the U.S. government's National Institutes of Health (the results were reported in 2002). The study showed that making healthful lifestyle changes could reduce the risk for developing (or slowing down for some with more of a predisposition to) mainly type 2 diabetes.

## What is the Blue Circle Test?

In order to better understand a person's risk for developing diabetes, the International Diabetes Federation (IDF) developed the Blue Circle Test (http://www.idf.org/worlddiabetesday/bluecircletest). Users click on the small circles surrounding a central question mark and choose the appropriate response in describing their status. Once the information is submitted, a report is generated indicating an individual's risk for developing diabetes. The blue circle is considered (by the IDF, which owns the rights to the blue circle for diabetes) to be the universal symbol for diabetes. The IDF chose the circle as it frequently occurs in nature and has been used by various cultures for centuries with a positive connotation and significance. The color blue represents the color of the sky and the flag of the United Nations. The icon was developed in response to the passage of United Nations Resolution 61/225 on December 20, 2006—"World Diabetes Day." This resolution was in response to what researchers have deemed a "diabetes epidemic" that they believe will eventually overwhelm health care resources all over the world.

# DIABETES EDUCATION ON THE INTERNET

## What is the *Living Textbook of Diabetes*?

The *Living Textbook of Diabetes* is truly a textbook of diabetes, presenting some of the basics as well as further details about diabetes. It presents itself as an "open-access, peer-reviewed, unbiased, and up-to-date knowledge base." It is written in an easy-to-follow format. The user can either join the site or register as a guest. It can be found at http://www .diapedia.org/.

## Do any online magazines (e-zines) feature information about diabetes?

Yes, several online magazines feature diabetes, and many of them are associated with print magazines. The following lists some of the more well-known e-zines:

- http://diabeticlivingonline.com/—This site, called Diabetic Living, is affiliated with Diabetic Living Magazine published by Meredith Corporation. It offers the same information as the print magazine but with more up-to-date news and information for people with diabetes.
- http://www.diabeticlifestyle.com/—Diabetic Lifestyle is an e-zine that offers information to people with diabetes, including the basics of diabetes, daily living with diabetes, and recipes.

- http://www.diabetesmonitor.com/—Diabetes Monitor is an e-zine that offers a good cross-section of information about diabetes, including downloadable guides to diabetes and up-to-date news about research in the field.
- http://diabetesdigest.com/—Diabetes Digest, from OmnichannelHealth Media, offers basic information about diabetes, along with recipes, free offers, and discounts for people who have diabetes.
- https://www.diabeteshealth.com/—Diabetes Health is an e-zine that offers resources and information to those who have just been diagnosed and those who have had diabetes for years.

## What websites concentrate on how genes affect a person with diabetes?

Because there often seems to be some genetic component to a person's developing diabetes, several websites educate the public about genes and diabetes.

- Diabetes Genes provides information for patients and professionals on research and clinical care in genetic types of diabetes—their website is at http://diabetesgenes .org. (For more about genes and diabetes—such as MODY, monogenic diabetes, and neonatal diabetes—see the chapter "Types of Diabetes.")
- Genetic and Rare Diseases (GARD) Information Center, PO Box 8126, Gaithersburg, MD 20898-8126, phone: (301) 251-4925, toll-free: (888) 205-2311, website: http://rarediseases.info.nih.gov/GARD/.

## What are some websites that help a person with diabetes plan for an emergency?

Many websites offer emergency plans for people with diabetes. The following lists some of the more well-known ones:

- The Centers for Disease Control and Prevention's site on emergency preparedness for people with diabetes is at www.cdc.gov/diabetes/living/preparedness.html.
- The American Diabetes Association lists some tips for dealing with an emergency for people with diabetes at www.diabetes.org/living-with-diabetes/treatment-and-care/medication/tips-for-emergency-preparedness.html.
- For information on how to store insulin during an emergency, the Food and Drug Administration (FDA) has a site called "insulin storage and switching between products in an emergency" at www.fda.gov/Drugs/EmergencyPreparedness/ucm085213.htm.

## What are some websites that offer dietary information to people with diabetes?

Many websites offer dietary help for people who have diabetes. The following lists some of the more well-known ones:

- National Institute of Diabetes and Digestive and Kidney Diseases has a great site to help people with diabetes eat more healthfully by breaking the topic down into guidelines on what to eat, when to eat, and how much to eat. It can be found at https://www.niddk.nih.gov/health-information/diabetes/diabetes-diet-eating.

- The Joslin Diabetes Center offers information about carbohydrate counting, a method often used by people with diabetes to keep track of eating and their blood glucose levels. The center also offers its own Diabetes Food Pyramid, similar to the old USDA food pyramid, which categorizes food according to carbohydrate content. It can be found at http://www.joslin.org/info/know_your_food_groups_with_diabetes.html.

- There are e-zines for people with diabetes who want to cook more healthfully. These include Diabetic Gourmet Magazine, which was started in 1995 and is now sponsored by CAPCO Marketing, New York. It can be found at http://diabeticgourmet.com/.

- The American Diabetes Association also offers information about eating for people with diabetes, including recipes and meal planners, found at http://www.diabetes.org/food-and-fitness/food.

- The Mayo Clinic also offers a plan for eating, including basic information about recommended foods for people with diabetes. It can be found at http://www.mayoclinic.org/diseases-conditions/diabetes/in-depth/diabetes-diet/art-20044295.

- Medline Plus, a website from the National Institutes of Health, offers information about diabetes, diet, and nutrition at https://medlineplus.gov/diabeticdiet.html.

- Among other offerings, the Diabetes Teaching Center in San Francisco has a good educational site, including information about diet, nutrition, and food exchanges, at https://dtc.ucsf.edu/.

## Are there websites that help a person with diabetes exercise?

Yes, several websites include information about how people with diabetes can best exercise. The following are some of the more well-known ones:

- The Joslin Diabetes Center offers information about how a person with diabetes can remain physically active, including articles with tips about exercise and even videos. It can be found at http://www.joslin.org/info/diabetes-and-exercise.html.

- The American Diabetes Association has a great website highlighting keeping physically active if a person has diabetes, including types of activities and how to stay safe and healthy while exercising. It can be found at http://www.diabetes.org/food-and-fitness/fitness/.

- For understanding how to cope with excessive heat and humidity when a person with diabetes is outdoor exercising (heat can raise blood sugar levels and leave a person dehydrated), see the National Weather Service's heat safety page at http://www.nws.noaa.gov/os/heat/.

## What websites help people with diabetes keep track of their daily blood glucose levels?

Several websites can help with tracking daily blood glucose levels. The following lists only a few (for more about keeping track of glucose, see the apps section of this chapter):

## Are any websites associated with television programs?

**Y**es, there are some websites for people with diabetes that are associated with television programs. For example, dLife, run by LifeMed Media, Inc., includes not only information about diabetes, diabetes apps, and recipes but also dLifeTV, the only web series dedicated to people with diabetes (it airs Sundays on dLifeTV.com, as of this writing, 7 P.M. Eastern Time, 4 P.M. Pacific Time). It can be found at http://www.dlife.com/.

*Sugar Stats*—This free website helps keep track of blood sugar levels at www.SugarStats.com.

*MyNetDiary Diabetes Tracker*—This is a pay-for website, but it does help a person with diabetes keep track of blood glucose levels through a computer or an app (see below for more apps). It can be found at http://www.mynetdiary.com/diabetes.html.

## What websites can help keep track of medications—diabetic or otherwise?

Several websites, many of them free, can help keep track of a person's medications—diabetic or otherwise. The following lists only a few:

*MedCoach*—This free website can be used to track blood glucose readings and other medications, found at www.medcoach.com.

*MedSimple*—This is also a free website that offers medication tracking, including blood glucose readings and diabetic medicines, found at www.medsimpleapp.com.

*My Medicine Tracker*—Another free website that can be used to keep track of diabetic medicines or other medications, found at www.mediguard.org.

## What are some websites that offer free diabetes risk assessment online?

Numerous websites offer free diabetes risk assessment online to "predict" the chances of a person's developing diabetes. (Note: Although these sites are interesting to try, they are based on statistical data on other people with diabetes; if a person suspects he or she may have diabetes, then it is best to be tested by a health care professional.)

*American Diabetes Association*—One of the easiest and simplest to use (and it's free) is from the American Diabetes Association's site. To take the risk assessment test, go online to www.diabetes.org. The test asks simple questions, such as about weight, age, family history, and other characteristics. If a person decides to take the risk assessment via phone, then he or she can call 1-800-DIABETES (1-800-342-2383; yes, there is an extra letter for a phone number—"S"—but just drop that number, which would be 7).

*Diabetes Forecast*—Another site is sponsored by the Diabetes Forecast publication (see magazines above) and is a similar assessment to the one offered by the American Diabetes Association. See http://www.diabetesforecast.org.

*National Institutes of Health* —The government has a risk-assessment test for seeing whether a person is at risk for developing type 2 diabetes. It is free to use at https://www.niddk.nih.gov/health-information/health-communication-programs /ndep/am-i-at-risk/diabetes-risk-test/Pages/diabetes-risk-test.aspx.

*Cleveland Clinic Foundation*—This group has a simple, free risk-assessment test. It can be found at http://www.clevelandclinic.org/health/interactive/diabetes.asp.

## What are some websites that help a diabetic find a dietitian?

Many websites help a diabetic person find a dietitian in his or her local area. The following lists several of the best places to learn about diabetes and diet:

- The Academy of Nutrition and Dietetics (formerly the American Dietetic Association) can help people with diabetes find a dietitian at http://www.eatrightpro.org/.
- There are also websites that offer a dietician professional in a person's area. For example, HealthProfs.com at https://www.healthprofs.com/cam can search a person's state for a dietitian who specializes in diabetes.

## Are any special days, weeks, or months set aside for diabetes awareness?

Yes, there are several days and periods—depending on the organization sponsoring the event—set aside for diabetes awareness. The following lists some of those days, weeks, and months:

*American Diabetes Association Alert Day*—This is usually celebrated on the fourth Tuesday in March and is when the association urges people to take the type 2 Diabetes

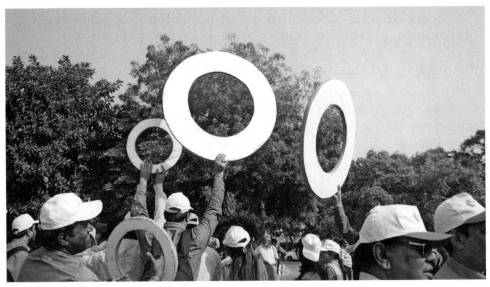

Participants hold up the blue circle symbol during a World Diabetes Day event. World Diabetes Day is held on November 14, the birthday of insulin co-discoverer Frederick Banting.

Risk Test. The test includes simple online questions, such as about age, gender, family history, weight, race, and ethnicity. It is used to help people realize not only the risks of type 2 diabetes but also to assess their own possible risk factors. Go to http://diabetes.org/risktest (or call 1-800-342-2383, or 1-800-DIABETES).

*National Diabetes Month and Diabetes Awareness Month*—November is National Diabetes Month, and according to the National Institutes of Health, the reason is "so individuals, health care professionals, organizations, and communities across the country can bring attention to diabetes and its impact on millions of Americans." Each year has a different theme. (Find out more at https://www.niddk.nih.gov/health-information/health-communication-programs/ndep/partnership-community-out-reach/national-diabetes-month/Pages/default.aspx). November is also considered Diabetes Awareness Month in many parts of the world in an effort to raise diabetes awareness.

*World Diabetes Day*—World Diabetes Day was started in 1991 by the International Diabetes Federation and World Health Organization in response to the increased number of people around the world who are developing diabetes. It is held on November 14 each year. More information can be found at http://www.idf.org/wdd-index/.

*American Diabetes Association's Tour de Cure*—According to the ADA, the Tour de Cure involves thousands of people across the United States who ride to support diabetes research. More information can be found at http://tour.diabetes.org/ (or call 1-800-342-2383, or 1-800-DIABETES).

## What are some organizations that train dogs to help people with diabetes?

Many organizations train dogs to help certain people with diabetes. Not everyone is a candidate for such an animal, nor is every dog a candidate to be trained, but there are several groups that can help educate people with diabetes about the possibilities. The following lists only some of those groups found on the Internet, with several linking to up-to-date information on their Facebook pages from their websites (for more information about dogs and people with diabetes, see the chapter "Taking Charge of Diabetes"). Please note that because such dogs are specially trained, many organizations have a long waiting list:

*Diabetic Alert Dogs of America*—DADA is a group that provides dogs and training, along with education about such animals; at www.diabeticalertdogsofamerica.com.

*Dogs 4 Diabetics*—This group has a very long waiting list and is mostly run by donations it receives; at http://dogs4diabetics.com.

*Canine Assistance, Rehabilitation, Education, and Services (CARES)*—This group provides diabetes alert dogs but, again, has a very long waiting list; at http://www.caresks.com.

*Diabetes Alert Dog Alliance*—This group has a listing of possible qualified trainers around the country; at http://www.diabetesalertdogalliance.org.

There are other places to investigate, too, including local adoption agencies such as the Society for the Prevention of Cruelty to Animals (SPCA) and the Humane Society. One group even offers training workshops around the country for people who want to train their own diabetes alert dogs (at www.Diabeticalertdoguniversity.com). Books and videos are also available, but be forewarned: Not all dogs qualify, and it may take a year or more to train a dog to become a diabetes alert dog.

# U.S. GOVERNMENT HELP
# ON THE INTERNET

### How is the Americans with Disabilities Act involved with diabetes?

The Americans with Disabilities Act (ADA) is a federal law enacted in 1990 (amended in 2008; in effect in 2009) that protects people with disabilities from discrimination. Under this law, diabetes can be considered a disability. Details about the ADA can be found at https://www.ada.gov/.

### Are there any government websites that offer educational material for people with diabetes?

Yes, many government websites do. Here are some of the more well-known sites:

*Centers for Disease Control and Prevention (CDC)*—This site, supported by the government as part of the U.S. Department of Health and Human Services, helps disseminate information about the basics of diabetes with plenty of up-to-date information. It also has educational information for people—children to adults—about diabetes, including the basics, statistics, and programs to help prevent diabetes. It can be found at http://www.cdc.gov/diabetes/home/.

*CDC Registry*—This site provides a national registry of recognized diabetes-prevention programs. It lists contact information for all CDC-recognized organizations that have type 2 diabetes-prevention programs in communities across the United States. (All of these programs have agreed to use a CDC-approved curriculum.) It can be found at https://nccd.cdc.gov/DDT_DPRP/Registry.aspx.

*National Diabetes Education Program* (under the Department of Human Health and Services' National Institute of Diabetes and Digestive and Kidney Diseases)—This site has a great deal of information, not only for the public, but also for health care professionals, found at https://www.niddk.nih.gov/health-information/health-communication-programs/ndep/Pages/index.aspx.

*The National Institute of Diabetes and Digestive and Kidney Diseases Health Information Center*—This center offers the public information, education, and the latest news about diabetes. It can be found at https://www.niddk.nih.gov/ health-information/diabetes.

*The Genetic and Rare Diseases (GARD) Information Center*—This center offers information on genetics and disease, including information on diabetes connections. It is at http://rarediseases.info.nih.gov/GARD/.

## What is the U.S. government's TrialNet program?

There is some help from the U.S. government when it comes to screening family members of people with type 1 diabetes and latent autoimmune diabetes in adults (LADA). The government-funded TrialNet program screens family members of people with the disease by measuring blood samples for auto-antibodies, which are considered to be strong indicators of someone's developing type 1 diabetes. Family members of type 1/LADA diabetes can also find information. (For more about type 1 diabetes and LADA, see the chapter "Prediabetes and Type 1 Diabetes.") See https://www.diabetestrialnet.org/.

# FAVORITE APPS

## Are there any free smartphone apps that help a person with diabetes?

Yes, there is a plethora of apps that help people with diabetes—too many to mention here (and more are being added every year, sometimes every month). The following lists some of the more well-known free and pay-for apps:

*Glucose Buddy*—This app tracks glucose readings, checking the daily highs, lows, and averages and presenting them on a graph. This feature allows users to understand trends as they go through the day and week. There are even more features on the web version. This is free and available for Apple and Android devices. It can be found at http://www.glucosebuddy.com/.

*Gomeals*—This app tracks restaurant offerings, listing carbohydrates and nutrition for menu items. It does this using GPS technology on smartphones, determining a person's location and showing menus for restaurants in the immediate area. It is free for Apple and Android devices. It can be found at https://www.gomeals.com/.

*Fitter Fitness Calculator*—For those interested in keeping their weight down or losing weight—especially if they have diabetes or are prediabetic—this app keeps track of a person's body mass index (BMI) and weight loss. It is free for Apple devices. (For more information about BMI, see the chapter "Diabetes and Obesity.") The app can be downloaded through iTunes, Google Play, and several other places on the Internet.

*Diabetes Companion*—This app, from mySugr, helps people with diabetes keep track of their blood glucose levels. Users enter information about the foods they're eating, how they're feeling, what activities they're doing, etc. The app then plots a graph, giving a seven-day average of how many hypo- and hyperglycemic episodes the person may have had; it even allows the person to print out the information for a health care provider. It can be found at https://mysugr.com/apps/.

### Are there any pay-for smartphone apps that help a person with diabetes?

Yes, there are many pay-for smartphone apps that help people with diabetes—again, too many to mention here (and more are frequently added). The following lists some of the more well-known ones:

*Diabetes App*—This app, put out by BHI technology, costs $6.99 at this writing and is available only for Apple devices. It tracks a person's carbohydrates consumed and holds such information as medications, activity, glucose readings, nutritional data, and weight. It can be purchased from iTunes.

*Sparkpeople*—This app is for Apple and Android devices and costs $3.99; for Black-Berry users, it is free. It is actually a diet and food tracker, so a person can keep track of calories, carbohydrates, protein, fats, weight, and blood glucose levels to help control blood glucose highs and lows. Information can be found at http://www.sparkpeople.com/mobile-apps.asp.

*Calorie King*—This app is from Calorie King Food Search and is free for Apple devices. There are also two other food apps, including Calorie King ControlMyWeight Calorie Counter ($4.99 for Apple devices) and Calorie King Create-a-Meal, which is free for Android devices. It is a good way to count calories and carbohydrates at a restaurant or to interpret food labels—giving a person with diabetes better control of blood glucose levels. It can be found at http://www.calorieking.com/.

*Little Bytes Software*—This company has a pay-for diabetes tracker that allows a person with diabetes to keep track of blood glucose levels via phone. It can be found at http://www.littlebytes.mobi/ (and sold in the Google Play store).

### What way of monitoring blood glucose levels came on the U.S. market in 2016?

In 2016, the Food and Drug Administration approved the sale of the Dario Blood Glucose Monitoring System, advertised as an "all-in-one" glucose meter. The unit, on sale in Europe since 2013, was developed by LabStyle Innovations Corporation of Israel and has a built-in lancing device, a meter, and test strips. It never needs a battery and uses a person's cell phone (iPhone or Android smartphones) to monitor blood glucose levels. Taking only six seconds for the process, the unit plugs into the cell phone's headphone socket, with an app automatically syncing with the meter. It also stores the data for reference in the future and allows the person to share the results of the monitor with anyone via phone. Overall, it is a good way for a person who needs to keep close track of blood glucose levels, especially in terms of how insulin and carbohydrates may affect the person while he or she is away from home.

# Appendix A: A Sampling of Food Exchanges

A "food exchange" is just what the words imply (exchange is also referred to as a choice, serving, or substitution). It allows a person to exchange one food for another on a list with any other food item on the same list, with each list having measured or weighed foods that have about the same nutritional level. For instance, looking at the samples below, a person can eat one small apple or half a mango—with either serving being 15 grams of carbohydrate and 60 calories. In order to determine how many calories, carbohydrates, proteins, and fats a person can eat at each meal, along with snacks, much larger lists are available (at places such as the University of California at San Francisco's Diabetes Teaching Center at https://dtc.ucsf.edu/living-with-diabetes/diet-and-nutrition/understanding-food/). Although there are books and Internet sites that offer listings and how to work with food exchanges, the American Diabetes Association also recommends that a registered dietitian be consulted in order to help the person with diabetes understand the complexity of such food exchanges—and to obtain better and more balanced nutritional information.

There are many lists of food exchanges on the Internet. The following is only a sampling of an exchange list, as per the U.S. Department of Health and Human Services' National Heart, Lung, and Blood Institute (to obtain more information about this listing link to https://www.nhlbi.nih.gov/health/educational/lose_wt/eat/fd_exch.htm):

**Vegetables** contain 25 calories and 5 grams of carbohydrate. One serving equals:

| | |
|---|---|
| ½ C | Cooked vegetables (carrots, broccoli, zucchini, cabbage, etc.) |
| 1 C | Raw vegetables or salad greens |

**Fat-Free and Very Low-Fat Milk** contain 90 calories per serving. One serving equals:

| | |
|---|---|
| 1 C | Milk, fat-free or 1% fat |
| ¾ C | Yogurt, plain nonfat or low-fat |

**Very Lean Protein** choices have 35 calories and 1 gram of fat per serving. One serving equals:

| | |
|---|---|
| 1 oz | Turkey breast or chicken breast, skin removed |
| 1 oz | Fish fillet (flounder, sole, scrod, cod, etc.) |
| 1 oz | Canned tuna in water |
| 2 | Egg whites |

**Fruits** contain 15 grams of carbohydrate and 60 calories. One serving equals:

| | |
|---|---|
| 1 small | Apple, banana, orange, nectarine |
| ½ | Grapefruit |
| ½ | Mango |
| 1 C | Fresh berries (strawberries, raspberries, or blueberries) |

**Lean Protein** choices have 55 calories and 2–3 grams of fat per serving. One serving equals:

| | |
|---|---|
| 1 oz | Chicken—dark meat, skin removed |
| 1 oz | Turkey—dark meat, skin removed |
| 1 oz | Salmon, swordfish, herring |
| 1 oz | Lean beef (flank steak, London broil, tenderloin, roast beef)* |
| 1 oz | Veal, roast, or lean chop* |
| 1 oz | Pork, tenderloin, or fresh ham* |

*Limit to 1–2 times per week

**Medium-Fat Proteins** have 75 calories and 5 grams of fat per serving. One serving equals:

| | |
|---|---|
| 1 oz | Beef (any prime cut), corned beef, ground beef* |
| 1 | Whole egg (medium)* |
| 1 oz | Mozzarella cheese |
| 4 oz | Tofu (note this is a heart healthy choice) |

*Choose these very infrequently

**Starches** contain 15 grams of carbohydrate and 80 calories per serving. One serving equals:

| | |
|---|---|
| 1 slice | Bread (white, pumpernickel, whole wheat, rye) |
| ½ | English muffin |
| ¾ C | Cold cereal |
| ⅓ C | Rice, brown or white, cooked |

**Fats** contain 45 calories and 5 grams of fat per serving. One serving equals:

| | |
|---|---|
| 1 tsp | Oil (vegetable, corn, canola, olive, etc.) |
| 1 tsp | Butter |
| 1 tsp | Mayonnaise |
| 1 tbsp | Salad dressing |

(Source: Based on American Dietetic Association Exchange Lists presented by the National Heart, Lung, and Blood Institute.)

# Appendix B: Examples of Glycemic Indexes

The following lists some of the glycemic indexes, glycemic loads, and net carbohydrates for some common foods (for more about glycemic indexes and loads, see the chapter "Shopping for Food and Eating Out"):

### GI and GL for Common Foods*

| Food | GI | Serving Size | Net Carbs | GL |
|------|-----|--------------|-----------|-----|
| Peanuts | 14 | 4 oz (113g) | 15 | 2 |
| Bean sprouts | 25 | 1 cup (104g) | 4 | 1 |
| Grapefruit | 25 | 1/2 large (166g) | 11 | 3 |
| Pizza | 30 | 2 slices (260g) | 42 | 13 |
| Lowfat yogurt | 33 | 1 cup (245g) | 47 | 16 |
| Apples | 38 | 1 medium (138g) | 16 | 6 |
| Spaghetti | 42 | 1 cup (140g) | 38 | 16 |
| Carrots | 47 | 1 large (72g) | 5 | 2 |
| Oranges | 48 | 1 medium (131g) | 12 | 6 |
| Bananas | 52 | 1 large (136g) | 27 | 14 |
| Potato chips | 54 | 4 oz (114g) | 55 | 30 |
| Snickers Bar | 55 | 1 bar (113g) | 64 | 35 |
| Brown rice | 55 | 1 cup (195g) | 42 | 23 |
| Honey | 55 | 1 tbsp (21g) | 17 | 9 |
| Oatmeal | 58 | 1 cup (234g) | 21 | 12 |
| Ice cream | 61 | 1 cup (72g) | 16 | 10 |
| Macaroni and cheese | 64 | 1 serving (166g) | 47 | 30 |
| Raisins | 64 | 1 small box (43g) | 32 | 20 |
| White rice | 64 | 1 cup (186g) | 52 | 33 |
| Sugar (sucrose) | 68 | 1 tbsp (12g) | 12 | 8 |
| White bread | 70 | 1 slice (30g) | 14 | 10 |
| Watermelon | 72 | 1 cup (154g) | 11 | 8 |
| Popcorn | 72 | 2 cups (16g) | 10 | 7 |
| Baked potato | 85 | 1 medium (173g) | 33 | 28 |
| Glucose | 100 | (50g) | 50 | 50 |

*GI = Glycemic Index; GL = Glycemic Load.

The following list, from the American Diabetes Association, lists the glycemic impact of many common foods:

### Glycemic Impact Levels of Various Foods

| Low Impact | Medium Impact | High Impact |
|---|---|---|
| **Breads, Cereals, Grains, and Pasta** | | |
| Whole-grain specialty breads | Whole-wheat bread | Bagel |
| Sourdough bread | White pita bread | English muffin |
| All-bran cereal | Tortilla | White Bread |
| Steel-cut oats/oatmeal | Shredded wheat | Cornflakes |
| Barley, bulgur wheat | Raisin bran | Instant oatmeal |
| | Brown rice, long-grain rice | Instant rice, short-grain rice |
| | Couscous, quinoa, pasta | Frozen waffles |
| **Fruit, Vegetables, and Legumes** | | |
| Lentils, dried beans | Cantaloupe, pineapple | Baked or boiled potatoes |
| Apples, peaches, oranges | Bananas, raisin | Instant mashed potatoes |
| Strawberries, blueberries | Watermelons | |
| Carrots, green peas | Corn, sweet potatoes | |
| Spinach, broccoli* | Plantains | |
| Lettuce, cucumbers* | | |
| **Dairy, Beverages, Other** | | |
| Milk, yogurt | | Sweetened soft drinks, sports beverages |
| Frozen desserts (ice milk, ice cream) | | |
| Nuts, seeds, peanut butter* | | |
| Eggs, low-fat cheeses* | | |
| Lean meats, fish* | | |
| Heart-healthy oils, vinegar* | | |

Source: Clinical Diabetes, 2011; 29(4): 161

*These items contain very little carbohydrates and have little effect on blood glucose.

# Glossary

**A1C**—A blood test that measures a person's average blood glucose over the past 2 to 3 months and is the best way to measure overall glucose control, especially for people with type 1 diabetes. It is recommended that it be measured two to four times a year, with a measurement goal of less than 6.5 (some say 7) percent.

**acanthosis nigricans**—Acanthosis nigricans (AN) is a condition in which the skin around the neck, armpits, or groin looks dark, thick, and velvety. It is most often a physical sign that a person has insulin resistance.

**ACE inhibitor (angiotensin-converting enzyme)**—An ACE inhibitor is a type of medication used to lower blood pressure. It is also used to help treat kidney problems that are related to diabetes.

**adrenaline**—Adrenaline (also called epinephrine) is a hormone that is secreted by the adrenal glands, especially in times of stress. It is often in reference to the body's "flight or fight" response, with the body experiencing an increase in blood circulation (particularly a faster heartbeat), breathing, and carbohydrate metabolism. This response prepares the muscles for exertion if needed, as the hormone causes the blood vessels to contract, redirecting blood to the major muscle groups, including the heart. It also causes the release of glucose, which is a concern to those who are under excessive stress and trying to control their blood glucose levels.

**antibodies**—Antibodies are natural proteins used by the immune system to identify and neutralize pathogens that invade the body. It is the way a person's body protects itself from foreign substances such as bacteria and viruses.

**autoimmune disease**—An autoimmune disease is characterized by the immune system mistakenly attacking and destroying body tissue that it believes to be foreign. For example, in type 1 diabetes (which is an autoimmune disease) the immune system attacks and destroys the insulin-producing beta cells in the pancreas.

**basal insulin**—Basal insulin is the long-acting or intermediate-acting insulin a person with type 1 diabetes injects once or twice a day. It is the insulin used to control the person's blood glucose levels overnight and between meals. (Also see bolus insulin.)

**basal/bolus insulin plan**—The basal/bolus insulin plan attempts to mimic the way the body's normally functioning pancreas produces insulin. A person with type 1 diabetes does this by using a certain combination of different insulin types in order to keep their blood glucose levels balanced during various times of the day, such as before, during, and after meals, when having snacks, during periods of physical activity, and throughout the night.

**beta cells**—Beta cells are the cells in the pancreas that produce insulin and are located within the islets of Langerhans in the organ.

**blood glucose level**—A person's blood glucose level (it is also called simply glucose level or sugar level) is the amount of glucose in the person's bloodstream at a certain time. The tell-tale sign of diabetes is if the blood glucose levels are too high (hyperglycemia), and for hypoglycemia, the blood glucose is too low.

**blood glucose meter**—There are many types of blood glucose meters. In general, they are a portable machine that measures a person's glucose in the blood at a certain time. After a person pricks their skin with a lancet to obtain a droplet of blood, it is put on a special test strip and then inserted in the blood glucose meter. From there, the machine presents a number on its digital display that represents a person's blood glucose level at that time.

**bolus insulin**—Bolus insulin is the rapid-acting or short-acting insulin a person with type 1 diabetes injects to cover carbohydrates eaten in a meal or snack. It is also used to lower blood glucose levels that are above the target number. (Also see basal insulin.)

**carbohydrate (carb) counting**—Carbohydrate counting is one of the popular meal planning approaches for children and adolescents who have diabetes. It involves calculating the number of grams of carbohydrates eaten at meals or snacks.

**carbohydrates (carbs)**—Carbohydrates are one of three sources of energy in the foods people eat (the other two are fats and protein). They are mainly sugars and starches that the body breaks down into glucose, with most of the carbohydrates raising the blood glucose levels. These include such foods as breads, crackers, and cereals; pasta, rice, and grains; vegetables; milk and yogurt; fruit, juice, and sweetened sodas; and table sugar, honey, syrup, and molasses, cakes, pies, and cookies.

**changing carbohydrate (carb) intake meal plan**—Changing carbohydrate intake meal plan is a way to help children and adolescents with diabetes who have to take multiple daily insulin injections or use an insulin pump. In this case, the young person does not have to eat the same amount of carbohydrates at every meal (or as a snack). But because of this, they have to adjust insulin doses (with either rapid- or short-acting insulin) to make up for the carbohydrates consumed. This is usually used with a basal/bolus insulin plan.

**cholesterol**—Cholesterol is a type of fat that is manufactured in the liver or intestines. It is also found in many of the foods consumed, especially animal foods, such as eggs, milk, cheese, liver, meat and poultry.

**continuous glucose monitor (CGM)**—A continuous glucose monitor records glucose levels for a person with diabetes through the day. The monitor works by inserting a small sensor (usually a small needle with the sensor attached) under the skin. The sensor measures glucose levels (the glucose found in the fluid between the cells) at regular intervals. The monitor collects the data wirelessly and sends the information to a pump or small monitor (some are even connected to a cellphone). If the levels are too high or low, an alarm is sounded so the person can manage the situation.

**conventional insulin therapy**—This type of insulin therapy is the most well-known and entails injecting insulin based on when a person eats, engages in physical activity, or other conditions.

**creatinine** —Creatinine is a waste product derived from the activity of the body's muscles. Healthy kidneys can remove this substance from the blood. But when the levels of creatinine rise, it usually means that the kidneys are beginning to not function normally or are definitely not functioning normally.

**diabetes educator**—A diabetes educator is a health care professional who has the skill and knowledge to teach a person with diabetes how to manage the condition. Diabetes educators can be listed as doctors, nurses, dietitians, mental health or fitness clinicians, and many have the credential initials CDE (Certified Diabetes Educator) after their name.

**diabetic ketoacidosis (also called ketoacidosis or DKA)**—Diabetic ketoacidosis is when the person (mainly with diabetes) has extremely high blood glucose levels along with a very low amount of insulin. This causes the body to breakdown fat reserves for energy and an accumulation of ketones in the blood and urine. It is a life-threatening condition that can lead to coma and death if not treated. The symptoms include nausea, stomach pain, vomiting, chest pain, rapid shallow breathing, and difficulty staying awake.

**diabetic macular edema**—Diabetic macular edema usually occurs when a person with diabetes has diabetic retinopathy, in which the fluid collects in the central part of the retina. The result is usually blurred vision, and is most often treated with laser surgery if the person's central vision is threatened.

**diuretic**—A diuretic is a chemical that increases urine output. Diuretics include alcohol and any beverages that contain caffeine (coffee, tea, colas). Diuretic medications are usually prescribed for patients with high blood pressure or congestive heart failure.

**epinephrine**—See adrenaline.

**fasting blood glucose test**—A fasting blood glucose tests involves taking a sample of a person's blood after they fast overnight. The blood is then analyzed for the amount of glucose in the blood.

**fructosamine test**—This blood test is used to detect overall changes in blood glucose over the past two or three weeks. The fructosamine test is usually used if there have been rapid changes in the person's diabetes treatment plan, or if the health care professional needs to see if other changes should be made in the short term.

**glucagon**—Glucagon is a natural hormone that raises the level of glucose in the blood. It is also injected in a person who is suffering from severe hypoglycemia.

glucose—Glucose is a simple form of sugar that is the main source of energy for the body. It is created when the body's digestive processes break down food. In general, glucose passes through the wall of the intestines, into the bloodstream to the liver, and eventually into the general bloodstream circulation. From there glucose enters individual cells or tissues throughout the body, which all use the sugar for energy.

glucose correction factor—The glucose correction factor is the amount of insulin a person with diabetes needs to lower their blood glucose to a target level.

glucose tablets (or gel)—Glucose tablets or gels are quick-acting forms of glucose. They are made of pure glucose (the tablets have a premeasured amount, while the gel is usually in a squeezable tube) and are often used to counteract an episode of hypoglycemia.

glucose tolerance test—The glucose tolerance test is a blood test to determine if a person has diabetes. After a person drinks a sugar-filled liquid, their blood is taken every hour or at a two-hour point after ingesting the liquid. After two hours, if the person's glucose is over 200 mg/dl (milligrams per deciliter), they are considered to be diabetic.

glycemic index (GI)—The glycemic index ranks foods containing equal amounts of carbohydrates based on how much they raise a person's blood glucose level. Each food has a certain high or low ranking. For example, the carbohydrate in a slice of 100 percent stone-ground whole wheat bread (a low glycemic index food) may have less impact on blood glucose than a slice of processed white bread (a high glycemic index food).

glycemic load (GL)—The glycemic load ranks the carbohydrates in foods and how much they raise a person's blood glucose level. It uses the glycemic index (GI) system's value and the carbohydrate content in an average serving of a food, a meal or a day's worth of food. It is considered to be a more accurate view of how carbohydrates affect a person's glucose values than the glycemic index.

glycogen—Glycogen is the glucose that is stored in muscles and liver.

hormone—A hormone is a natural chemical produced by an organ in the body. In most cases, a hormone travels in the blood and affects other organs and cells.

hyperglycemia—Hyperglycemia means a person has high blood glucose levels. A high reading is usually considered 160 mg/dl (milligrams/deciliter) or above a person's individual blood glucose target.

hyperosmolar hyperglycemic state (HHS)—Hyperosmolar hyperglycemic state (HHS) is considered to be a serious (but uncommon) condition resulting from extremely high levels of blood glucose. Symptoms include excessive urination and severe dehydration (but it is not associated with ketones in the blood or urine).

hypertension—In general, hypertension is also called high blood pressure (blood flows through the blood vessels with a greater than normal force). Although there is disagreement, it is defined as a blood pressure equal to or greater than 140/90 mm Hg (systolic over diastolic pressures). It also is associated with adults who have diabetes, and increases the risk of heart attacks, strokes, and kidney problems.

hypoglycemia—Hypoglycemia is an often serious condition in which a person's blood glucose drops below 80 mg/dl (milligrams per deciliter) with or without symptoms or below 90 mg/dl with symptoms. Symptoms can include confusion, sweating, heart palpitations, shaking, anxiety, and many other conditions, many of which the person who is having the attack is not even aware of the lower glucose levels. Such low blood glucose levels can occur for a multitude of reasons, such as during or after exercise, if too much insulin is present, or not enough food is consumed.

hypoglycemia unawareness—Hypoglycemia unawareness is a complication of diabetes in which a person is not aware that their blood glucose levels are dropping. This occurs because the usual trigger—a drop in the glucose that causes the secretion of epinephrine, or adrenaline—does not occur. Because of this, none of the "usual" symptoms of a hypoglycemic event are generated, such as sweating, heart palpitations, and/or shaking.

impaired fasting glucose (IFG)—Impaired fasting glucose means a person's fasting glucose level is between 100 mg/dl and 125 mg/dl. If a person has a fasting blood test and the results are between these levels, it usually means that they have prediabetes.

impaired glucose tolerance (IGT)—The impaired glucose tolerance is often used as another term for prediabetes. It means a person's blood glucose level, after a two-hour glucose tolerance test, is between 140 and 199 mg/dl. This is usually an indication that the person has prediabetes.

insulin—In the body, insulin is a natural hormone produced by the pancreas that helps glucose pass into the cells. In the cells, it is used to create energy for the body.

insulin pen—The insulin pen is an insulin delivery method that looks like a writing pen. It is a customized syringe used to inject insulin into a person with diabetes.

insulin pump—An insulin pump (usually computerized) is an insulin delivery system. It is usually a small mechanical device, typically the size of a beeper or small cell phone. It works by releasing insulin into the tissues of the body through a combination of tubing and a needle.

insulin reaction—An insulin reaction is when a person has low blood glucose (hypoglycemia) resulting from either too much insulin, too much activity, or too little food.

insulin resistance—Insulin resistance is a condition that makes it harder for cells to properly use insulin; it also means the body does not respond normally to the action of insulin. People who have insulin resistance can develop type 2 diabetes.

insulin sensitivity factor—Also called the correction factor or supplemental factor, the insulin sensitivity factor is the amount of blood glucose measured in milligrams per deciliter that can be lowered by taking one unit of rapid-acting or regular insulin. The insulin sensitivity factor is used to calculate the amount of insulin a person with diabetes needs to return blood glucose levels to within their target range.

insulin-to-carbohydrate ratio—The insulin-to-carbohydrate ratio is a method to determine how much rapid-acting insulin is needed to cover the carbohydrate ingested at a meal or snack.

**islet cell transplantation**—Islet cell transplantation is when beta cells that produce insulin are donated from a person who has healthy cells into a person whose pancreas no longer produces insulin.

**islet cells**—The islet cells found in the pancreas make insulin and are also called pancreatic beta cells.

**ketoacidosis**—See diabetic ketoacidosis.

**ketones**—Ketones are chemicals made by the body when there is not enough insulin in the blood. Thus, the body must break down fat for energy, which produces ketones. They are usually associated with high blood glucose, but also may occur if a person is ill and blood glucose levels fall below the person's target range. See also diabetic ketoacidosis (DKA).

**ketonuria**—Ketonuria is the presence of ketones in the urine.

**ketosis**—Ketosis is the excessive formation of ketones in the blood. Signs of ketosis are often nausea, vomiting, and stomach pain.

**lancet**—A lancet is a small needle (most often inserted in a spring-loaded device) that is used to prick the skin and obtain a drop of blood for checking blood glucose levels.

**metabolic syndrome**—Metabolic syndrome is a combination of conditions that increase the risk of developing vascular disease (heart disease, strokes, and peripheral vascular disease). This syndrome is characterized by abdominal obesity, high blood pressure (or hypertension), high triglycerides, low HDL (the "good" cholesterol), and glucose intolerance.

**metabolism**—Metabolism is a process in the body by which the cells change food to be used for energy. This also helps to build and maintain cells and tissues throughout the body.

**neuropathy**—Neuropathy is another word for nerve damage. It can affect certain areas of the body or even organs throughout the body. Nerve damage can be caused by many medical conditions, including uncontrolled high blood glucose levels common in people with diabetes

**nocturnal hypoglycemia**—Nocturnal hypoglycemia is when a person's blood glucose drops in the middle of the night.

**nonproliferative retinopathy**—Nonproliferative retinopathy is the initial stage in diabetic retinopathy. It is caused by high levels of blood glucose that eventually damage the blood vessels in the retina. This causes the blood vessels to leak fluid, which can collect and cause the retina to swell.

**oral glucose-lowering medications**—Oral glucose-lowering medications (also referred to as oral antidiabetes medications) refer to the pills taken by people with diabetes (usually type 2). They are usually used in combination with lifestyle changes (especially meals and exercise) and sometimes with other ways of controlling blood glucose levels (such as combinations of oral medications).

pancreas—The pancreas is a small gland located below and just behind the stomach that is responsible for producing the hormone insulin.

peak effect time—The peak effect time is when insulin has its major impact on reducing blood glucose levels in the body.

prediabetes—Prediabetes is a condition in which either a person's fasting or two-hour post-meal blood glucose levels are higher than normal, but not high enough for a diagnosis of type 2 diabetes.

proliferative retinopathy—Proliferative retinopathy is considered a serious stage of diabetic retinopathy in which there is a greater loss of vision or even total blindness. During this stage, abnormal blood vessels grow over the surface of the retina. (Also see nonproliferative retinopathy.)

protein—Proteins are some of the main nutrients from food, along with carbohydrates and fats. The body uses protein to build and repair the body, including muscles, organs, bones, skin, and many of the hormones in the body are made from protein.

quick-acting glucose—Quick-acting glucose is considered to be foods or sugar products that are used to quickly raise a person's blood glucose levels during a hypoglycemic episode. For example, glucose tablets or gels are often used to raise blood glucose levels.

rapid-acting insulin—Rapid-acting insulin lowers a person's blood glucose levels within 10 to 30 minutes and works hardest 30 minutes to 3 hours after injection.

rebound hyperglycemia—Rebound hyperglycemia (also called high blood glucose or the Somogyi phenomenon) is a result of too low a level of glucose and stress hormones cause the liver to release too much glucose.

retinopathy—Retinopathy refers to damage to the eye's retina, the thin, light-sensitive inner lining in the back of the eye. In a person with diabetes, this usually occurs when there is damage to the small blood vessels in the retina from high blood glucose levels.

short-acting insulin—Short-acting insulin is a type of insulin that begins to work to lower blood glucose within 30 to 60 minutes and works hardest 1 to 5 hours after injection. The common form of short-acting insulin is called "regular."

single dose—Single dose refers to an injection that contains one type of insulin.

syringe—A syringe is a device used to inject medications such as insulin into body tissue.

test strips—Test strips are specially designed strips used in blood glucose meters to check blood glucose levels, or in urine testing for ketones.

triglycerides—Triglycerides are a type of fat stored in fat cells as body fat and burned for energy. High levels of triglycerides are linked with an increased risk of heart and blood vessel disease.

# Index

(Note: italicized page numbers indicates main entry.)